KU-546-395

WITHDRAWN

Cardiac Care
An introductory text

Cardiac Care

An introductory text

Edited by

IAN JONES RN, NFESC

President, British Association for Nursing in
Cardiac Care and Lecturer in Cardiac Nursing,
School of Nursing, University of Salford, Salford, UK

W

WHURR PUBLISHERS

LONDON AND PHILADELPHIA

Copyright © 2006   Whurr Publishers Limited (a subsidiary of John Wiley & Sons Ltd)
The Atrium, Southern Gate, Chichester,
West Sussex PO19 8SQ, England
Telephone   (+44) 1243 779777

Email (for orders and customer service enquiries): cs-books@wiley.co.uk
Visit our Home Page on www.wiley.com

All Rights Reserved. No part of this publication may be reproduced, stored in a retrieval system or transmitted in any form or by any means, electronic, mechanical, photocopying, recording, scanning or otherwise, except under the terms of the Copyright, Designs and Patents Act 1988 or under the terms of a licence issued by the Copyright Licensing Agency Ltd, 90 Tottenham Court Road, London W1T 4LP, UK, without the permission in writing of the Publisher. Requests to the Publisher should be addressed to the Permissions Department, John Wiley & Sons Ltd, The Atrium, Southern Gate, Chichester, West Sussex PO19 8SQ, England, or emailed to permreq@wiley.co.uk, or faxed to (+44) 1243 770620.

Designations used by companies to distinguish their products are often claimed as trademarks. All brand names and product names used in this book are trade names, service marks, trademarks or registered trademarks of their respective owners. The Publisher is not associated with any product or vendor mentioned in this book.

This publication is designed to provide accurate and authoritative information in regard to the subject matter covered. It is sold on the understanding that the Publisher is not engaged in rendering professional services. If professional advice or other expert assistance is required, the services of a competent professional should be sought.

Other Wiley Editorial Offices

John Wiley & Sons Inc., 111 River Street, Hoboken, NJ 07030, USA

Jossey-Bass, 989 Market Street, San Francisco, CA 94103-1741, USA

Wiley-VCH Verlag GmbH, Boschstr. 12, D-69469 Weinheim, Germany

John Wiley & Sons Australia Ltd, 42 McDougall Street, Milton, Queensland 4064, Australia

John Wiley & Sons (Asia) Pte Ltd, 2 Clementi Loop #02-01, Jin Xing Distripark, Singapore 129809

John Wiley & Sons Canada Ltd, 22 Worcester Road, Etobicoke, Ontario, Canada M9W 1L1

Wiley also publishes its books in a variety of electronic formats. Some content that appears in print may not be available in electronic books.

A catalogue record for this book is available from the British Library

ISBN -13   978-1-86156-471-9
ISBN -10   1-86156-471-6

Printed and bound in Great Britain by TJ International Ltd, Padstow, Cornwall

This book is printed on acid-free paper responsibly manufactured from sustainable forestry in which at least two trees are planted for each one used for paper production.

Contents

Preface

Although this book has been written predominantly for nurses, the information presented serves as a comprehensive clinical resource for any nurse, doctor or allied health professional new to cardiac care.

The aim of the book is to provide a quick and simple reference guide for clinicians to enable them to provide effective and evidence-based practice. Coronary heart disease (CHD) remains the biggest killer and cause of disability in the western world. The improvement in the acute management of these patients and subsequent reduction in mortality will mean that all health professionals will care for patients with CHD at some time in their professional careers.

I have spent most of my adult life caring for patients with CHD. I have witnessed the misery and suffering that this awful disease can cause. Historically cardiac textbooks have concentrated on developing the knowledge base of staff working within the coronary care unit and although this development is vital it is important to recognize that most people suffering from CHD are cared for outside specialist units.

It is very difficult for clinicians new to cardiac care to ensure an adequate knowledge base in all areas. This book has been written by experienced clinicians who are able to take the reader step by step through the patient journey, providing an overview of the fundamental aspects of cardiac care.

Ian Jones

Contributors

Paula Bithell, MA, RN, Consultant Nurse in Cardiology, Pennine Acute Trust, Rochdale, UK

Gillian Blanchard, RN, Cardiology Interventional Specialist Nurse, Central Manchester NHS Trust, Manchester UK

Anne Dormer, BSc, RN, Specialist Nurse in Heart failure, Pennine Acute Trust, Oldham, UK

Frances Gascoigne, RN, MSc, MA, Lecturer in Nursing, School of Nursing, University of Salford, Salford, UK

Miriam Gaston, MSc, RN, PGDipEd, Lecturer in Nursing, School of Nursing, University of Salford, Salford, UK

Barbara Hastings-Asatourian, BNurs, MSc, RN, RHV, Lecturer in Nursing, School of Nursing, University of Salford, Salford, UK

Ian Jones, BSc, PGCLT, RN, NFESC, President, British Association for Nursing in Cardiac Care and Lecturer in Cardiac Nursing, School of Nursing, University of Salford, Salford, UK

Jan Keenan, MSc, PGDip, RN, Nurse Consultant in Cardiology, John Radcliffe Hospital, Oxford, UK

Mike Lappin, MSc, PGCE, RN, Lecturer in Nursing, School of Nursing, University of Salford, Salford, UK

Elizabeth Lawson, RN, Lecturer in Nursing, School of Nursing, University of Salford, Salford, UK

Denis Parkinson, MSc, RN, Lecturer in Nursing, School of Nursing, University of Salford, Salford, UK

Brian Parr, BA, RN, DipN, Cardiac Nurse Specialist, Hope Hospital, Salford, UK

Catherine Rimmer, BA, RN, Cardiac Nurse Specialist, Cardiac Surgery, Central Manchester NHS Trust, Manchester, UK

Andrea Saycell, RN, DipN, Nurse Specialist in Chest Pain, Pennine Acute Trust, Oldham, UK

Shonagh Senior, RN, Cardiac Nurse Specialist, Cardiac Surgery, Central Manchester NHS Trust, Manchester, UK

Debra Vickers, BSc, RN, Thrombolysis Co-ordinator, Pennine Acute Trust, Rochdale, UK

Acknowledgements

The authors would like to thank colleagues, friends and family who have supported them through this venture and without whom they could not have realized their ambitions.

The publishers and authors would like to thank all the people who have supported and assisted them through this process, including Professor Martin Johnson, Professor Tom Quinn and Mrs Jill Wild.

In particular a special mention and thank-you must go to my wife, Diane, without whose support I would not have been able to commit to such a task, and to our children Christopher, Matthew, Adam, Sophie and Carys, who, despite their young age, have demonstrated great patience and understanding throughout the writing and editing of this book. Finally I wish to thank my parents who have always believed in me.

CHAPTER ONE

The physiology and pathophysiology of the cardiovascular system

FRANCES GASCOIGNE

This chapter centres on the structure and functioning of the heart and blood vessels along with the transport media, blood and plasma. The structure of the cell and the principles of homoeostasis are discussed because the concepts play a significant role in the understanding of the pathophysiology *of the circulatory system* and the relevant drug therapy. The pathophysiology is presented in boxes within the main text, which details the anatomy and physiology.

The primary function of the circulatory system is transportation, with its secondary function being a contribution towards maintaining homoeostasis and cellular function. Blood serves as the transport medium for delivering and removing respiratory gases, nutritive molecules and metabolic waste products to and from the body cells. In addition, the blood also plays a part in the protection of body cells along with the regulation and integration of cellular function by carrying protective elements, enzymes and hormones. Cellular function is crucial for cellular tissue and therefore for organ survival.

The heart acts as a central pump and creates the pressure to push the blood around the body in a circuit of channels called blood vessels, which leads to and from the heart. The heart and blood vessels comprise the circulatory system (Figure 1.1).

Anatomy of the heart and circulatory system

Structure of the heart

The human heart is a four-chambered muscular organ, cone shaped and with a size that is roughly the same as the clenched fist of the person whose heart it is. It lies in the mediastinum between the lungs, with about two-thirds of its mass to the left of the midline of the body and one-third to the right.

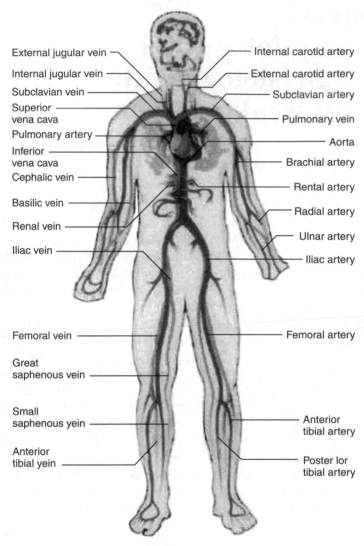

External jugular vein

Internal jugular vein

Subclavian vein

Superior
vena cava

Pulmonary artery

Inferior
vena cava

Cephalic vein

Basilic vein

Renal vein

Iliac vein

Femoral vein

Great
saphenous vein

Small
saphenous yein

Anterior
tibial yein

Internal carotid artery

External carotid artery

Subclavian artery

Pulmonary vein

Aorta

Brachial artery

Rental artery

Radial artery

Ulnar artery

Iliac artery

Femoral artery

Anterior
tibial artery

Poster lor
tibial artery

Figure 1.1 The circulatory system showing the heart and major blood vessels.

To count the apical beat of the heart, a stethoscope is placed directly over the apex, in the space between the fifth and sixth ribs – the fifth intercostal space – on a line with the midpoint of the left clavicle. The upper border of the heart, the base of the cone shape, lies just below the second rib (Parker Anthony 1944). The boundaries (Figure 1.2), which indicate the size of the heart, are clinically significant and are measured when diagnosing heart disorders, such as dilated cardiomyopathy when the heart becomes enlarged, termed 'cardiomegaly' (Figure 1.3).

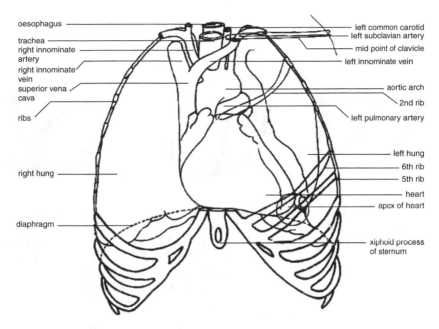

oesophagus
trachea
right innominate artery
right innominate vein
superior vena cava
ribs
right hung
diaphragm

left common carotid
left subclavian artery
mid point of clavicle
left innominate vein
aortic arch
2nd rib
left pulmonary artery
left hung
6th rib
5th rib
heart
apex of heart
xiphoid process of sternum

Figure 1.2 The blunt pointed end of the cone-shaped heart, called the apex, is located downwards and forwards, and points towards the left of the chest, just above the diaphragm. The positioning of the stethoscope is represented by the circle.

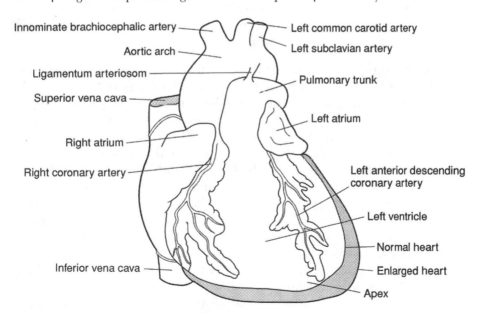

Innominate brachiocephalic artery
Aortic arch
Ligamentum arteriosom
Superior vena cava
Right atrium
Right coronary artery
Inferior vena cava

Left common carotid artery
Left subclavian artery
Pulmonary trunk
Left atrium
Left anterior descending coronary artery
Left ventricle
Normal heart
Enlarged heart
Apex

Figure 1.3 External view of the heart showing the borders in a normal and enlarged heart.

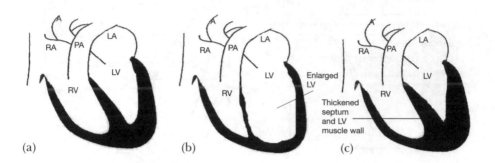

(a)   (b)   (c)

Figure 1.4 Cardiomyopathy: (a) the heart, normal left ventricular muscle; (b) dilated cardiomyopathy: enlarged left ventricle with weak muscle wall resulting in a reduction in the strength of the contractility; and (c) hypertrophic cardiomyopathy: thickened septum and left ventricular wall – the end-diastolic volume is reduced as the muscle is unable to stretch and relax as normal. A, aorta; LA, left atrium; LV, left ventricle; PA, pulmonary artery; RA, right atrium; RV, right ventricle.

Cardiomyopathy (as shown in Figure 1.4) occurs when the heart is enlarged and the muscle walls of the heart, the myocardium, has become enlarged, thickened or stiffened, and is classified as either primary or secondary. No specific cause is identified in primary cardiomyopathy, whereas secondary cardiomyopathy is attributed to a specific cause. There are three main types of cardiomyopathy:

1. Dilated congested cardiomyopathy is a disorder of myocardial function with heart failure in which there is an overall enlargement of the four heart chambers, especially the ventricles. There are several aetiologies, including myocardial ischaemia as a result of coronary artery disease (CAD), which lead to dilated cardiomyopathy. With ischaemia the ventricular myocardium is deprived of essential nutrients and gases, functions without an adequate fuel supply and becomes weak. In this weakened state the muscles overwork in an attempt to compensate for their poor contractility, which leads to dilatation, thinning and hypertrophy of the myocardium. This altered structure of the ventricles causes mitral or tricuspid regurgitation and atrial dilatation.
2. Hypertrophic cardiomyopathy is characterized by left ventricular hypertrophy. Aetiology includes hereditary disorders and acromegaly. There are two forms of hypertrophic cardiomyopathy: in one the intraventricular septum becomes enlarged and obstructs the blood flow from the left ventricle and is known as hypertrophic obstructive cardiomyopathy (HOCM) or idiopathic hypertrophic subaortic stenosis (IHSS); in the

other the outflow tract is not obstructed and is referred to as non-obstructive hypertrophic cardiomyopathy (Steinbis 2003)
3. Restrictive cardiomyopathy presents with rigid, non-compliant ventricular walls, which resist being stretched during ventricular diastole and ventricular filling with oxygen. Aetiologies include diffuse systemic sclerosis and endocardial fibrosis.

The thoracic cage provides protection to the mediastinal structures and the heart is further protected because it is enclosed within the pericardium, often referred to as a pericardial sac. The pericardial sac consists of two portions: an outer fibrous pericardium and an inner serous pericardium (Figure 1.5).

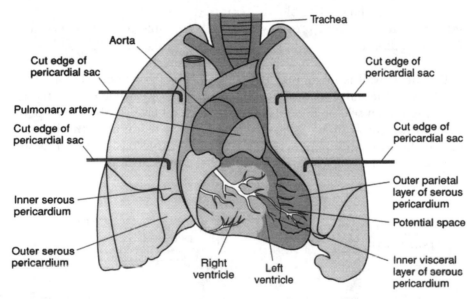

Figure 1.5 View of the pericardial sac cut open at the front to expose the mediastinal structures. The inner and outer layers of the pericardium are visible. The serous layer consists of two layers separated by the potential space, which contains pericardial fluid.

The serous portion is divided into an outer parietal layer, which lines the fibrous pericardium, and an inner visceral layer or epicardium, which covers the heart and blood vessels. These two serous layers are connected by a cavity filled with pericardial fluid. This fluid is essentially an ultrafiltrate of plasma arising from the visceral layer and serves as a lubricator preventing friction between the two pericardial portions as the heart pumps. The heart moves easily in this inextensible 'loose fitting jacket'. As it cannot be stretched it may, in some clinical conditions, cause constriction and inhibit myocardial function.

Pericarditis and cardiac tamponade are clinical problems involving the potential space surrounding the heart or pericardium. Inflammation of the pericardial tissue is known as pericarditis and is often painful because the two layers move against each other when the heart beats (Menet et al. 2001). Acute pericarditis may be an early consequence of acute myocardial infarction (MI) (10–15% of cases). The syndrome that occurs late after an MI (Dressler's syndrome) usually occurs within 10 days to 2 months after an MI, and is characterized by fever, pericarditis with friction rub, pericardial effusion, pleurisy, pleural effusions and joint pain. Occasionally, the heart may rupture after an MI, causing haemopericardium. This usually occurs 1–10 days after an MI and is more common in women.

In cardiac tamponade, cardiac surgery may be complicated by postoperative haemorrhage. The blood is trapped inside the pericardial sac; it squeezes the heart and prevents it from being able to beat (Beers and Berkow 1999).

The heart wall is made up three distinct layers of tissue (Figure 1.6). The bulk of the wall consists of the myocardium or cardiac muscle tissue. Covering the muscle on the outside is the visceral layer of the serous pericardium (or epicardium). A layer of endothelial tissue lines the interior wall of the myocardium. There are ridge-like projections, known as the papillary muscles, on the inner surface of the myocardium.

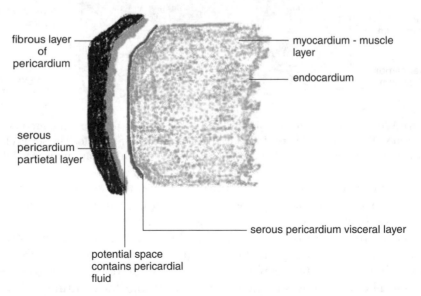

Figure 1.6 Section of the heart wall showing the components of the outer pericardium, muscle layer and inner lining of the heart.

The papillary muscles attach to the lower portion of the interior wall of the ventricles. They connect to the chordae tendineae, tendons that link these papillary muscles to the tricuspid valve in the right ventricle and the mitral valve in the left ventricle. As the papillary muscles contract and relax, the chordae tendineae transmit the resulting increase and decrease in tension to the respective valves, causing them to open and close (Figure 1.7). The chordae tendineae are string like in appearance and sometimes referred to as 'heart strings' (Parker Anthony 1944).

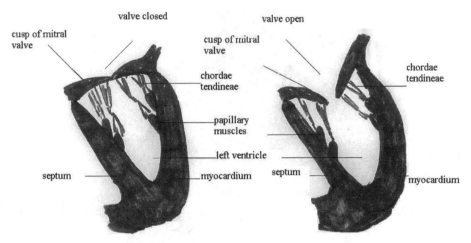

Figure 1.7 Papillary muscles and chordae tendineae with the action of the mitral valve: (a) valve closed; (b) valve open.

Rupture or dysfunction of chordae tendinae or of papillary muscles occurs secondary to ischaemia and myocardial infarction and leads to mitral valve regurgitation/malfunction.

The internal structure of the heart consists of two linked halves: the right half is separated from the left half by a wall of muscular tissue called the septum. Each half has two chambers, the two upper chambers being termed the 'left and right atria separated by the atrial septum' and the two lower chambers the 'right and left ventricles separated by the ventricular septum'.

The ventricles are considerably larger than the atria and the left ventricle has thicker muscle walls in comparison to the right ventricle. These structural differences reflect the work that the chambers have to do in order to pump the blood around the respective circuits. A layer of dense connective tissue, known as the fibrous skeleton of the heart, lies between the atria and the ventricles.

There are four valves at specific locations in this dense connective barrier which act as gates through which the blood can flow either into or out of the ventricles. An atrioventricular (AV) valve separates each atrium from each ventricle. A semilunar valve separates each ventricle from its connecting artery – these structures are visible in Figure 1.8.

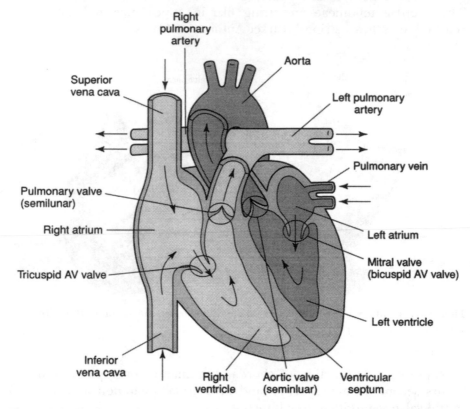

Figure 1.8 The internal structures of the heart. The arrows indicate the direction of the flow of blood to and from the heart and through the heart. AV, atrioventricular.

The heart functions as two separate halves with two distinct pressure circuits (Figure 1.9) working simultaneously; the right side is known as the pulmonary circulation and the left as the systemic circulation:

- Deoxygenated blood returns to the right atrium via the superior and inferior cavae.
- From the right atrium, the blood flows through the tricuspid valve into the right ventricle, which then pumps the blood through the pulmonary valve into the pulmonary trunk and pulmonary arteries, and to the lungs to be oxygenated.

- From the lungs, the oxygenated blood is returned to the left atrium via the pulmonary veins.
- The oxygenated blood then flows from the left atrium through the mitral valve into the left ventricle. From the left ventricle, it is pumped through the aortic valve into the aorta and to the body tissues via the blood vessels.

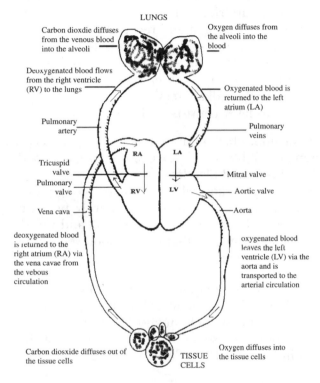

LUNGS

Carbon dioxdie diffuses from the venous blood into the alveoli

Oxygen diffuses from the alveoli into the blood

Deuxygenated blood flows from the right ventricle (RV) to the lungs

Oxygenated blood is returned to the left atrium (LA)

Pulmonary artery

Pulmonary veins

RA LA

Tricuspid valve

Mitral valve

Pulmonary valve

RV LV

Aortic valve

Vena cava

Aorta

deoxygenated blood is returned to the right atrium (RA) via the vena cavae from the vebous circulation

oxygenated blood leaves the left ventricle (LV) via the aorta and is transported to the arterial circulation

Carbon diosxide diffuses out of the tissue cells

TISSUE CELLS

Oxygen diffuses into the tissue cells

Figure 1.9 The two distinct pressure circuits in the heart – the light grey represents oxygenated blood and the dark grey deoxygenated blood.

Blood vessels

The blood vessels form a tubular network of channels in which the blood is transported around the body. Blood leaving the heart passes through vessels of progressively smaller diameter referred to as the arterial system. Capillaries link the smallest arterial vessels, the arterioles, to the smallest venous vessels, the venules, thus linking arterial flow to the venous flow. Blood returning to the heart from the capillaries passes through vessels of progressively larger diameter referred to as the venous system (Fox 2004).

The walls of both arteries and veins have three layers that surround the lumen:

1. Tunica adventitia: the outermost layer made primarily of loose connective tissue. This anchors the blood vessel to the surrounding tissue.
2. Tunica media: the middle layer, which consists primarily of smooth muscle. The larger arteries contain numerous layers of elastin fibres, which facilitate the expansion and recoil ability of larger arteries. This ability to recoil creates the smoother, less pulsatile flow of blood in the smaller arteries and arterioles. The smaller vessels create the greatest resistance because they are less elastic and have a thicker layer of smooth muscle for their diameters.
3. Tunica intima: this layer consists of three sublayers:

   – the endothelium, which is an inner simple squamous layer that lines the lumina of all blood vessels and provides a smooth surface that repels blood cells and platelets
   – the basement membrane, which is made up of glycoproteins overlying connective tissue; it acts as a selectively permeable barrier to blood solutes and secretes vasoconstrictors and vasodilators; it also provides a smooth surface that repels blood cells and platelets
   – a layer of elastic fibres.

The walls of *arterioles* are composed of a layer of simple squamous epithelium or endothelium, which facilitates diffusion and osmosis. The walls of *venules* are made up of endothelium and fibrous tissue.

The diameter of the vessel and the composition of the blood vessel wall, as shown in Figure 1.10, reflect the volume and pressure of blood flow.

Capillaries

Capillaries are the smallest vessels in the tubular network and they are the most abundant. The total volume of this system is roughly 5 litres, the same as the total volume of blood. However, if the heart and major vessels are to be kept filled, all the capillaries cannot be filled at once. So a continual redirection of blood from organ to organ takes place in response to the changing needs of the body. During vigorous exercise, for example, capillary beds in the skeletal muscles open at the expense of those in the viscera. The reverse occurs after a heavy meal (Tortora et al. 2003). This control of the capillary is regulated by the actions of precapillary sphincter muscles, as shown in Figure 1.10.

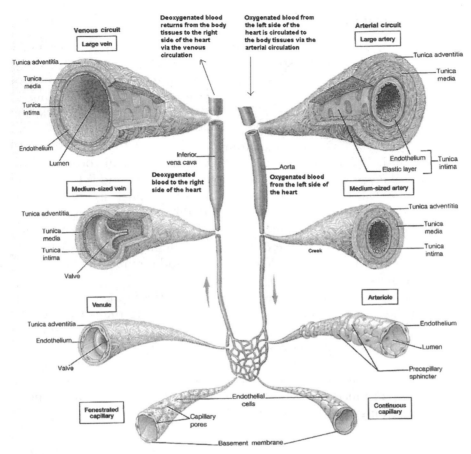

Figure 1.10 The structure composition of blood vessels and capillaries.

Three different types of capillaries are denoted by the nature of the endothelial lining, which is continuous, fenestrated or discontinuous:

1. In continuous capillaries the adjacent endothelial cells are closely joined together so they lack intercellular channels. They are found in muscles, lungs, adipose tissue and the central nervous system (CNS). The lack of intercellular channels in the CNS is a significant feature of the blood–brain barrier.
2. The kidneys, endocrine glands and intestines have fenestrated capillaries, which are characterized by intercellular pores covered by a layer of glycoprotein.
3. In the liver, bone marrow and spleen, the gap between endothelial cells is so large that the lining appears sporadic and the vessels are termed 'discontinuous capillaries'. The gaps are seen as little cavities called sinusoids in the liver.

Coronary blood flow

A reduction in blood supply to myocardial cells leads rapidly to cellular damage. Cardiac muscle tissue demands a constant supply of O_2 and nutrients. The coronary arteries as shown in Figure 1.3 are the network of blood vessels that carry O_2- and nutrient-rich blood to the cardiac muscle tissue. The blood leaving the left ventricle exits through the aorta, the body's main artery. Two coronary arteries, referred to as the 'left' and 'right' coronary arteries, emerge from the root of the aorta. The initial segment of the left coronary artery is called the left main coronary. This blood vessel is approximately the width of a soda straw and is less than an inch (2.5 cm) long. It branches into two slightly smaller arteries: the left anterior descending coronary artery and the left circumflex coronary artery. The left anterior descending coronary artery, or LAD, is embedded in the surface of the front side of the heart. The left circumflex coronary artery circles around the left side of the heart and is embedded in the surface of the back of the heart (Marieb 2004).

Just like branches on a tree, the coronary arteries branch into progressively smaller vessels. The larger vessels travel along the surface of the heart and the smaller branches penetrate the heart muscle. The smallest branches, capillaries, are narrow which results in the red blood cells moving in single file. In the capillaries, the red blood cells provide O_2 and nutrients to the cardiac muscle tissue and bond with CO_2 and other metabolic waste products, taking them away from the heart for disposal through the lungs, kidneys and liver (Levick 2003).

When the flow of blood through a coronary artery is reduced or interrupted, the cardiac muscle tissue fed by the coronary artery beyond the point of the blockage is deprived of O_2 and nutrients. This area of cardiac muscle tissue ceases to function properly because supply does not meet demand. Damage to the cardiac muscle tissue itself is called a myocardial infarction (MI). During exercise the flow through these arteries is up to five times the normal flow. Blocked flow in coronary arteries can result in death of heart muscle, leading to a heart attack.

Blockage of coronary arteries is usually the result of gradual build-up of lipids and cholesterol in the inner wall of the coronary artery. Occasional chest pain, angina pectoris, can result during periods of stress or physical exertion. Angina indicates that O_2 demands are greater than the capacity to deliver it and that an MI may occur. As heart muscle cells do not divide and replicate, damaged or dead myocardial cells are not replaced.

Cardiac muscle

Cardiac muscle is striated and the muscle cells consist of myofibrils (Figure 1.11) surrounded by sarcoplasmic reticulum (for calcium release and uptake) and mitochondria (for generation of adenosine triphosphate [ATP], the energy source for contraction) contained within the sarcolemma.

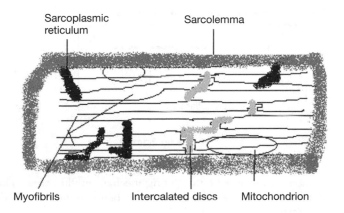

Figure 1.11 Longitudinal section of cardiac muscle showing myofibrils surrounded by sarcolemma. The muscle is striated similarly to skeletal muscle but is adapted for the rhythmic contractions required for the heart to function. Note the transverse bands called intercalated discs, which are junctions that allow for communication between the individual muscle cells, myofibrils. These gap junctions enable the rapid passage of electrical impulses (action potentials) from one cell to another and thus the simultaneous contraction of the atria and ventricles.

Each myofibril is made up of a number of sarcomeres, which are short, branched and interconnected longitudinally by dense attachments between the sarcomeres at the Z band (the insertion site of the actin filament). The intercalated discs represent gap junctions that are passages between the myofibril or myocardial cells, and permit the rapid transmission of electrical impulses, action potentials, from one myocardial cell to another. It is these gap junctions that enable the simultaneous contraction of the heart muscle in the two upper chambers and then in the two lower chambers, creating the essential rhythmic contractions.

Each sarcomere contains thick myosin filaments and thin actin filaments that slide over each other. The sliding mechanism that pulls the Z bands closer to each other (Figure 1.12), and thus brings about the *contraction* of the muscle, is energized by ATP. When the muscle relaxes actin filaments slide back into their original position in relation to the myosin filaments and the distance between the Z bands is returned. To bring about

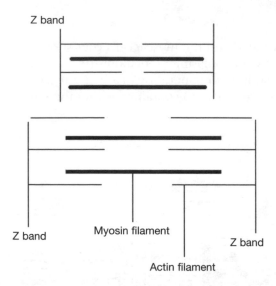

Figure 1.12 A single sarcomere with the sliding mechanism illustrated. The actin filaments move towards each other and the distance between the Z bands decreases as the muscle contracts.

this sliding mechanism the myosin filament interacts with the actin filaments in the following way:

- Each myosin molecule has a head which, when energized by hydrolysis of ATP (by an ATPase that is part of the myosin molecule), stands out at right angles to the myosin filament – as shown in Figure 1.13.
- Each myosin filament is surrounded by six actin filaments.
- There are a number of active protein-binding sites along the actin filaments that can interact with the myosin heads.
- In the resting state, these active sites on the actin filaments are covered by another protein, tropomyosin. Attached to the tropomyosin is a third protein, called troponin.
- When calcium combines with one of the protein subunits of troponin, the tropomyosin undergoes a conformational change such that these binding sites become available to the myosin head.
- The myosin head then interacts with the actin-binding site and forms a cross-bridge, which then facilitates the pushing of the actin filament longitudinally along the myosin filament – as shown in Figure 1.14.
- The higher the number of cross-bridges formed the stronger the contraction.
- The energy stored in the myosin heads is used to power this pushing mechanism.

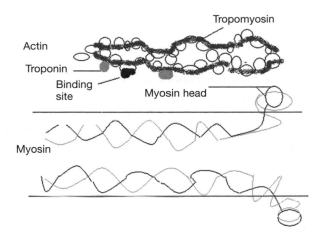

Figure 1.13 The structure of myosin and actin, showing the binding site for the myosin head. Note the position of the tropomyosin.

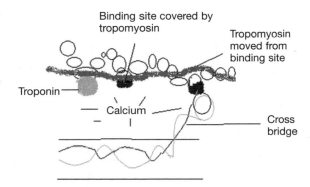

Figure 1.14 The movement of tropomyosin from the binding site when calcium interacts with the troponin. Note the formation of the cross-bridge.

At the end of the power push, which is likened to the stroke of an oar with the myosin filament represented by the oar, an uncoupling of the myosin head from the actin site occurs, and the myosin head is re-energized and moved back into a 'cocked' position by hydrolysis of another molecule of ATP.

The myosin heads then act in a wave-like fashion, interacting and uncoupling with each consecutive binding site and sweeping the actin filaments along, thus moving the Z lines closer together.

The strength of the myocardial contraction appears to be mediated primarily by the degree of uncovering of the actin active sites, as tropomyosin is pulled away from the active sites through the combination of troponin and calcium. The magnitude of this effect depends on the affinity of troponin for calcium and the availability of Ca^{2+} ions

When Ca^{2+} is removed from the cell at the termination of the action potential a conformational change reoccurs with disengagement of the actin filament from the myosin filament and tropomyosin, recovering the actin-active sites. This results in the relaxation of the sarcomere. As the removal of Ca^{2+} from the cytosol, by the huge number of ATP-dependent Ca^{2+} pumps in the sarcotubular system, is an energy-dependent process, relaxation therefore needs energy in the form of ATP.

Electrophysiology

Action potential

The term 'action potential', as seen in Figure 1.15, is the language of the nervous system and is the conductance of an electrical impulse that brings

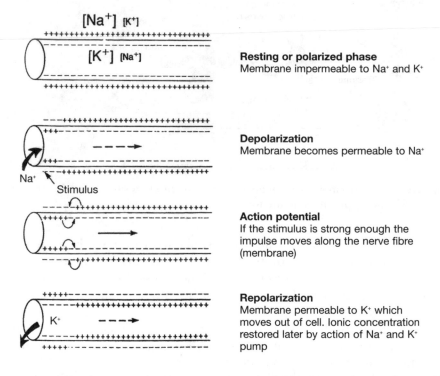

Resting or polarized phase
Membrane impermeable to Na^+ and K^+

Depolarization
Membrane becomes permeable to Na^+

Action potential
If the stimulus is strong enough the impulse moves along the nerve fibre (membrane)

Repolarization
Membrane permeable to K^+ which moves out of cell. Ionic concentration restored later by action of Na^+ and K^+ pump

Figure 1.15 The depolarization and repolarization along the cell membrane with the change of electrical gradients that occurs during the generation of an action potential.

about the contraction of the cardiac muscle. The electrocardiogram (ECG) reflects the electrical activity of cardiac tissue. This electrical activity relies on several essential factors as described in the following paragraph.

The cardiac cells, similar to all cells, have different concentrations of extracellular and intracellular ions, which create a chemical concentration gradient across the cell membrane, e.g. there is a high concentration of intracellular potassium (K^+) in comparison to the extracellular compartment, resulting in a chemical gradient for K^+ to diffuse out of the cell. The opposite situation is found with sodium (Na^+) where a high concentration of extracellular Na^+ is found in comparison to the intracellular concentration and the diffusion gradient is towards the inside of the cell (Figure 1.16).

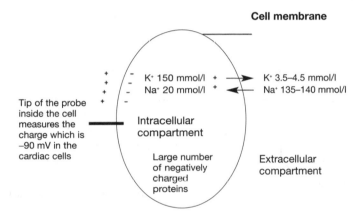

Figure 1.16 The cell indicating the intra- and extracellular ion concentrations which create the diffusion gradients, as indicated by the arrows, for Na^+ and K^+. Note the large number of negatively charged proteins inside the cell, which create the overall negative charge along the inner lining of the cell membrane.

There are also negatively charged proteins in the cell that cannot cross the cell membrane and collect along the inner cell membrane, and it is the collection of these negatively charged proteins that creates the overall negative charge of –90 mV (millivolts) across the cell membrane when measured from inside the cell (Shamroth 1957). This electrical difference that exists across the cell membrane is called the 'membrane potential'. Potential is described as the possibility/potential of the cardiac muscle cell having the capability/potential to contract forcefully.

Membrane potentials are determined primarily by:

- the concentration of intracellular and extracellular Na^+ and K^+ as indicated in Figure 1.16
- the concentration of intracellular and extracellular Ca^{2+}

- the permeability of the cell membrane to these ions
- the activity of the Na^+/K^+ ATPase and the Ca^{2+} transport pumps that maintain the concentrations of these ions across the membrane.

At rest when the heart is in between heart beats, the *resting potential* (Figure 1.17a) for a myocardial muscle cell is about −90 mV which is near the equilibrium potential for K^+. As the equilibrium potential for K^+ is −96 mV and the resting membrane potential is −90 mV, there is a net driving force of 6 mV acting on the K^+ to cause it to diffuse out of the cell. Therefore, as the resting cell has a finite permeability to K^+ and there is a small net outward driving force acting on K^+, there is a slow outward leak of K^+ from the cell.

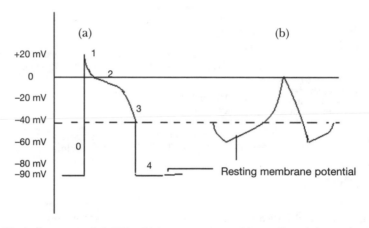

Figure 1.17 Action potential (AP) of (a) a non-pacemaking cell and (b) a pacemaking cell. The AP of the non-pacemaking cardiac cell begins with an initial rapid depolarization – the abrupt upstroke that is labelled phase 0 and brought about by the opening of the Na^+ gates and the inward flux of sodium. Phase 1 represents the early rapid repolarization followed by a phase of slow repolarization (phase 2) which is termed the plateau. Phase 3 is the terminal phase of relatively rapid repolarization. Phase 4 is the resting phase.

If the extracellular K^+ (serum K^+) concentration were increased from 4 to 7 millimoles (mmol) the chemical gradient for diffusion out of the cell would be reduced, and therefore the membrane potential required to maintain electrochemical equilibrium would be less negative, which brings the membrane potential nearer to zero and makes the cardiac tissue irritable. This irritability leads to arrhythmias, e.g. ventricular ectopics.

As the Na^+ concentration is higher outside the cell Na^+ ions diffuse down their chemical gradient into the cell. To prevent this inward flux of Na^+, there would need to be a large positive charge inside the cell (relative to the outside) in order to balance out the chemical diffusion forces. At rest, however, the permeability of the membrane to Na^+ is very low, so that only a small amount Na^+ leaks into the cell (Marieb 2004).

Although the resting potential of non-pacemaking cells is stable at −90 mV, until depolarization by a propagated impulse results in its abrupt reversal towards positive: phase 0 on an external reference electrode (Figure 1.17). The resting potential of pacemaking cells, as found in the sinoatrial node (SAN), is not recorded as a true resting phase. These cells have a so-called resting membrane potential of between −60 mV and −70 mV which is seen on an external reference electrode (Figure 1.17b) as a continuous slow spontaneous depolarization during the resting diastole caused by the relatively slow, inward diffusion of Ca^{2+} from the extracellular compartment through slow Ca^{2+} channels. When this spontaneous depolarization reaches the action potential threshold of −40 mV large amounts of additional Ca^{2+} ions stored in the sarcoplasmic reticulum are released and diffuse, via fast Ca^{2+} channels, which are opened in response to the depolarization (change in the concentration and distribution of ions) into the sarcomere. This rapid inward flux of Ca^{2+} ions opens the Na^+ voltage gates, which contributes towards the upshoot of the action potential (phase 0 on Figure 1.17a) which peaks at a measurement of about +20 mV (Figure 1.18).

The cycle of myocardial contraction and relaxation is directly related to cytosolic Ca^{2+} concentration. As the concentration of intracellular Ca^{2+} increases so more Ca^{2+} ions attach to the troponin proteins, causing the

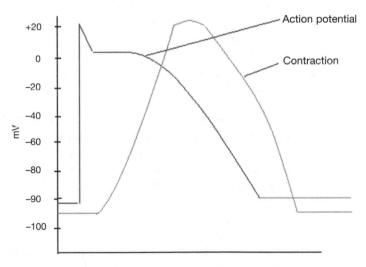

Figure 1.18 Action potential and contraction illustrating the change of voltage as measured across the cell membrane. The contraction occurs very rapidly after the heart muscle receives the message to contract.

tropomyosin proteins to move away from the binding sites on the actin filaments, thus enabling the formation of the cross-bridges (Romero et al.
2003). Once the muscle has contracted, relaxation is facilitated by the rapid
active transport of about 90% of the intracellular Ca^{2+} out of the sarcoplasm
by the Ca^{2+} ATPase pump in the sarcoplasmic reticulum and the rest by
Na^+/Ca^{2+} exchange and other mechanisms (Morgan and Morgan 1984).

As the initial movement of Ca^{2+} through the channels is not rapid, the
rate of depolarization (slope of phase 0 as shown in Figure 1.17) is much
slower than found in other non-pacemaker cardiac cells such as the
Purkinje cells and ventricular cells. When these cells are rapidly depolarized to the threshold of −70 mV by the conduction of another action
potential, there is a rapid depolarization to peak at +20 mV.

Although pacemaker activity is spontaneously generated by SAN cells
that give the inherent heart rate, the rate of this activity can be modified
significantly by external factors such as by autonomic nerves, hormones,
ions and ischaemia/hypoxia.

Repolarization follows depolarization and is caused by the opening of K^+
voltage gates and the outward diffusion of K^+ until the membrane potential is restored to between −60 mV and −70 mV. This repolarization is
divided into three phases (Figure 1.17):

1. Phase 1 represents an initial early and rapid movement of K^+ ions.
2. Phase 2 is termed the plateau, which results from the slow inward flux
   of Ca^{2+} ions that balances the outward flow of the K^+ ions and repolarization is delayed. This inward Ca^{2+} movement is through long-lasting
   (L-type) Ca^{2+} channels that open up when the membrane potential
   depolarizes to about −40 mV.
3. Phase 3 is the terminal phase which occurs as the concentration gradients of Ca^{2+} and K^+ are changing and K^+ ions continue to diffuse
   relatively rapidly outwards through the open voltage gates.

During phases 0, 1, 2 and part of 3 there is a period of time called the
effective refractory period (ERP), when the cell is incapable of responding
to the initiation of new action potentials This acts as a protective mechanism by limiting the frequency of action potentials and reducing preload.

Although the ECG shows heart rate and rhythm and can indicate myocardial damage, it gives no information on the adequacy of contraction.
Normal electrical complexes can exist in the absence of cardiac output, a
state known as pulseless electrical activity or electromechanical dissociation

Whenever an action potential is generated, Na^+ enters and K^+ leaves
the cell. Although the number of ions moving across the membrane of the
cell in a single action potential is very small, relative to the total number
of ions, after several action potentials there would be a significant change
in the inter- and intracellular concentrations. To maintain the chemical

concentration gradients, there is an ATP energy-dependent pump system, Na^+/K^+ ATPase, in the cell membrane that pumps three Na^+ ions out of the cell for every two K^+ ions entering the cell (Figure 1.19).

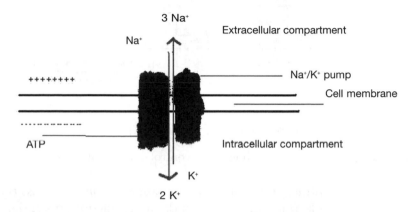

Figure 1.19 The Na^+/K^+ pump that is responsible for maintaining the chemical concentration gradients across the cell membrane. The ATP is fuelled by O_2 and glucose in cell respiration.

By pumping more positive changes out of the cell than into the cell, the pump activity creates a negative potential within the cell. As Ca^{2+} enters the cell during action potentials, it is necessary to maintain its concentration gradient. This is accomplished by Ca^{2+} transport pumps on the cell membrane. If the Na^+/K^+ pump ceases to function, such as in anoxic conditions when ATP is not generated, Na^+ accumulates intracellularly and intracellular K^+ falls, causing depolarization of the resting membrane potential which may be up to -10 mV. Cardiac muscle has a much richer supply of mitochondria than skeletal muscle, which reflects its greater dependence on cellular respiration for ATP and, as cardiac muscle has little glycogen, it gets limited benefit from glycolysis in anoxic conditions.

When Ca^{2+} enters the cell it leads to the actin–myosin interaction as described earlier. Energy is expended as the myosin heads are re-energized after each movement, and energy is expended in the removal of calcium from the cell back into the extracellular compartment by the Ca^{2+} pumps.

The conduction system

Heart rate is determined by the rate of spontaneous depolarization at the SAN but can be modified by the autonomic nervous system. The vagus nerve acts on muscarinic receptors to slow the heart, whereas the cardiac sympathetic fibres stimulate β-adrenergic receptors and increase heart rate as seen in the flow chart in Figure 1.20 (Main and Tucker 1993).

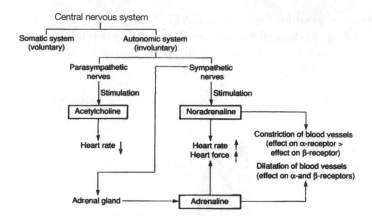

Figure 1.20 The factors contributing to the control of heart rate and blood vessels.

Myocardial contraction results from a change in voltage across the cell membrane (depolarization), which leads to an action potential and, although a contraction may happen spontaneously, it is normally in response to an electrical impulse. The action potential that drives contraction of the heart passes from fibre to fibre through gap junctions structured as intercalated discs (see Figure 1.11), which enable all the muscle fibres to contract in a synchronous wave.

This impulse starts in the SAN, a collection of pacemaker cells located at the junction of the right atrium and the superior vena cava. These specialized cells depolarize spontaneously, and generate electrical impulses that are conducted by special conducting tissue to the atrioventricular node (AVN). This causes a wave of contraction to pass across the atria.

On reaching the AVN, located between the atria and ventricles, the electrical impulse is relayed down conducting tissue (the bundle of His), which branches into pathways that supply the right and left ventricles. These paths are called the right bundle branch (RBB) and the left bundle branch (LBB), respectively. The impulses are then generated through the ventricular muscle via the Purkinje fibres.

Electrical impulses generated in the SAN cause the right and left atria to contract first, which is depicted by the 'P' wave. Depolarization occurs almost simultaneously in the right and left ventricles one- to two-tenths of a second after atrial depolarization. The entire sequence of depolarization, from beginning to end (for one heart beat), takes two- to three-tenths of a second and is depicted by the 'QRS' complex. The T wave represents repolarization of the ventricles and the return of the ventricles to the resting membrane potential. Repolarization of the atria is not pre-presented because it occurs while the ventricles are contracting and is hidden in the electrical recording. The R, QRS and T waves are illustrated in Figures 1.21 and 1.22.

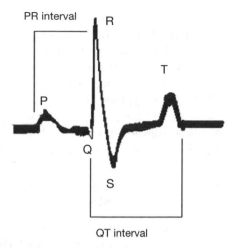

Figure 1.21 The basic waves of the electrocardiogram (ECG) illustrating the three distinct ECG waves designated P, QRS and T, which represent changes in potential between two regions on the surface of the heart. They are produced by the fused effects of action potentials in numerous myocardial cells (Shamroth 1957).

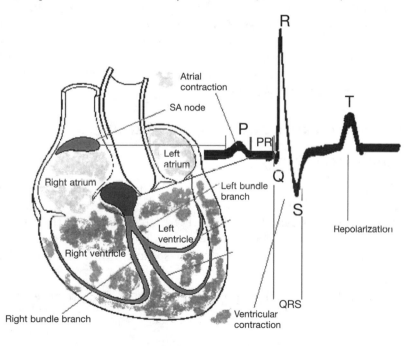

Figure 1.22 The relationship between the conduction system and the ECG: the first wave, called the P wave, records the electrical activity of the atria; the second wave, called the QRS complex, records the electrical activity of the septum; and the third wave, called the T wave, records repolarization. SA, sinoatrial.

The SAN is known as the 'heart's pacemaker' because electrical impulses are normally generated there. At rest the SAN usually produces 60–70 signals a minute. It is the SAN that increases its rate as a result of stimuli such as exercise, stimulant drugs or fever. If the SAN fails to produce impulses, the AVN can take over. The resting rate of the AVN is slower, generating 40–60 beats/min. The AVN and remaining parts of the conducting system are less capable of increasing heart rate as a result of stimuli previously mentioned than the SAN. The bundle of His can generate 30–40 signals a minute. Ventricular muscle cells may generate 20–30 signals a minute.

Heart rates below 35–40 beats/min for a prolonged period usually cause problems resulting from not enough blood flow to vital organs.

Problems with signal conduction, caused by disease or abnormalities of the conducting system, can occur at any point along the heart's conduction pathway. Abnormally conducted signals, resulting in alterations of the heart's normal beating, are called arrhythmias or dysrhythmias.

Cardiac arrhythmias can be caused by acute ischaemia (O_2 deprivation), sympathetic nervous system activation and myocardial scarring. Disorders in electrophysiology can include: (1) changes in automaticity (i.e. the ability of the heart to contract without external stimuli – resulting from the presence of its inherent pacemaker, the SAN) and (2) changes in conductivity (the ability to transmit an electrical impulse from cell to cell) caused by myocardial damage.

Blood pressure and cardiac output

Cardiac cycle

The cardiac cycle refers to a complete heart beat, which consists of a pattern of contraction and relaxation of both atria and ventricles. The phase of contraction is called systole and the phase of relaxation diastole. The cycle is described in a series of events that are called phases (see below) and are linked to the ECG. These five phases are shown in Figures 1.23–1.27.

Blood will flow only from point A to point B if the pressure at point A is greater than that at point B.

The heart is resting, all the chambers are in diastole and all the valves are closed. Blood is being returned into the atria as a result of the muscular pump and the negative intrapulmonary and intrapleural pressures. The ECG is represented as a straight isovolumetric line and is termed the

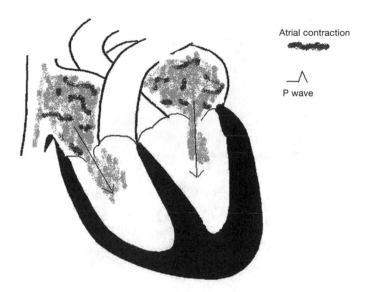

Figure 1.23 Phase 1 of the cardiac cycle: atrioventricular valves open and semilunar valves remain closed.

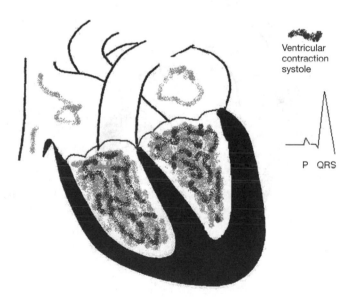

Figure 1.24 Phase 2 of the cardiac cycle: isovolumetric contraction – all valves closed.

'isovolumetric relaxation phase'. As the pressure in the atria rises above the pressure in the ventricles, the AV valves are pushed open and the blood flows from the atria into the ventricles down the pressure gradient – this may be called passive filling of the ventricles and accounts for between

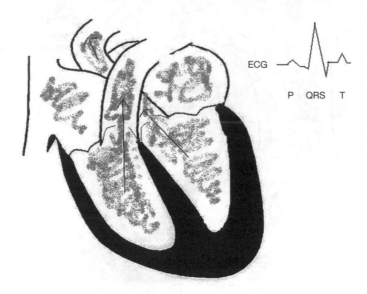

Figure 1.25 Phase 3 of the cardiac cycle: ventricular ejection – atrioventricular valves closed and semilunar valves open.

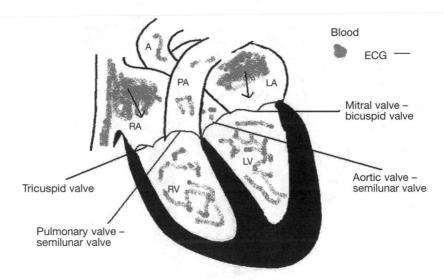

Figure 1.26 Phase 4 of the cardiac cycle: isovolumetric phase – the heart is in diastole and all valves close. A, aorta; LA, left atrium; LV, left ventricle; PA, pulmonary artery; RA, right atrium; RV, right ventricle.

70 and 90% of ventricular filling (the amount of blood returned into the ventricles). When the ventricles begin to fill, it occurs rapidly because the atrial pressure gradient is at its highest although, as the blood flows into

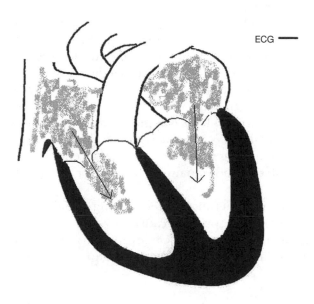

ECG ▬

Figure 1.27 Phase 5 of the cardiac cycle: ventricular filling – the valves open and the blood flows passively down its pressure gradient into the ventricle.

the ventricles, this pressure starts to even out across the AV valves and the flow into the ventricles starts to slow down – ventricular filling rate decreases – this phase is denoted as phase 5. Towards the end of ventricular filling the SAN depolarizes.

Phase 1: atrial systole, AV valves open, semilunar valves closed

- This is the first phase of the cardiac cycle because it is initiated by the P wave of the ECG which represents electrical depolarization of the atria. Atrial depolarization then causes contraction of the atrial musculature.
- The ventricles are in diastole.
- As the atria contract, the pressure in the atrial chambers increases so that a pressure gradient is built up again across the open (AV) valves, which causes a rapid flow of blood into the ventricles and completes the ventricular filling. This may be called active filling of the ventricles and accounts for between 10 and 30% of the amount of blood in the ventricles. When a person is at rest, most of the ventricular filling occurs before the atria contract and is therefore passive. However, if the heart rate is very high (e.g. during exercise), the atrial contraction may account for up to 40% of ventricular filling. This is sometimes referred to as the 'atrial kick'. Atrial contribution to ventricular filling varies inversely with duration of ventricular diastole and directly with atrial contractility.

- Blood is prevented from flowing backwards into the vena cavae by venous return and the wave of contraction throughout the atria.
- After atrial contraction is complete, the atrial pressure begins to fall below that in the ventricles, which causes the AV valves to float upward (pre-position) before closure. At this time, the ventricular volumes are maximal, which is termed the end-diastolic volume or EDV. The left ventricular EDV (LVEDV), which is typically about 120 ml, comprises the ventricular preload and is associated with end-diastolic pressures of 8–12 mmHg and 3–6 mmHg in the left and right ventricles, respectively.
- The atria repolarize and remain in diastole for the duration of the cardiac cycle.
  A heart sound is sometimes noted during atrial contraction (fourth heart sound, S4). This sound is caused by vibration of the ventricular wall during atrial contraction. Generally, it is noted when the ventricle compliance is reduced ('stiff' ventricle), as occurs in ventricular hypertrophy.

Phase 2: isovolumetric contraction, all valves closed

- This phase of the cardiac cycle is initiated by the QRS complex of the ECG, which represents ventricular depolarization–contraction–systole.
- The abrupt rise in pressure causes the AV valves to close because intraventricular pressure exceeds atrial pressure. Contraction of the papillary muscles with attached chordae tendineae prevents the AV valve leaflets from bulging back into the atria and becoming incompetent (i.e. 'leaky').
- Closure of the AV valves results in the first heart sound LUB; this sound is normally split because mitral valve closure precedes tricuspid closure.
- During the time period between the closure of the AV valves and the opening of the semilunar valves, ventricular pressure rises rapidly without a change in ventricular volume (i.e. no ejection occurs). Contraction is, therefore, said to be 'isovolumic' or 'isovolumetric'.

Phase 3: ventricular ejection, AV valves closed, semi-lunar valves open

- When the intraventricular pressures exceed the pressures within the aorta and pulmonary artery, the aortic and pulmonic valves are pushed open and blood is ejected out of the ventricles into the outflow tracts, i.e. the pulmonary artery and the aorta. The pressure in the left ventricle is typically about 120 mmHg and about 25 mmHg in the right ventricle. It is important to note that the ventricles are not emptied completely and the residual volume is called the end-systolic volume or ESV. No heart sounds are noted during ejection because the opening of healthy valves is silent. The presence of sounds during ejection (i.e. ejection murmurs) indicates valve disease or intracardiac shunts.

- Atrial pressure initially decreases as the atrial base is pulled downward, expanding the atrial chamber. Blood continues to flow into the atria from their respective venous inflow tracts.
- After the QRS complex, which represents ventricular systole, is completed ventricular repolarization occurs (T wave). As the ventricles relax with ventricular diastole, the intraventricular pressures fall below those in the pulmonary arteries and aorta. The higher pressures in the outflow tracts cause the aortic and pulmonic valves to close as a result of the back pressure. The closing of the semilunar valves causes the second heart sound – DUP.

Murmur: abnormal heart sound caused by a malfunctioning valve.

Stenosis: narrowing of the opening of a valve often caused by the stiffening of valve cusps resulting from scar tissue formation. In aortic stenosis, there is a narrowing of the aortic semilunar valve. This makes it harder for the left ventricle to push the required amount of blood through. Thus, the workload of the left ventricle has increased. The left ventricle will adapt by hypertrophying, i.e. getting larger, so that its greater muscle mass will be able to generate the force now necessary.

Prolapse: malfunction where one or more valve flaps bulge backwards into the atria.

Phase 4: isovolumetric relaxation, all valves closed

- Ventricular pressures decrease; however, volumes remain constant because all valves are closed so we have isovolumetric relaxation.
- The ESV is about 50 ml in the left ventricle (LVESV). The difference between the EDV and the ESV is about 70 ml and represents the stroke volume.
- Atrial pressures continue to rise as a result of venous return.
  The ESV provides a reserve volume for an increase in ventricular ejection with an increase in the force of myocardial contraction.

Phase 5: ventricular filling, AV valves open

- When the ventricular pressures fall below atrial pressures, the AV valves open and ventricular filling begins.
- The cardiac cycle is complete and returns to phase 1 to start again with the next heart beat.

Figure 1.28 shows the relationship of the ECG, intraventricular pressure changes and heart sounds during the phases of the cardiac cycle.

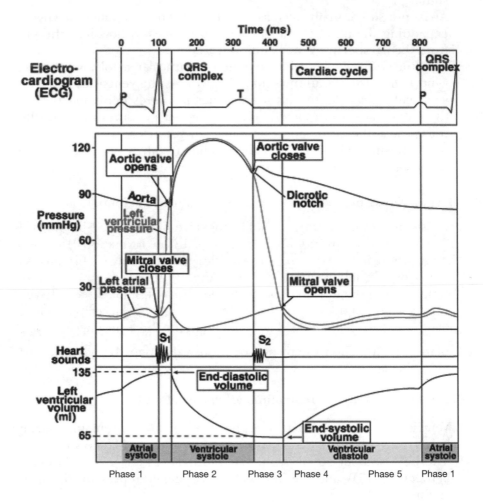

Figure 1.28 The interrelationship of the ECG, intraventricular pressure changes and heart sounds during the phases of the cardiac cycle described in the text.

Blood pressure

The flow of blood through the heart is a controlled pattern of contraction and relaxation known as the cardiac cycle. The main function of the heart is to pump blood around the body at an optimum pressure. This optimum pressure is measured as blood pressure.

Blood pressure is expressed as two numbers, e.g. 120/80. The first is the pressure during systole and units of measurement are millimetres of mercury (mmHg) or torr. In this example, the pressure is equivalent to that produced by a column of mercury 120 mm high. The second number is the pressure at diastole. The sounds heard are known as Korotkoff's sounds, the first sound being heard as blood passes in a turbulent flow through the constricted opening. This sound continues to be heard at every systole until the cuff pressure equalizes with the diastolic pressure and the sounds stop; in some people the sound does not disappear but alters in quality at the diastolic pressure.

Although blood pressure can vary greatly in an individual, when it is consistently above 140/90 it is diagnosed as hypertension. Causes of hypertension in most cases are unknown, although stress, obesity, high salt intake and smoking can add to a genetic predisposition. In these cases it is known as primary or essential hypertension. Hypertension that occurs as a result of known diseases is termed 'secondary hypertension' (Beers and Berkow 1999).

Blood leaves the heart via the large arteries, which divide into their terminal branches, the arterioles. Capillaries link the arterioles to the tributaries of the venous vessels, the venules, from where the blood is carried to the veins and returned to the heart. The blood vessels are structured in a closed circuit within which the blood circulates down a pressure gradient.

The initial force in the circuits is created by the simultaneous contraction of the ventricles. The ejection of blood that occurs at each contraction is transmitted through the elastic walls of the arterial system and is detected as the pulse. The pressure of arterial blood is largely dissipated when the blood enters the capillaries.

Murray's law predicts the manner in which arteries, vessels and capillaries should taper to progressively smaller diameters to optimize the circulatory system's efficiency in moving blood through the body with a minimal amount of friction (Zhou et al. 1999). Capillaries are tiny vessels with a diameter that is just about that of a red blood cell (7.5 μm). Although the diameter of a single capillary is quite small, the number of capillaries supplied by a single arteriole is so great that the total cross-sectional area available for the flow of blood is much higher. Therefore, the pressure of the blood decreases as it enters the capillaries.

When blood leaves the capillaries and enters the venules and veins, little pressure remains to force it along. Blood in the veins below the heart is helped back up to the heart by the muscle pump, which is simply the squeezing effect on the veins of contracting muscles running through them. The negative intrapleural and intrapulmonary pressures created on inspiration also act to pull blood back to the heart. One-way flow to the heart is achieved via valves within the veins.

Inserting an underwater drain may decrease the effect of the intrapleural negative pressure in the chest and reduce venous return, resulting in
peripheral oedema.

Blood pressure (BP) is affected by the heart rate (HR) and the stroke
volume (SV), which in turn is determined primarily by the blood volume
and total peripheral resistance (TPR).

Cardiac output and peripheral resistance are considered to be the two
most significant variables, with cardiac output over a minute expressed as
stroke volume times heart rate (Figure 1.29).

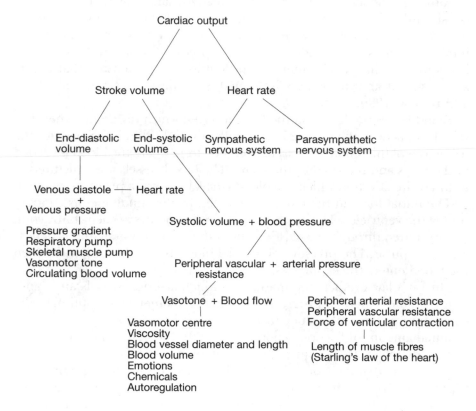

Figure 1.29 Flow chart summarizing the factors that contribute towards cardiac output.

Cardiac output is defined as the amount of blood pumped out of the
right ventricle into the pulmonary artery and out of the left ventricle into
the aorta with each heart beat simultaneously. This can be written as:

Cardiac output = Heart rate × Stroke volume
i.e. CO = HR × SV.

The decrease in heart rate corresponds with increased age and an elevation in the stroke volume.

If the heart rate is 70 beats/minute and the stroke volume is 70 ml, the cardiac output will be 70×70, which gives a cardiac output of 4.9 l/min or 4900 ml/min. For a 70-kg man, these are the normal values, so the cardiac output is about 5 l/min. Factors that alter the rate of the heart beat or the stroke volume will alter the cardiac output and therefore the blood pressure. An increase in heart rate is compensated for by a decrease in stroke volume, and vice versa, e.g. if the heart rate is 50 beats/min, to compensate for the reduced rate and maintain the cardiac output, and thus tissue perfusion, the stroke volume will increase to 95–100 ml. The cardiac index is the cardiac output per square metre of body surface area – normal values range from 2.5 to 4.0 l/min per m².

Cardiac output

Stroke volume is measured as the amount of blood pumped out of the ventricle with each heart beat or contraction. The stronger the contraction the greater the stroke volume tends to be. Stroke volume is measured by subtracting the amount of blood left in each ventricle at the end of each ventricular contraction (ESV) from the total amount in the ventricle before ventricular contraction (EDV):

SV = EDV – ESV.

The ejection fraction is determined by measuring the amount of blood ejected from the left ventricle with each beat as a fraction of the total EDV. If contraction strength is sufficient to eject 70–80 ml out of a total EDV of between 110 and 130 ml, the ejection fraction is about 60%. The ejection fraction will decrease with myocardial damage if the myocardial cells are unable to contract as efficiently.

Stroke volume is determined by three main factors: preload, contrachility and afterload (Figure 1.30).

Preload

End-diastolic volume is the workload imposed on the ventricles before they contract and is referred to as preload, which is determined by the length of ventricular diastole (how long ventricular filling time is) and venous return (how much blood is returned to the heart with which to fill the ventricles):

• Ventricular diastole is reliant on heart rate. If the heart rate is increased venous filling time is reduced, which in turn can affect cardiac output.

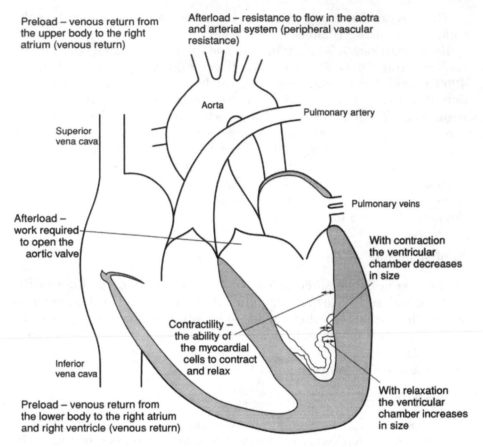

Figure 1.30 Summary of preload, contractility and afterload.

- Venous return is determined by the pressure gradient, which relies on the respiratory pump and the intrathoracic pressures, the skeletal muscle pump, the balance of constriction and dilatation in the venous system, and the circulating blood volume.

The stroke volume is directly proportional to preload or EDV. An increase in the EDV results in an increase in the stroke volume.

The Frank–Starling law of the heart demonstrates that the strength of the ventricular contraction varies directly with the EDV. When the EDV is increased within physiological limits, the ventricular myocardial muscle cells are stretched and the force of the contraction is increased in strength. Thus an increase in venous return increases stroke volume, which in turn raises cardiac output and BP. The parameters of stretch are significant here because, if the ventricle is overstretched beyond the length of the sarcomere, the myosin heads are dislodged and the cross-bridges disengage and the force of contraction may be significantly weakened with a reduction in stroke volume.

The stroke volume is also directly proportional to contractility, which is defined as the force with which the myocardial muscle cells contract.

Contractility

The most important influence on contractility is the sympathetic nervous system and the adrenal gland. β-Adrenergic receptors are stimulated by noradrenaline (norepinephrine) released from sympathetic nerve endings, and contractility increases. A similar effect is seen with circulating adrenaline (epinephrine) from the adrenal medulla. This response is termed a 'positive inotropic effect' and is a result of an increase in the amount of calcium made available to the sarcomeres. Contractility is reduced by acidosis, myocardial ischaemia, and the use of β-blocking and anti-arrhythmic agents.

To eject blood into the outflow tracts, the right and left ventricular systolic pressures must be higher than the pressures in the pulmonary artery and aorta.

Afterload

This is the resistance to ventricular ejection and is determined by the resistance to flow in the pulmonary and systemic circulations, which are referred to as the pulmonary and systemic vascular resistance, respectively. In a healthy circulation the resistance is characterized by the diameter of the arterioles and pre-capillary sphincters: the narrower or more constricted the blood vessel, the higher the resistance. The level of systemic vascular resistance is controlled by the sympathetic system which, in turn, controls the tone of the muscle in the wall of the arteriole, and hence the diameter. The flow of blood through the arterial blood vessels can be significantly reduced by disease processes as a result of which the lumen is narrowed or clogged, as in atherosclerosis.

If the left ventricle spends 70% of its contractile force building up enough pressure to open the aortic semilunar valve, it would have 30% of its contractile force to eject blood. If the pressure in the aorta is significantly higher, the left ventricle has to expend 85% of its contractile force to open the valve and so it has only 15% remaining for the ejection of blood. With an increase in the aortic blood pressure caused by narrowing, occlusion or peripheral arterial disease, which results in back pressure, the afterload increases and stroke volume must decrease. The left ventricle then has to work harder and harder to pump the blood into the aorta, which results in hypertrophy in response to the high afterload.

Tissue perfusion

The internal environment, which is made up of the plasma and interstitial fluid, provides all the requirements for cell functioning and survival by delivering essential ingredients to the cell and removing harmful waste from it. The phospholipid bilayer, which makes up the cell membrane, acts as the barrier between the interstitial fluid and the intracellular matrix and organelles. Cell requirements such as O_2 and sugar are transported across the cell membrane by a variety of routes, which, for example, involve passive diffusion and active transport processes. Substances such as CO_2 can diffuse out of cells and into the interstitial fluid.

The interstitial fluid is in continuous circulation at a flow determined by cardiac output. When the blood arrives in the capillaries fresh supplies of the glucose, O_2 and other plasma solutes are filtered through tiny endothelial channels in the capillary walls.

Control of the heart rate and blood pressure

Autonomic control

The nervous system coordinates many of the body's functions, as indicated in Figure 1.20. The sympathetic nervous system, in conjunction with the parasympathetic nervous system, helps regulate the heart rate and blood pressure in a negative feedback mechanism to compensate for deviations, as shown in Figures 1.31 and 1.32. In the heart, stimulation of the parasympathetic nerves (vagi) leads to a reduction in heart rate whereas stimulation of the sympathetic nerves increases the rate and force of contraction.

The response of the heart to a given situation is governed by a fine balance between these two systems. Neural impulses along the parasympathetic or sympathetic nerves achieve their effect by the release of chemical messengers, the neurotransmitters acetylcholine and noradrenaline (norepinephrine), which bind to the respective receptors (Figure 1.33). These pathways of neural messages elicit biochemical reactions, which are seen as physiological responses as indicated in Figures 1.31 and 1.32.

The smooth muscle cells of the blood vessels receive sympathetic adrenergic innervations and the tone of most blood vessels is directly related to the level of sympathetic activity. Impulses pass over the adrenergic receptors (Figure 1.33) and keep the blood vessels in a constant state of moderate constriction. An increase in the number of impulses reaching the muscle fibres raises the tone of the vasculature and increases tone, and therefore blood pressure, whereas a reduction in the number of impulses leads to a relaxation of the smooth muscle and vasodilatation, and

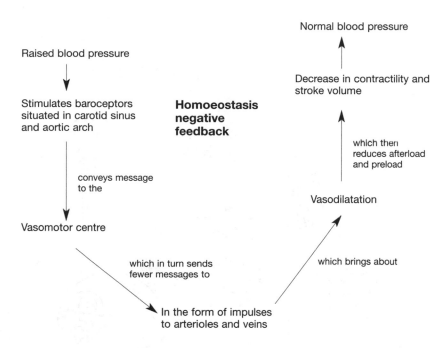

Figure 1.31 The negative feedback with raised blood pressure.

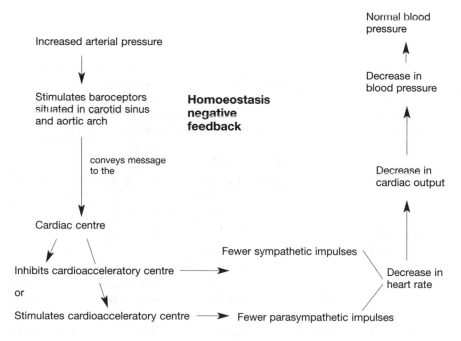

Figure 1.32 The negative feedback with raised arterial pressure.

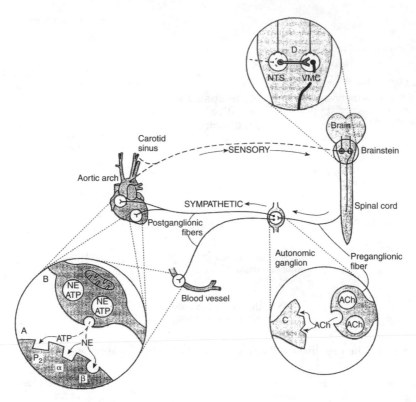

Figure 1.33 Schematic representations of the sympathetic arc involved in blood pressure regulation and sites where drugs may act to influence the system: (a) receptors on effector cells; (b) adrenergic varicosity: (c) nicotinic receptors (postganglionic fibres); (d) brain-stem nuclei. NTS, nucleus of the tractus solitarius; VMC, vasomotor centre: ACh, acetylcholine; NE, noradrenaline (norepinephrine); α, α-adrenoreceptors; β, β-adrenoreceptors; P₂, P₂ purinoceptors; ATP, adenosine triphosphate (adrenergic and cholinergic synapses). (From Westfall 1994.)

therefore blood pressure. The increased constriction manifests as cold peripheries, often termed 'peripheral shutdown'. With vasodilatation the peripheries may be warm and appear to be well perfused.

Baroreceptors, situated in the carotid artery and aortic arch, detect and relay the increased pressure message via afferent nerve fibres such as the vagus nerve to the cardiac (NTS – nucleus tractus solitarius) and cardio-vascular (vasomotor) centres in the medulla oblongata. Sympathetic activity via efferent fibres is reduced, bringing about a slowing of the heart rate and a decrease in stroke volume, resulting in a reduction in cardiac output and hence a lowered BP. There is also a reduction in the number of impulses to the blood vessels, causing vasodilatation, which reduces venous return and cardiac output. The homoeostatic responses to increased blood pressure and arterial pressure are illustrated in Figures 1.31 and 1.32.

Conversely, the baroreceptors relay a drop in blood pressure and sympathetic stimulation increases and raises the cardiac output, directly by increasing the heart rate and stroke volume and indirectly by vasoconstriction. By constricting the peripheral vessels the preload is increased which, according to Starling's law, will increase the stroke volume in a relatively healthy heart (Tortora et al. 2003). The peripheral vasotone is maintained at a constant state of moderate constriction for normal venous return by a steady number of adrenergic impulses.

Renal control of blood pressure

In response to a drop in the systemic blood pressure with a reduction in renal perfusion pressure, a chain of physiological events is triggered in order to restore the systemic blood pressure:

- Granular cells in the juxtaglomerular apparatus secrete the proteolytic enzyme, renin, directly into the bloodstream.
- Renin acts on angiotensinogen, a plasma globulin made in the liver, and cleaves off part of this peptide to produce angiotensin I.
- Angiotensin I is converted into angiotensin II by a peptidase, angiotensin-converting enzyme (ACE), which is an enzyme found in vascular endothelium, particularly the blood vessels in the lungs.
- Angiotensin II is a vasoconstrictor and acts by constricting the walls of arterioles and closing down capillary beds, hence raising blood pressure.
- Angiotensin II stimulates the proximal tubules in the kidney to reabsorb sodium ions, thus reducing the amount of water excreted and the volume of urine, hence increasing the circulating blood volume and in turn raising the blood pressure.
- Angiotensin II stimulates the adrenal cortex to release a hormone called aldosterone.
- Aldosterone causes the kidneys to reclaim still more sodium and therefore water.
- Angiotensin II can be broken down by enzymes – aminopeptidases A and N – into angiotensin III and IV.
- Angiotensin III stimulates aldosterone secretion and stimulates the thirst centres in the hypothalamus that make a person thirsty.
- Angiotensin IV activates the release of plasminogen activator inhibitor-1 (PAI-1) from the endothelium.

In addition to a fall in blood pressure, the release of renin is activated by prostaglandins, sympathetic nerve activity and circulating catecholamines. Blood pressure can also be sensed by stretch receptors on the afferent arterioles (Figure 1.34), which activate the renin–angiotensinogen system.

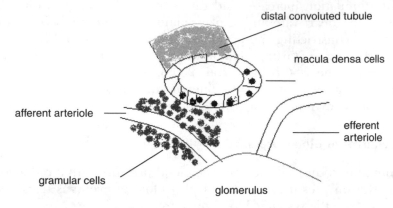

Figure 1.34 Juxtaglomerular apparatus.

In response to an increase in circulating blood volume there are mechanisms to increase urine output:

- Stretch receptors in the right atrium activate an inhibition of anti-diuretic hormone (ADH), which promotes a reduction in circulating blood volume by increasing urine production (natriuresis).
- Receptors in the right atrium detect the increased right atrial pressure and produce a hormone, atrial natriuretic factor (ANF), which promotes salt and water excretion in the kidney.

Atrial natriuretic factor antagonizes various actions of angiotensin II: it inhibits the secretion of aldosterone and renin, and promotes vasodilatation.

Blood

As a transport medium

Blood is a viscous fluid connective tissue that consists of cells and cell fragments suspended within a yellow fluid called plasma; this is the medium in which dissolved gases, nutrients, hormones and waste products are transported.

Gases

Blood, along with the heart and the blood vessels (e.g. veins and arteries), comprise the circulatory system of the body. The circulatory system helps in maintaining balanced conditions within the body (i.e. homoeostasis), e.g. O_2 is picked up by blood as it passes through the lungs; this blood in turn flows through successively narrower blood vessels – from arteries to arteriolcs and finally the capillaries – where the O_2-rich blood delivers its O_2 to the cells. O_2 is taken from the lungs to the cells of the body and CO_2 from the cells to the lungs.

Nutrients

Nutrients are taken from the gastrointestinal tract to the cells and waste products from the cells to the lungs, kidneys and bowel.

Hormones

Hormones are taken from glands to the cells.

Other

Essential elements such as white blood cells are taken to sites of invasion by foreign micro-organisms.

Blood also regulates pH – the acidity and alkalinity of the blood.

The role of blood is not just for the transportation of substances within the body. The white blood cells are a vital source of defence against external organisms. White blood cells also serve as 'health maintenance engineers' cleaning up dead cells and tissue debris which would otherwise accumulate and lead to problems.

The different specialized cells found in blood suspended in the plasma are:

- red blood cells – erythrocytes
- platelets – thrombocytes
- white blood cells (five different classes)
- granulocytes, which are subdivided into:
  - neutrophils
  - eosinophils
  - basophils – all contain granules
- agranulocytes, which are subdivided into lymphocytes and monocytes, which do not contain granules.

About 90% of plasma is water – blood's solvent – with the rest composed of dissolved substances, primarily proteins (e.g. albumin, globulin and fibrinogen).

Plasma typically accounts for 55% by volume of blood; of the remaining 45% the greatest contribution is from the red blood cells.

Red blood cells

These are flexible, biconcave discs, which make up 99% of the cells in the blood. They are formed by a process called erythropoiesis which starts in red bone marrow of certain bones, including the vertebrae, ribs, breast bones, skull bones and long bones. Red blood cells do not have a nucleus and can neither reproduce nor undertake metabolic activities. They are the principal carriers of the red-coloured haemoglobin molecules. Flexibility is vital in order for them to be able to pass through blood vessels to reach other cells. The average lifespan of a human red blood cell is 120 days. Every second, 2.4 million red blood cells are destroyed. The dead red cells are removed through the liver and spleen, where phagocytes engulf them, removing them from circulation. The number of red blood cells destroyed must be replaced by producing more.

Haemoglobin is an iron-containing protein which binds about 97% of all O_2 in the body. O_2 is not very soluble in water hence if O_2 were simply dissolved in the fluid of blood not much could be carried by the bloodstream. The unique surface shape of red blood cells is nature's design to maximize surface area in order to facilitate absorption and release of O_2.

People's blood is not all the same. The cell membrane of red blood cells contains different proteins, which are responsible for different types of blood. There are primarily two types of proteins found in the cell membrane of red blood cells: protein A and B. Different combinations of these proteins and their antibodies result in four types of blood:

1. Type A: have protein A and antibodies to B protein
2. Type B: have protein B and antibodies to A protein
3. Type AB: have both proteins A and B but neither of the antibodies
4. Type O: have neither protein but have both the antibodies.

Type AB is called 'universal acceptor' and type O is called 'universal donor' because of the ability of people with these blood groups to accept blood or donate blood to all other blood groups, respectively.

White blood cells

Also known as leukocytes, white blood cells (WBCs) have nuclei and are used to defend the human body against harmful bacteria. These blood cells are amoeba-like cells that can move against the current of the bloodstream. Some can penetrate through the walls of blood vessels and enter the tissues.

The different kinds of WBCs are formed in various sites. Granular leukocytes develop from red bone marrow and contain distinct granules, e.g.:

- Neutrophils ingest micro-organisms and contain enzymes that destroy these foreign invaders, e.g. bacteria, by a process called phagocytosis. They also ingest dead tissue cells that remain after an injury or surgery.
- Eosinophils increase in numbers and become active in the presence of certain infections and allergies.
- Basophils, which secrete heparin and histamine. They have similar functions to eosinophils. They contain a large amount of the chemical histamine, which is released during an allergic response and in injured tissues. Basophils also play a role in preventing clotting in the body. They release an anti-clotting chemical called heparin, which prevents blood from clotting within blood vessels.

There are two kinds of non-granular leukocytes: lymphocytes and the less numerous monocytes, both of which are associated with the immune system. Lymphocytes are formed in the thymus, the lymph glands and other lymphatic tissue. They have an important role in producing antibodies and in cellular immunity. Monocytes are formed initially in the bone marrow and spend the first 24 hours in the bloodstream; thereafter they leave the blood for further development in the spleen, liver, lymph nodes and other organs. They differentiate into macrophages which are phagocytic, and digest foreign substances, and any cellular debris, acting as a back-up for neutrophils in infections.

Humans can find out if they have any sort of bacterial infections through knowledge of their WBC count. The normal amount of WBCs is 7000/mm³ of blood (about one for every 700 red blood cells). If the count increases, the individual has some kind of bacterial infection.

Thrombocytes or platelets

These are small, round, non-nucleated bodies with a diameter about one-third that of red blood cells. They are formed in the bone marrow by the fragmentation of cells called megakaryocytes. Thrombocytes adhere to the walls of blood vessels at the site of an injury and thus plug the defect in the vascular wall. As they disintegrate, they release clotting agents which leads to the local formation of thromboplastin; this helps to form a blood clot, the first step in the healing of an injury.

Blood formation and reactions

All blood cells originate from cells in the bone marrow called pluripotent stem cells. Pluripotent means that they are capable of becoming many different things. Pluripotent stem cells give rise to two different types of cells: lymphoid stem cells, which migrate to the lymphatic tissue, and myeloid stem cells, which remain in the bone marrow. These cells then divide by mitosis to produce all the other kinds of blood cells.

Of current interest is the replacement of stem cells by either donor or cloned cells.

Plasma and platelets in clotting

If damage occurs to a blood vessel, circulating platelets immediately get trapped at the injury site. On accumulating, the platelets 'plug' the leak in the vessel providing a first step in damage control. This mechanism is supplemented by 'blood coagulation', or clotting, which is the most important means of defence against bleeding.

Plasma contains several dissolved proteins:

- Fibrinogen is a rod-shaped soluble protein which, in the presence of the catalyst thrombin, gets converted to an insoluble protein fibrin.
- Fibrin molecules make a tangled net of fibres by adhering end to end and side to side, which immobilizes the fluid portion of blood (causing it to solidify) and also traps the red blood cells.

The combined action of the platelets and 'fibrin web' is sufficient to prevent a dangerous loss of blood. In cases where the formation of fibrin and hence formation of a clot is impaired for some reason (e.g. a genetic disorder as in haemophilia), the person is at great risk of bleeding to death.

Blood clotting means the conversion of fluid blood to a solid clot (Rang et al. 1999), with the soluble fibrinogen becoming an insoluble fibrin mesh. This process is an enzyme-driven one with the proteolytic enzymes and co-factors creating a complex cascade of events, resulting in the formation of a clot. There are two main pathways:

1. The intrinsic pathway, which occurs when the plasma is exposed to a negatively charged surface such as the glass of a test tube or to collagen in damaged blood vessels.
2. The extrinsic pathway, which is initiated by a substance called 'tissue factor'. This is the cellular receptor and co-factor for factor VII, which is the starting point for a 'shortcut' formation of fibrin.

Inactive precursors are activated in a series of steps, each vital for the next stage in the cascade. These pathways overlap as both result in the activation of thrombin, which converts fibrinogen into the fibrin mesh (Figure 1.35).

Blood clotting is controlled by enzyme inhibitors such as anti-thrombin III and fibrinolysis. Dissolution of the clots is brought about by the molecule kallikrein, which catalyses the conversion of inactive plasminogen into the

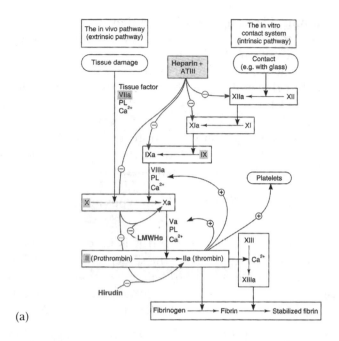

(a)

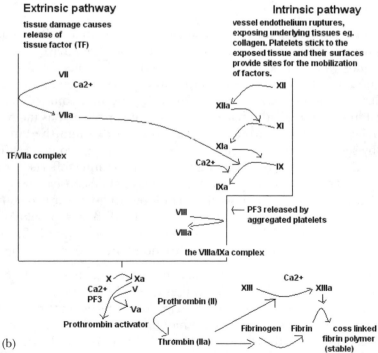

(b)

Figure 1.35 (a) The blood clotting pathways. (b) The events that lead to platelet aggregation. ATIII, anti-thrombin III; PL, phospholipid.

active molecule plasmin. Plasmin is an enzyme that digests fibrin. As the damaged blood vessel is repaired, activated factor XII promotes the activation of the proteolytic enzyme kallikrein.

Anti-thrombin III is activated by heparin, a mucoprotein produced in the liver. Anti-thrombin III combines with and inactivates thrombin.

Vitamin K is required for the conversion of the amino acid, glutamic acid, which is an ingredient of several of the clotting factor proteins, into γ-carboxyglutamic acid. This derivative is more effective than glutamic acid at binding to calcium, which is needed for the correct functioning of a number of the clotting factors such as factors II, VII, IX and X.

The human adrenoceptor (see Figure 1.33) subtypes are classified as: α_1, α_2, β_1, β_2 and β_3.

The subdivision of adrenoceptors into α and β is based on the relative potencies of various adrenergic agonists and the susceptibility of blockade by specific drugs: the catecholamines, noradrenaline, adrenaline and isoproterenol stimulate α-adrenergic receptors in a descending order of sensitivity: adrenaline > noradrenaline > isoproterenol (Hieble et al. 1995a).

In contrast β-adrenergic receptors are stimulated most potently by: isoproterenol > adrenaline > noradrenaline.

Propranolol is a competitive β-adrenergic antagonist that is devoid of agonist activity. Efforts to generate additional antagonists have resulted in compounds that can be distinguished by relative affinity for β_1- and β_2-receptors, blockade of α-adrenergic receptors, capacity to induce vasodilatation and general pharmacokinetic properties. Some of these distinguishing characteristics have clinical significance such as tachycardia and increased cardiac output. These are further distinguished into subtypes by selective and non-selective agonists and antagonists. Different β-antagonistic agents caused varying degrees of unwanted effects, e.g. some of the β blockers such as propranolol caused bronchial constriction in some individuals, along with the desired effect of lowering the cardiac output by slowing the heart rate – termed non-selective (binds β_1 and β_2 subtype) – as opposed to atenolol, which is selective because it binds with the β_1 subtype only and does not cause bronchial constriction (Hieble et al. 1995b).

Carvedilol is a non-selective β blocker that slows the heart rate. In addition carvedilol is an α blocker that causes arterial dilatation. This reduces the arterial resistance (afterload), which in turn reduces ventricular systolic pressure (systolic blood pressure). Both of these actions reduce myocardial metabolic activity and thus the demand for O_2 and nutrients. It is used when supply does not meet demand as in atherosclerosis of the coronary arteries, which has caused left ventricular failure or heart failure.

Cardiac enzymes or biochemical markers

These are molecules released into the circulation as a consequence of cardiac injury. They are used in the diagnosis of MI, but elevations are not synonymous with an ischaemic mechanism of injury and results should be interpreted in the context of clinical and ECG findings.

It is important to note that cardiac enzymes such as creatine kinase (CK), aspartate aminotransferase (AST) and lactate dehydrogenase (LDH) are of variable specificity to cardiac muscle.

Cardiac troponins T and I are the preferred markers for the diagnosis of myocardial injury. These markers are more sensitive and more specific than measuring CK, AST or LDH. Some authorities believe that these latter assays should no longer be used to evaluate cardiovascular disease (Beers and Berkow 1999). It is accepted, however, that total CK may have a role in trials to allow comparison with previous data and also that measurement of the variant CK-MB may help clarify whether a cardiac event has occurred within the preceding 48 hours. Cardiac enzymes include:

- cardiac troponin T and I, CK: earliest to rise
- AST: second to rise
- LDH: latest to rise.

Peaks tend to occur earlier and are often higher after successful thrombolytic therapy. This is attributed to the 'wash-out' of enzymes from the infarcted area immediately after re-perfusion occurs.

Pathology

Coronary artery disease

Partial occlusion of the coronary blood vessels by atheromatous deposits has important consequences for the functioning of the heart. The disease process of atherosclerosis is largely asymptomatic.

Atherosclerosis affects mainly medium and large arteries and the two main coronary arteries, and is characterized by patchy thickening and hardening of the blood vessel wall. This thickening then encroaches into the lumen of the blood vessel. The diameter of the vessel and the degree of intrusion will determine the degree of stenosis, or total occlusion may result.

Deposits of intracellular and extracellular fatty substances and cholesterol, calcium, intimal smooth muscle cells and connective tissue along with cellular waste products build up in the inner lining of an artery. This build-up is called plaque or atheroma and may grow slowly and over several decades. With time the plaque becomes calcified (Woodcock 1989). Although the plaques can grow large enough to reduce the blood flow

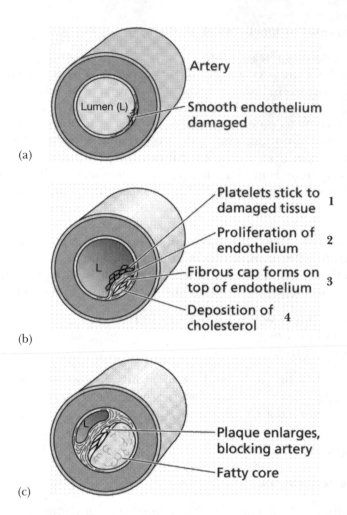

Figure 1.36 The development of a plaque from damaged endothelial lining of blood vessel. The sequence of events, 1–4, are shown in (b). The fatty core in (c) is referred to as a foam cell.

through an artery significantly, most of the damage occurs when they become fragile and rupture.

Plaque stability

Some plaques are deemed unstable or vulnerable. The plaques (Figure 1.36) are rich in lipids and inflammatory cells (e.g. macrophages) and covered by a thin fibrous cap; they undergo spontaneous fissure or rupture, exposing the plaque contents to flowing blood. Plaques that rupture cause blood clots to form which can block blood flow or break off and become an embolus and travel to another part of the body. If either happens and blocks a blood vessel that feeds the heart muscle, it causes an acute myocardial ischaemic event. The blood clot may gradually become incorporated into the plaque, contributing to its stepwise growth.

After atherosclerotic plaque rupture a sequence of events is triggered as detailed in Figure 1.35b. Platelets adhere to the subendothelial cells and become activated. Collagen, thrombin, ADP and thromboxane A_2 (TxA$_2$) are some of the stimuli able to induce and then perpetuate full platelet activation. Collagen acts primarily through a glycoprotein VI and thrombin, ADP and TxA$_2$ function through G-protein-coupled receptors.

Once activated, platelets:

- change from smooth discs to spiny spheres with protruding pseudopods, which facilitates their mobility and activations
- secrete granule contents which include the platelet agonist, ADP, coagulation factors and platelet-derived growth factors
- biosynthesize mediators, platelet-activating factor and TxA$_2$
- mediate platelet aggregation by fibrinogen–fibrinogen connects the platelets by bridging complexes of glycoprotein IIb/IIIa on adjacent platelets. Each platelet contains about 50 000–80 000 glycoprotein IIb/IIIa (GPIIb/IIIa) molecules on its surface.

The rapid formation of a 'platelet plug' at sites of vascular injury is the main mechanism of primary haemostasis; however, when platelets become activated after the rupture of atherosclerotic plaques or in regions of disturbed blood flow, the sequence of events leads to thromboembolic complications that underlie thrombotic events such as myocardial infarction.

Thromboxane A_2 is produced by activated platelets by the sequential conversion of arachidonic acid by phospholipase A_2, cyclo-oxygenase-1 (COX-1) and thromboxane synthase (see Figure 1.35b). In vascular endothelial cells, COX-1 is involved in the generation of prostacyclin which inhibits platelet activation and leads to vasodilatation.

There are two main hypotheses proposed to explain the development of the atherosclerotic plaque: the lipid hypothesis and the chronic endothelial injury hypothesis.

The lipid hypothesis

An elevation in plasma low-density lipid (LDL) levels results in the following:

- Penetration of LDL into the arterial wall, leading to lipid accumulation in smooth muscle cells and in macrophages.

- LDL augments smooth muscle cell hyperplasia and migration into the subintimal and intimal region, in response to growth factors.
- LDL is oxidized in this environment which make it more atherogenic.
- The modified LDL is chemotactic to monocytes, promoting their migration into the intima, their early appearance in the fatty streak, and their transformation and retention in the subintimal compartment as macrophages.
- Scavenger receptors on the surface of macrophages facilitate the entry of oxidized LDLs into these cells, transferring them into lipid-laden macrophages called foam cells. Normally macrophages protect the body by ingesting invading micro-organisms and toxic substances, including oxidized lipids. In fatty plaques the macrophages become so engorged with the LDLs that they migrate between the interna, where they are transformed into foam cells and lose their scavenging ability.
- Oxidized LDL is also cytotoxic to endothelial cells and may be responsible for their dysfunction or loss from the more advanced lesion.

The proliferating smooth muscle cells accumulate lipid. As the fatty streak and fibrous plaque enlarge and bulge into the lumen, the subendothelium becomes exposed to the blood at sites of endothelial retraction or tear, and platelet aggregates and mural thrombi form. Release of growth factors from the aggregated platelets may increase smooth muscle proliferation in the intima. Alternatively, organization and incorporation of the thrombus into the atherosclerotic plaque may contribute to its growth (Woodcock 1989).

Cholesterol is a soft, waxy substance found among the lipids (fats) in the bloodstream and in all the body's cells. It is part of a healthy body because it is used to form cell membranes and some hormones, and is needed for other functions. However, a high level of cholesterol in the blood – hypercholesterolaemia – is a major risk factor for coronary heart disease (CHD), which leads to myocardial infarction.

Cholesterol and other fats cannot dissolve in the blood. They have to be transported to and from the cells by special carriers called lipoproteins. Although there here are several kinds of lipoproteins, the significant two are LDL and high-density lipoprotein (HDL).

Low-density lipoprotein is the major cholesterol carrier in the blood. In excess it contributes towards the formation of atheromas or plaques. Excessive cholesterol may be released from cells and travel in the blood as HDL which is the removed by the liver. The cholesterol in HDL is not taken into the arterial wall because these cells lack the membrane receptor required for endocytosis of the HDL particles. Some say that HDL is beneficial because the cholesterol is travelling away from the arterial walls.

Lipoprotein a [Lp(a)] is a genetic variation of plasma LDL and delivers cholesterol to sites where tissues is being repaired, e.g. damaged endothelium.

A high level of Lp(a) is an important risk factor for developing atherosclerosis prematurely because it is thought to promote mitosis of the cells in the vessel wall. In addition, it resembles plasminogen so it can assist with blood clot formation but is not capable of dissolving clots. It therefore competes against the 'clot busters' activity of plasminogen and may prevent the disposal of undesirable clots.

The chronic endothelial injury hypothesis

This hypothesis suggests that endothelial injury by various mechanisms produces loss of endothelium which initiates an inflammatory reaction with:

- adhesion of platelets to subendothelium
- aggregation of platelets
- chemotaxis of monocytes and T-cell lymphocytes, and release of platelet-derived and monocyte-derived growth factors which induce migration of smooth muscle cells from the media into the intima, where they replicate, synthesize connective tissue and proteoglycans, and form a fibrous plaque
- other cells, which include macrophages and endothelial cells also produce growth factors that can contribute to smooth muscle hyperplasia and extracellular matrix production (Beers and Berkow 1999).

Causes of damage to the arterial wall and exacerbation of atherosclerosis include:

- elevated levels of cholesterol and triglyceride
- high blood pressure
- tobacco smoke
- diabetes.

Research also suggests that inflammation in the circulating blood may play an important role in triggering heart attacks and strokes. Inflammation is the body's response to injury, and blood clotting is often part of that response. Blood clots, as described above, can slow down or stop blood flow in the arteries.

Plaque rupture and acute coronary syndromes

After acute plaque rupture thrombosis ensues. This thrombosis can partially or completely occlude the affected coronary artery. In addition to this clotting cascade, Maseri et al. (1978) suggest that vasoconstriction may also play an important role. The extent of the occlusion and subsequent vasoconstriction can be classified to some degree with differing diagnosis. Most practitioners are now familiar with the umbrella term acute coronary syndromes – it reflects not only the commonality in pathophysiology but also its usage as a discharge diagnosis, although it may also reflect the current difficulty in diagnosing the various manifestations.

Unstable angina occupies the beginning of this spectrum, causing disability and risk greater than stable angina but less than that of non-Q-wave MI (Braunwald et al. 1994). The risk of death or non-fatal MI complicating unstable angina ranges from 8% to 16% at the 1-month follow-up (Bertrand et al. 2000). Although non-Q-wave MI was for many years thought to have a similar prognosis to unstable angina some studies indicate that the prognosis for this group is similar to ST-elevation MI (Aguire et al. 1995).

In unstable angina a platelet-rich thrombosis at the site of plaque rupture occurs, resulting in temporary occlusion of the affected artery lasting around 10–20 minutes. Vasoconstriction may also occur further reducing coronary flow (Willerson et al. 1989). This temporary occlusion produces areas of ischaemia in the surrounding myocardium and manifests itself on the ECG as ST depression (Jones 2003). In non-ST elevation MI a more severe plaque damage may occur, resulting in thrombus formation and coronary occlusion for up to 1 h (Fuster et al. 1992). If coronary blood flow is obstructed for longer than 20 min, a growing area of cell necrosis develops in the affected part of the muscle (Jones 2003). Coronary flow can be disturbed in excess of 1 h without full-thickness infarct developing, if collateral circulation is sufficient, and so at this point full-thickness infarct is avoided. Resolution of vasoconstriction and spontaneous thrombolysis may also play a role in the limitation of this process (Theroux and Fuster 1998). In ST-elevation MI, larger plaque fissures result in the formation of a fixed and persistent thrombus (Fuster et al. 1992). This thrombus will often be fibrin rich, which traps circulating blood cells and encapsulates them in a thick mesh. This stubborn clot leads to coronary occlusion in excess of 2 h (unless thrombolysis occurs), resulting in transmural or fullthickness MI (Willerson et al. 1986).

References

Aguire FV, Younis LL, Chaitman BR et al. (1995) Early and 1 year clinical outcome of patients evolving non-Q wave and Q wave MI after thrombolysis: results from the TIMI II study. Circulation 91: 2541–8.

Beers M, Berkow R (eds) (1999) The Merck Manual of Diagnosis and Therapy, 17th edn. Whitehouse Station, NJ: Merck Research Laboratories.

Bertrand ME, Simoons ML, Fox KAA et al. (2000) Management of acute coronary syndromes: acute coronary syndromes without persistent ST segment elevation.

Recommendations of the Task Force of the European Society of Cardiology. Eur Heart J 21: 1406–32.

Braunwald E, Jones RH, Mark DB et al. (1994) Diagnosing and managing unstable angina. Circulation 90: 613–22.

Fox S (2004) Human Physiology, 7th edn. London: WmC Brown.

Fuster V, Badimon L, Badimon JJ, Chesebro JH (1992) The pathogenesis of coronary artery disease and the acute coronary syndromes. N Engl J Med 326: 242–50, 310–18.

Hieble P, Ruffolo R, Bondinell W (1995a) Alpha- and beta adrenoceptors: From the gene to the clinic. 2. Structure–activity relationships and therapeutic applications. J Med Chem 38: 18.

Hieble P, Ruffolo R, Bondinell W (1995b) An overview of the current status of α- and β-adrenoceptor pharmacology and medicinal chemistry. 2nd part. J Med Chem 38: 19.

Jones I (2003) Acute coronary syndromes: Identification and patient care. Professional Nurse 18: 289–92.

Levick J (2003) An Introduction to Cardiovascular Physiology, 4th edn. London: Arnold.

Main B, Tucker H (1993) Medicinal Chemistry, 2nd edn. New York: Academic Press.

Marieb E (2004) Human Anatomy and Physiology, 6th edn. London: Pearson Benjamin Cummings.

Maseri A, L'Abbate A, Baroldi G et al. (1978) Coronary vasospasm as a possible cause of myocardial infarction: a conclusion derived from the study of pre-infarction angina. N Engl J Med 299: 1271–7.

Menet E, Corbi P, Ancey C et al. (2001) Interleukin-6(IL-6) synthesis and gp130 expression by human pericardium. Eur Cytokine Network 12: 639–46.

Morgan J, Morgan K (1984) Calcium and cardiovascular function. Intracellular calcium levels during contraction and relaxation of mammalian cardiac and vascular smooth muscle as detected with aequorin. Am J Med 77(5A): 33–46.

Parker Anthony C (1944) Textbook of Anatomy and Physiology, 7th edn. St Louis, MO: Mosby.

Rang H, Dale M, Ritter J (1999) Pharmacology, 4th edn. London: Churchill Livingstone.

Romero M, Sanchez I, Pujol M (2003) New advances in the field of calcium channel antagonists: cardiovascular effects and structure–activity relationships. Curr Med Chem – Cardiovasc Hematol Agents 1: 113–41.

Shamroth L (1957) An Introduction to Electrocardiography, 6th edn. London: Blackwell.

Steinbis S (2003) Hypertropic obstructive cardiomyopathy and septal ablation. Crit Care Nurse 23: 47–50.

Theroux P, Fuster V (1998) Acute coronary syndromes: Unstable angina and non Q wave myocardial infarction. Circulation 97: 1195–206.

Tortora G, Grabowski N, Reynolds S (2003) Principles of Anatomy and Physiology: Vol. 1: Organization of the Human Body, 10th edn. New York: Wiley & Sons.

Westfall D (1994) Antihypertensive drugs. In: Craig C, Stitzer R (eds), Modern Pharmacology. London: Lippincott-Raven.

Willerson JT, Hillis LD, Winniford MD, Buja M (1986) Speculations regarding mechanisms responsible for acute ischaemic heart disease syndromes. J Am Coll Cardiol 8: 245–50.

Willerson JT, Golino P, Eidt J, Campbell WB, Buja M (1989) Specific platelet mediators and unstable coronary artery lesions. Experimental evidence and potential clinical implications. Circulation 80: 198–205.

Woodcock J (1989) Characterisation of the atheromatous plaque in the carotid arteries. J Clin Physiol 10: 445–9.

Zhou Y, Kassab G, Molloi S (1999) On the design of the coronary arterial tree: a generalization of Murray's law. Physics Med Biol 44: 2929–45.

CHAPTER TWO

Primary prevention

BARBARA HASTINGS-ASATOURIAN

> Good health is the bedrock on which social progress is built. A nation of healthy people can do those things that make life worthwhile, and as the level of health increases so does the potential for happiness.
>
> Lalonde (1974)

The number of deaths from coronary heart disease (CHD) has been consistently declining since the 1970s. However, CHD remains the biggest killer especially among middle-aged men. Heart attacks usually result from a blood clot in a coronary artery already damaged by atherosclerosis. A number of predisposing biological, psychological social and societal risk factors can be used to predict who will develop CHD. Although, as far back as 1976, McKeown criticized the medical model as too individualized and disease oriented, ignoring the wider social, economic and environmental influences on health, progress from traditional medicine in this direction has been very slow. The perspective taken here recognizes how inextricably bound are individual behaviour and wider politics, using current data that demonstrate overwhelmingly that the poorer people in society are often exposed to the highest risks.

This chapter provides an overview of public health policy pertinent to primary prevention of CHD, and highlights and discusses the concept of 'social capital' as one means of addressing inequity.

A brief resumé of current epidemiological data and international comparisons is drawn from the latest national statistics, and includes visual representations of the trends based on current statistics (British Heart Foundation 2003).

The role of the government, the community and the individual is identified. There is also some detail of how these models can be and have been integrated into community intervention strategies, and how agencies and professions have worked and can work together.

The lifestyle factors associated with the development and progression of CHD are discussed individually with consideration of the social and financial impacts, and human rights issues of health promotion.

Three recognized levels of prevention most commonly used to describe public health initiatives are referred to throughout. Readers may come across the term 'secondary prevention' in medical management as referring not to screening and early detection but to drug therapy after a myocardial infarction (MI):

1. Here we describe primary prevention as involving measures that ensure total avoidance of a condition. An example of this in the prevention of CHD would be enabling a whole population to access the prerequisites for health as stated in the Ottawa Charter of Health Promotion (WHO 1986) on a societal scale, or receives five portions of fresh fruit or vegetables each day on an individual level (Acheson 1998).
2. Secondary prevention here refers to early detection through screening for it. Opportunistic measurement of blood pressure, or a programme of well person screening of blood lipids, is an example of this. In medical management this often refers to giving drug therapy to post-event patients, e.g. after an MI.
3. Tertiary prevention here refers to preventing further deterioration in people with a diagnosed condition. Treating a person with hyperlipidaemia and ensuring attention to other risk factors would fall into this category, although at the other extreme coronary artery bypass grafts are also tertiary prevention.

Public health policy

According to the World Health Organization (WHO), the main aim of healthy public policy is to create a supportive environment to make it possible for people to lead healthy lives, thus making healthy choices possible or easier. Creation of that supportive environment is a vast undertaking, achievable only by addressing each and all of the determinants of health shown in the box.

Determinants of health

Fixed determinants: genes, sex, ageing
Social and economic determinants: poverty, employment, social exclusion
Environmental determinants: air quality, housing, water quality, social environment
Lifestyle determinants: diet, physical activity, smoking, alcohol, sexual behaviour, drugs
Access to services: education, NHS, social services, transport, leisure

Adapted from Select Committee on Health Second Report (DoH 2001)

The WHO (1986) Ottawa Charter of Health Promotion listed the following as prerequisites for health:

> . . . peace, shelter, education, food, income, a stable ecosystem, sustainable resources, social justice and equity. Improvement in health requires a secure foundation in these basic prerequisites
>
> (WHO on www.euro.who.int/AboutWHO/Policy/20010827_2)

The Sundsvall Declaration (WHO 1991) went on to call for the creation of supportive environments, allowing for broad community involvement and control through education, food, housing, social support and care, work and transport in order to expand their capabilities and develop self-reliance.

Health inequalities data in recent decades (Black 1980, Acheson 1998) have repeatedly highlighted that, the poorer a community is, the higher the levels of chronic disease. Without exception the responsibility for health improvement on a large scale points at national policy, with Acheson (1998) drawing distinction between the dramatic impact of 'upstream' governmental interventions and the moderate impact of the 'downstream', more individually targeted activities at a secondary level (Acheson 1998). Contemporary national and international evidence confirms that a combination of interventions aimed at an individual and a population, including active public participation and community development initiatives, is the most effective at impacting on behaviour and therefore health outcomes. Population approaches address underlying causes of CHD in the population, thereby preventing the development of new cases, whereas the 'high-risk' individual approach targets individuals to raise their awareness of their personal risk, in order to provoke a change in behaviour (Rose 1981).

Lifestyle choices are paradoxically heavily influenced by socioeconomic circumstances. Health improvements are unlikely to occur if social needs remain unmet. However, if the prevailing culture believes in the benefits of an intervention or change, then any preventive actions taken are more likely to be supported and sustained by that community. The health settings approach of installing positive health values into an environment, e.g. 'healthy schools', emerged from Ottawa (WHO 1986), highlighting how much home, workplace and study environment can affect health and well-being. This concept has been carried forward in the UK through the *Health of the Nation* (DoH 1992) and later *Saving Lives: Our healthier nation* (DoH 1998a). Use of a health-setting approach provides an ideal opportunity to begin addressing health in the younger generation early enough for them to establish health habits and lifestyles, and prevent coronary artery damage.

Some may say that complete avoidance of a disease means never taking up habits or behaviours likely to result in the disease. New politics in the UK do not welcome high levels of state intervention. Nevertheless, criticism has been levelled at the British government for not taking a top-down approach to tackle heart disease 'upstream'. Arguments advanced against top-down control hinge on the ethics of choice and human rights.

Examples of 'upstream' approaches

Banning tobacco advertising
Banning advertising of unhealthy foods at children's TV viewing times
Promoting healthy foods at children's TV viewing times
Enforcing a reduction in fat and salt content of foods by manufacturers
Providing companies with incentives for promoting healthy snacks with
    healthy messages
Heavily subsidizing the cost of fruit and vegetables
Restricting large corporate traders of high fat- or high salt-containing
    foods from sponsoring sporting events

Although there is evidence that public health practitioners are working both with communities and with a population focus, general practitioners nationally are currently largely working downstream, and at the levels of secondary and tertiary prevention. The implementation at general practice level of the National Service Framework (NSF) recommended screening programmes for CHD has so far demanded disproportionate effort at individual level, with no significant immediate gains (Hippisley-Cox and Pringle 2001). However, as is the case with many preventive activities and initiatives, evaluation of longer-term effects of interventions cannot be predicted at this early stage.

The WHO (1986 – on www.euro.who.int/AboutWHO/Policy/ 20010827_2) proposed that health promotion does not belong to traditional health professions, but rather is the responsibility of the following long list of organizations including governments, health and other social and econom-ic sectors, non-governmental and voluntary organizations, local authorities, industry, media, individuals, families and communities. The Ottawa Charter further states that health promotion should take into account different social, cultural and economic systems.

In spite of these very clear messages of governmental responsibility suc-cessive British government health policies have vacillated between state and individual, and between upstream and downstream foci. The Department of Health and Social Security (DHSS 1976) visibly identified how risk fac-tors for CHD inter-relate: smokers are often also overweight; obese people take less exercise. The Conservative governments that followed placed a stronger emphasis on the responsibility of the individual (DoH 1992). During the Thatcher and Major years the inequalities data of the Black Report were not publicized or utilized in *The Health of the Nation*. The Labour governments of 1997 and 2001 moved into a more central position. By 2004 the British Labour government was showing a strong emphasis on collaboration, partnership and tripartite contract of state, general public and individual, acknowledging the responsibility that the government has in addressing inequalities, recognizing and informing individuals of actions that they can take for themselves to improve their health and well-being, e.g. 'Ten tips for better health' in the box, and featuring public participation and consultation as key features of positive health policy.

Ten tips for better health
 1. Don't smoke. If you can, stop. If you can't, cut down.
 2. Follow a balanced diet with plenty of fruit and vegetables.
 3. Keep physically active.
 4. Manage stress by, for example, talking things through and making time to relax.
 5. If you drink alcohol, do so in moderation.
 6. Cover up in the sun, and protect children from sunburn.
 7. Practise safer sex.
 8. Take up cancer screening opportunities.
 9. Be safe on the roads: follow the Highway Code.
10. Learn the first aid ABC – airways, breathing, circulation.

Source: Department of Health (1999)
(www.archive.official-documents.co.uk/document/cm43/4386/4386-tp.htm)

A major international example of a collaborative community-wide approach can be drawn from one study in north Karelia in Finland (Puska et al. 1983). This project was a response to Finland's having the highest mortality rates from heart disease in the 1960s. It involved health service, mass media, social services, the business community, voluntary organizations, trades unions, sports organizations and local political leaders.

North Karelia produced the seven-point plan in the box to help individuals modify their behaviour, and enlisted 1000 'lay leaders' from the local community to deliver health messages.

Seven-point plan

1. Improved preventive services to identify risk factors.
2. Information to educate the population about behaviour and health.
3. Persuasion to motivate people to adopt healthy actions.
4. Training to increase skills of self-management, environmental control and necessary action.
5. Social support to help people maintain the initial action.

6. Environmental change to create opportunities for healthy actions and improve unfavourable conditions.
7. Community organization to mobilize the community for broad range changes.

Source: adapted from Tones et al. (1991, p. 26).

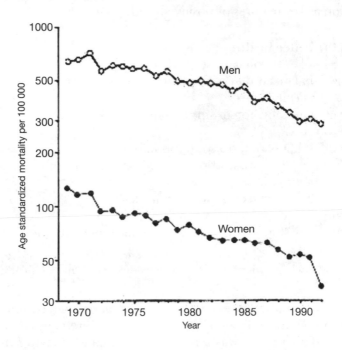

Figure 2.1 Statistics from north Karelia in Finland 1970–1992. (From Puska et al. 1983.)

North Karelia and the Framingham Study in the USA showed marked decline in other major diseases, not only CHD, as a result of lifestyle adaptations. Cancer mortality also reduced in the course of Framingham's community heart disease prevention programme (Kannel et al. 1961, Kannel 1991).

An inter-relationship between determinants has also been demonstrated, e.g. the social class differences in mortality, stress levels, environment, fat and alcohol intakes and physical inactivity. Isolated interventions on, say, smoking behaviour described by Acheson as 'downstream' are not as effective as early primary prevention interventions, which can result in much wider health impact on populations, e.g. banning smoking in public places.

Epidemiology

The NSF for Coronary Heart Disease documented more than 110 000 deaths from CHD in England in 1 year in 1998, including more than 41 000 under the age of 75 years (DoH 2000).

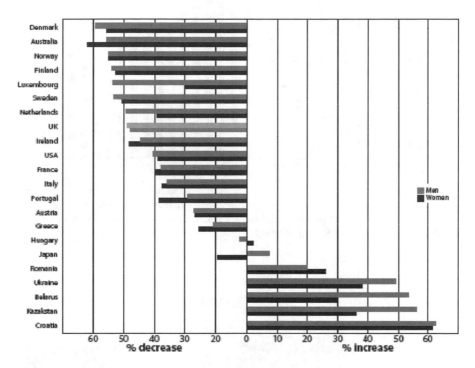

Figure 2.2 Changes in the death rates from coronary heart disease, men and women aged 35–74, between 1988 and 1998, selected countries. (Source British Heart Foundation Statistics 2003.)

Winning the War on Heart Disease (DoH 2004) states that deaths from cardiovascular disease have fallen by 23% since 1995. Deaths have fallen by 4% per annum since the 1970s (Figure 2.3), but are still high in comparison with many other countries (see Figure 2.2).

Although the trend in heart disease prevalence is down, heart disease rates are still the predominant cause of death in the UK, accounting for 40% of all deaths:

- 22% of female deaths in England and Wales
- 30% of male deaths in England and Wales
- about 40% of deaths of men aged 55 and 64 in England and Wales.

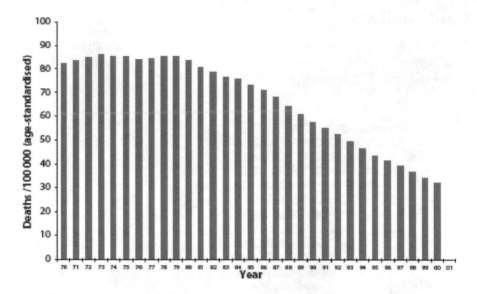

Figure 2.3 Trend in UK deaths from coronary heart disease: death rates from coronary heart disease for people aged under 65, 1970–2000, England. (Source British Heart Foundation Statistics 2003.)

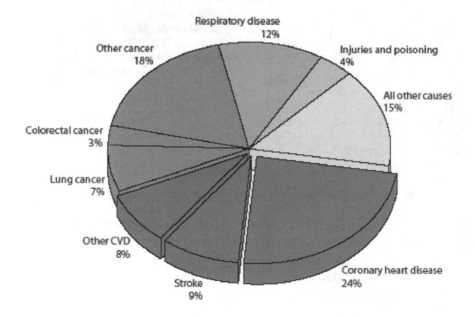

Figure 2.4 Death by causes in men, 2001, UK. (Source British Heart Foundation Statistics 2003.)

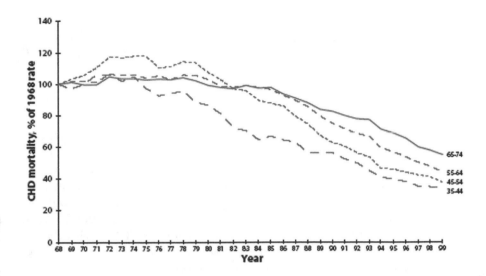

Figure 2.5 Age-specific death rates from coronary heart disease in men, 1968–1999, UK, plotted as a percentage of the rate in 1968. (Source British Heart Foundation Statistics 2003.)

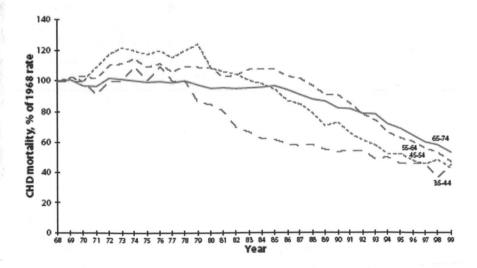

Figure 2.6 Age-specific death rates from coronary heart disease in women, 1968–1999, UK, plotted as a percentage of the rate in 1968. (Source British Heart Foundation Statistics 2003.)

The main proposed explanation for the declining trend is reduced prevalence of known risk factors among the population, reduced prevalence of risk factors in people with CHD, and improved response rates from and treatments of people who have an event, leading to better survival rates

Risk factors, however, are not universally predictive. In some countries, e.g. in eastern Europe and the former Soviet Union, mortality for cardiovascular disease has recently been found to be higher in people at young ages than in England and Wales. Deaths are also more likely to be sudden, and many people who die show little evidence of the expected coronary artery lesions (Landsbergis and Klumbiene 2003). Risk factors identified in western epidemiological research, such as smoking, lipid levels and physical activity, have little value. One important consideration, especially if working in a multi-ethnic population, is that lipid metabolism appears to differ between different races and ethnic groups, so traditional screening for risk factors may not be relevant in every community. The impact of binge alcohol drinking, used as a means of easing stress, should not be overlooked.

Other factors involved in the development of CHD – smoking, dietary fat and low fruit and vegetable intake – undoubtedly do lend themselves to interventions 'upstream', e.g. free school fruit schemes and legislation around permitted amounts in foodstuffs, smoking in public places and alcohol advertising strategies.

However, as soon as risks are sought out, the definition of the level of prevention shifts from primary (complete avoidance) to secondary (early detection). Screening enables secondary prevention. Early detection here does not refer to detection of CHD itself, but rather to the early detection of the presence of a predisposing risk factor or factors that once reduced or eradicated may bring about complete avoidance of CHD, so in that respect the use of such interventions might be perceived as primary prevention.

Using heart charts

The impact of risk factor detection has been detailed in the Framingham study (Kannel et al. 1961, Kannel 1987) which reported a 10-year follow-up of about 5000 residents of Framingham, Massachusetts, USA from the late 1960s. Subsequent studies have shown that the Framingham equations can predict coronary risk with reasonably accuracy in white men and women in the UK. However, little is known about chart validity in other ethnic minorities.

Heart charts estimate the risk of CHD for individuals who have not developed symptoms, not for patients with existing disease. To estimate an individual's absolute 10-year risk of developing CHD, variables such as

neonatal mortality and morbidity in the early twentieth century. They implicated poor maternal health and diet. Body weight of less than 8 kg (18 lb) at 1 year was suggested as being predictive of heart disease in later life. Adult height has also been found to be significant as a risk measure for heart disease (Floud et al. 1990, Marmot et al. 1991).

Prevention of poverty and deprivation are huge and multifactoral, and an example of an initiative designed to tackle inequalities and improve health in the early years of life is Sure Start, a multi-sector initiative, part of which targets the compete prevention of heart disease in later life by including efforts to help women reduce smoking in pregnancy and improve the nutrition of their children.

Gender

Up to the age of 45 years, CHD is much more prevalent in men than in women. Women in their reproductive years have relatively high levels of HDL-cholesterol and are therefore relatively protected before the menopause. This protection declines postmenopausally so that by the age of 75 the incidence of CHD is equal in both sexes.

Although the prevalence of smoking among both men and women has been declining overall since the mid-1970s, the decline is slower in women. In western societies since the early 1990s, women have been adopting smoking and drinking behaviour formerly associated with men. The longer-term effect of this is that life expectancy differences may narrow because there may be a rising level of smoking-related mortality among women. Reinforcement of health messages through educational interventions at primary, secondary, further and higher education are required, but as young people are often avid followers of television soaps a concurrent message via this mass media may also help to embed a healthy message.

Men are still much less likely to seek medical help than women when they are unwell, and are most unlikely to consult about preventive issues (Carroll 1995). In *Community Practitioner* (Editorial 2004) there was a report from a developing patient partnership survey that 24% of men surveyed would seek advice from their mother, 48% would ask their partner, and 3% would use a pharmacy in the current non-private climate in pharmacies.

Men carry, in general, more risk factors than women. Figures from the British Heart Foundation show that 28% of men smoke and 39% of men drink too much. One survey found that two of five men were drinking more than 3-4 units of alcohol per day. Moreover, 60% of men are defined as overweight, 17% as obese and 4% as being underweight. Men are also one and a half times more likely to develop diabetes.

A strategy to address this might attempt to provide services where men feel more comfortable – in the workplace, or a leisure facility, e.g. the gym or the local pub. Women care for men – they often shop, cook and prepare foods – and are therefore frequently in control of dietary intakes and habits, how much fat is taken in and how much salt is added. Men can be reached indirectly via those women who do the shopping and cooking.

Women using oral contraceptives are more at risk of thrombosis, and there is a dose-dependent increase in fibrinogen and factor VII in contraceptive pill users, although the risk is increased significantly in obese women who smoke (Bloemenkamp et al. 2002). These women should already be receiving screening and advice when they attend at least at the time they collect their pill prescription.

A further example of primary prevention here could be the provision of free exercise facilities or walking groups for women. The 2004 initiative, organized in conjunction with the food manufacturer Kellogg, enables individuals to collect a free pedometer. Further involvement of the food industry could extend to giving healthy messages in their products, including promotion of fat, sugar and salt reduction, e.g. the interest now being shown by fast food outlets in offering salad alternatives.

Some insights from geographical and cultural differences

Italian and French populations suffer relatively little CHD. It is believed that the high consumption of monounsaturated fats such as olive oil and antioxidants may be responsible for the low rates of CHD in Italy. In France, the CHD mortality rate remains very low and it has been postulated that this is the result of high consumption of alcohol, in particular wine, and a diet rich in garlic and fresh vegetables.

In New Zealand a 54% fall in mortality rate could be attributed to risk reduction (smoking 30%, cholesterol 12%, population blood pressure 8% and unidentified factors 4%). Between 38 and 51% of this decrease in mortality from CHD could be accounted for by reduced blood cholesterol levels and smoking between 1968 and 1980 (Capewell et al. 2000).

In Finland the decline in deaths from CHD over the past years was almost entirely predicted by the changes in serum cholesterol, blood pressure, and smoking in both women and men in a population approach (Puska et al. 1983).

Mortality from CHD in Iceland has decreased by 17–18% since 1970. During 1981–86 the rate of heart attacks in men aged under 75 decreased by 23%. A decrease occurred in the level of all three major risk factors after 1968. The fall in the serum cholesterol concentration coincided with a reduction in consumption of dairy fat and margarine. The reduction in mortality from CHD was caused substantially by a decreased incidence of myocardial infarction and could be attributed largely to the reduction in risk factors. Data from Iceland illustrate that the predicted 35% decrease in risk was mirrored by a decrease in mortality from CHD (Sigfusson et al. 1991).

A decrease in smoking and better control of hypertension in Japan contributed to the decrease in mortality from CHD between 1968 and 1978. In Australia the decrease in mortality is compatible with the improved nutrition and reduced tobacco consumption.

In Russia the greatest increases in mortality were in regions experiencing the most rapid economic transition. Men with poor education have experienced higher mortality than those who were well educated, the main difference between the two groups being external causes and cardiovascular diseases. Other correlations have been drawn from lack of control over life circumstances and poor social support. The increase in mortality in men in central and eastern Europe in the 1980s was greatest among unmarried men, partly attributed to the psychological factors associated with men's sense of economic failure, which was not mirrored by the experience of women, who were more able to report having fulfilling roles within the home. Poor nutrition, high rates of smoking and the availability of cheap alcohol provide a long-term risk of premature death (Landsbergis and Klumbiene 2003).

The strategies that would be most needed in societies undergoing such a dramatic economic transition would be those that helped in the management of change, stress management and state or community level prevention of adverse circumstances.

An individual's response to the circumstances is highly significant in CHD, with those with a strong internal 'locus of control' much less likely to experience CHD. Rotter (1966) described locus of control as the extent to which people believe they have control over their circumstances. The continuum of internal to external locus of control ranges from feeling very strongly in control to disempowered or victimized by external circumstances. A locus of control assessment is available on-line at www.psych.uncc.edu/pagoolka/LocusofControl-intro.html. An individual's response to the circumstances is highly significant in CHD, with those with a strong internal locus of control much less likely to experience CHD. Clearly strategies that help shift an individual from external to internal locus of control will have a positive impact.

Seasonal and climate differences

Plasma fibrinogen levels and plasma viscosity have been found to be higher and HDL-cholesterol lower in the winter than in the summer, and there is

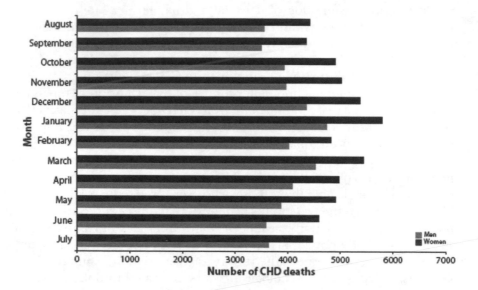

Figure 2.7 Deaths from coronary heart disease by month, 2000–1, England and Wales. (Source British Heart Foundation Statistics 2003.)

a higher incidence of MI and stroke in winter (Stout and Crawford 1991) (Figure 2.7). The increase in MI in the winter has also been associated with changes in plasma vitamin D levels, because the metabolite of vitamin D can affect the contractility of the heart (Scragg et al. 1990). Mortality is higher in the cooler, northern parts of the UK, although this is contentious because there are clearly economic factors to be considered in the north–south divide.

Cholesterol

Lowering serum cholesterol concentrations in a population is critical in reducing mortality from CHD. Law's work (Law et al. 1994) concludes that the combined evidence from the 10 largest cohort studies, 3 international (ecological) studies and 28 randomized trials confirms that a 10% reduction in serum cholesterol concentration reduces CHD by 50% at age 40, 40% by age 50, 30% by age 60 and 20% by age 70. The greater part of the benefit is realized after 2 years and the full benefit after 5 years.

Wider action such as health education, food labelling and improved food policies will be required in addition to individually targeted and population screening approaches.

Diet and obesity

Diet appears to affect heart health in a number of ways. Obesity is not an independent risk factor, but predisposes to hypertension and diabetes, and obesity has also been seen to correlate with higher fibrinogen levels. There is evidence from population data that a diet high in saturated fat, low in fruit and vegetables, high in salt and low in antioxidants is associated with CHD mortality.

Current prices encourage consumption of cholesterol-raising foods, particularly among poorer people. Marshall (2000) recommends that, by adding tax to the main sources of dietary saturated fat, between 900 and 1000 premature deaths per annum could be avoided and the revenue generated could finance compensatory measures to raise income for low-income groups. He further recommends that econometric and health policy research should measure the effects of price changes on diet and health.

It has also been suggested that fish oils may protect against both arrhythmias and clotting.

North–south divide

The north–south divide in relation to CHD is best illustrated graphically (Figure 2.8). Although small inner city areas nationally do demonstrate patterns of deprivation that predispose to CHD, the picture of death rates from CHD nationally points to a north–south divide.

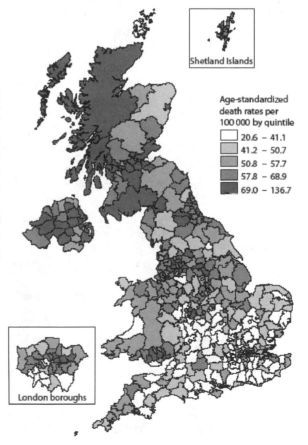

Figure 2.8 Age-standardized death rates per 10 000 population from coronary heart disease for men under 65 by local authority, 1998–2000, UK. (Source British Heart Foundation Statistics database: www.heartstats.org.)

There is also a north–south divide in protective vitamin C intake, with the north-west region (47 mg) and Scotland (49 mg) having the lowest daily average and the south-west and south-east regions the highest (60 mg vitamin C).

Smoking

According to the WHO tobacco is the second major cause of death in the world and is responsible for the death of one in ten adults worldwide (about 5 million deaths each year). If current smoking patterns continue, it will cause some 10 million deaths each year by 2025. Half of today's smokers, about 650 million people, will eventually be killed by tobacco.

In the UK in 2001, 28% of men and 26% of women in the UK smoked cigarettes. The 2002 UK General Household Survey (National Statistics 2002) found around 13 million adult cigarette smokers. Smoking prevalence is slightly higher among men than among women. In the youngest age group, those aged 16–19 years, women have a higher smoking rate (31% for women and 25% for men) but about equal rates in the over-50s.

Highest smoking rates are in the 20- to 24-year age range (40% in men and 35% in women). Rates are lowest in those aged 60 and above (16% in men and 17% in women). Before the 1980s, smoking prevalence was overall very similar. This reflects the trend for men and women aged 35 and over who have given up smoking.

Interventions at individual and structural levels were proposed by the UK Department of Health in *Smoking Kills* (DoH 1998b) – some are health public policy and some more individually targeted. Some of these are outlined in Figure 2.9.

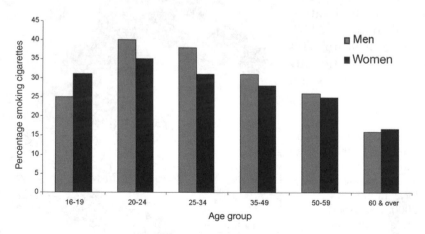

Figure 2.9 Prevalence of cigarette smoking by sex and age, 2001, UK. (Source: British Heart Foundation Statistics database: www.heartstats.org.)

Healthy public policy in respect of smoking

Healthy public policy can be introduced internationally, nationally, regionally and locally. It is just as appropriate at the WHO as in a local young people's centre. Such policies might include:

- Economic and fiscal measures, e.g. adding tax, removing any subsidies from tobacco companies.
- Control of product information, e.g. packet warnings, advertising bans, disallowing sponsorship.
- Control of availability, e.g. legislation about age of use, local policies.
- Control of use or related behaviours, e.g. smoke-free areas, no promotion of glamour.
- Environmental modification, e.g. ventilation.
- Product modification – banning toxic additives.

Interventions at international level

A worldwide effort was launched in May 2004 by the WHO – World No Tobacco Day 'Tobacco and Poverty: a vicious circle' (WHO 2004) – to emphasize the economic cost of tobacco use and cultivation to families, communities and countries. The slogan 'a vicious circle' explains the link that exists between tobacco and poverty, and how the use of tobacco is especially by poorer people who consume this product the most. The poorest and least educated people tend to smoke the most and bear most of the disease burden. A recent study published by Action on Smoking and Health (2004) in Brazil concluded that smoking prevalence among people with 4 or fewer years of education is 26%, compared with 17% for those with 9 or more years education. Poorer people spend a higher percentage of their household income on tobacco products, to the detriment of food, health care or education. In Bangladesh, for example, 10.5 million people currently malnourished would have an adequate diet if two-thirds of the money spent on tobacco in the country were spent on food. The World Bank estimates that high-income countries spend currently between 6% and 15% of their total health-care costs to treat tobacco-related diseases.

The effects of smoking on individual health

Smokers die younger than non-smokers. Smokers also die younger than ex-smokers. The effects of smoking are attributed to carbon monoxide and nicotine. Carbon monoxide levels are raised and there is a correlation between raised fibrinogen levels and carboxyhaemoglobin levels. Both blood fibrinogen levels and blood viscosity are raised in hyperlipidaemia. Carbon monoxide reduces the oxygen available to heart muscle, and the stimulating effect of nicotine increases the work undertaken by the heart. Both have an impact on blood clotting. Cigarette smoking directly reduces blood levels of vitamin C, vitamin E and β-carotene. Smokers are doubly affected if they are also consuming fewer portions of fruit and vegetables than non-smokers (Cade and Margetts 1991). For smokers under the age of 50 years, the risk of developing CHD is 10 times greater than for non-smokers of the same age.

The longer-term effects of smoking on the heart become apparent only after many years. Evidence from the Framingham study showed how smoking raises fibrinogen levels in the blood of smokers in a dose-related way, increasing the risk of clot formation (Kannel et al. 1961, Kannel 1988). The levels begin to fall once a person stops smoking, but it can take 5 years to return to non-smoker levels.

Blood viscosity, which impacts on blood pressure and white cell counts, is also raised in smokers and can remain raised for 10 years after stopping (Meade et al. 1993). Tobacco contributes substantially to the sex difference in mortality: cigarette smoking approximately doubles the risk of morbidity and mortality from CHD compared with a lifetime of not smoking, and the risk is related to the duration and amount of smoking. The risk of morbidity and mortality associated with cigarette smoking falls immediately after stopping smoking, although it may be more than 20 years, if at all, before the risk associated with smoking is completely reversed.

Smoking cessation interventions

Evidence suggests that the longer an individual practitioner spends with a smoker in smoking cessation activities and the more support offered, the more successful the intervention:

- up to 3 minutes' advice has been found to be 2% better than no advice
- up to 10 minutes' advice has been found to be 3% better than no advice
- up to 10 minutes' advice plus nicotine replacement has been found to be 6% better than advice alone

The following are vital components in a smoking cessation strategy:

- Regular enquiry into a person's smoking status
- Regular advice to stop smoking with the offer of interventions to aid abstinence
- Consistent follow-up
  Particularly effective interventions include the following:
- Setting a date to stop smoking completely
- Enlisting family support
- Analysing past behaviour and attempts
- Planning strategies to deal with difficult situations
- Trying smoking cessation products, e.g. nicotine replacement.

Alcohol

Binge drinking is particularly associated with a marked increase in the risk of heart disease death, and in particular sudden death, pointing to different levels of risk associated with different patterns of drinking. It is, however, important not to consider alcohol in isolation because heart disease in heavy drinkers may be multivariate. Heavy and binge drinking, for example, may be an indicator of stress. Poor diet is also associated with alcohol consumption in two ways: first heavy drinkers often have low intake of dietary micronutrients from fruit and vegetables and, second, poor absorption of vitamins, both of which would provide a protective effect. Research continues into the long-term positive impact of low doses of alcohol, when compared with total abstainers.

Stress

It has been suggested that acute stressful life events and chronic stressful life situations increase susceptibility to heart disease (Krantz and Raisen 1988). However, social support buffers have also been identified such as having a spouse, family friends and other social networks.

Type A personality was first identified in the 1950s as a possible contributor to heart disease because a type A personality drives competitiveness, aggression, speed, impatience, urgency, and an increased potential for anger and hostility. There is evidence that the stress factors contributing to CHD are mediated by the activity of the sympathetic adrenal medullary and pituitary adrenocortical systems (Krantz and Manuck 1984). Anger and hostility have been identified to predict future coronary events. It has been concluded that the environment and pressures are not the key predictors, but rather how a person reacts to those circumstances.

Primary prevention of heart disease would once again favour self-management strategies that shift the locus of control (Rotter 1966) of a person identified as 'type A' from external to internal. Associated with this are relaxation and mind–body techniques such as yoga, t'ai chi and other forms of meditation, and a discipline that makes a small space for these every day.

Physical activity

Other forms of physical activity have also been found to improve well-being, reduce stress, and help prevent obesity and hypertension. An early study (Morris et al. 1980, 1990) found that London's former bus conductors on double-decker buses had fewer heart attacks than drivers. Postmen were found to have fewer heart attacks than telephonists and post office clerks. Nowadays physical activity is largely seen as something to do in leisure time, because work has become less and less physical. Regular and vigorous exercise has been found to protect against heart disease – including brisk walking, jogging, cycling, gardening, DIY and housework. 'Regular' now means on most days, and vigorous means sufficient to take the heart and respiratory rates up, creating a feeling of increased body heat, energy and well-being.

Intervention strategies

Theories and models of attitude and behaviour change warrant a chapter in their own right, and might focus on creating cognitive dissonance or shifting the locus of control (Rotter 1966). How this is achieved and sustained largely falls into two categories: prescriptive and facilitative interventions. Some of these are outlined below.

Social learning theory

Individuals are most likely to model the behaviour they see in people they admire, especially if they feel an emotional attachment to that person. As far as children and young people are concerned their first contact is with parents/carers, and there is significant evidence to suggest modelling parents'/carers' behaviour. Not every parent is aware of this. Clearly there is a public health role to raise the awareness of parents that this is a powerful mechanism, and that modifications in their behaviour may have longer-term health benefits for their children.

Use of the mass media

Many television programmes depict unhealthy behaviour and dramatic representations of people engaging in unhealthy activities. It has only recently been realized how much impact the behaviour of soap opera characters can have.

It is now widely recognized that using the mass media is a powerful mechanism for awareness raising, and should therefore have a key function in any serious health campaign. One important reason for this is that many people who may be at risk and unlikely to seek conventional health services may spend a lot of time watching television or listening to the radio. Downie et al. (1991) give evidence that a media campaign supported by community intervention enhances the effectiveness of interventions, but it is the sustained and personal feedback and encouragement that are required in the community to help in the maintenance of healthy behaviour.

There is, however, now a growing body of evidence to suggest that such activity is too heavily labour intensive for most health service settings. Hippisley-Cox and Pringle (2001) report on a study of 18 computerized general practices which estimates that the workload involved in meeting the expectations of the NSF is matched by the benefits gained.

The EUROASPIRE I and II follow-up studies of secondary prevention (Wood 2002) illustrate the size of the gap between what is and what could be done in secondary prevention. Lipid-lowering prescribing of β blockers and angiotensin-converting enzyme (ACE) inhibitor prescribing improved, whereas smoking and obesity, i.e. the factors under control of the patients, did not.

Seedhouse (2001, p. 124) asserts:

> People must be allowed to exercise choice, and the fullest choice can come only from possession of the fullest relevant information.

The Oxcheck (1991) study (analysed by Wonderling et al. 1996) study employed nurses to run special clinics in general practices and showed modest reductions in cholesterol and blood pressure sustained over 3 years. The resource requirements led the authors to conclude: 'The benefits of health promotion through primary care must be weighed against their costs, and in relation to other priorities.'

The British Family Heart Study (Family Heart Study Group 1994) used nurse-run clinics and showed a 12% relative risk reduction in coronary risk scores. It estimated that a practice with 1000 men aged 40–55 would need to employ four full-time nurses over 18 months and concluded that alternative strategies were needed.

This suggests that these interventions are costly, complex and hard to measure, and still mainly focus on individual change. Moreover, for screening to be ethical, there should be adequate and equitable facilities for diagnosis and treatment.

It may be that a shift in the belief that primary prevention and screening interventions needs to be undertaken in those conventional health settings. Population-based approaches to promote primary prevention, using similar advertising techniques to the tobacco and food industry, could be equally if not more cost-effective at encouraging healthy lifestyles than general population screening and counselling. Investigation of policy initiatives is equally important in promoting lifestyle change in society.

Conclusion

Among the ethics and human rights issues that are raised by intervening in the lives of individuals, Lupton (1997) perceives one of the problems to be that health promotion constrains individual freedom and blames the individual for not being healthy.

Initiatives that have no immediate relevance to the participants will not be taken up. Seedhouse (2001) cites Professor Michael Oliver, once president of the British Cardiac Society, who rejected 'one policy fits all' as too simplistic. He maintained that heart disease is so complex, and its causes so diverse, that health promotion can never be a matter of following policies without thinking.

Advocating change – steps to achievement requires

A champion
Identification of an issue
Support – from a working group
Needs assessment – get to know your community
Development of an action plan
Participation – work towards success
Communication with the public through the media
Implementation of the change
Monitoring/evaluation/adjustment

Source: *Making Public Policy Healthy*, a heart health programme available in Labrador, Canada (www.infonet.st-johns.nf.ca/providers/nhhp/docs/policy.html)

In reality primary prevention of CHD demands dramatic political events and strategies, and requires uprooting from the confines of traditional curative medicine. To reduce the social class disparity, governments must provide resources that enable communities to be rid of poverty and other financial inequalities, improve maternal nutrition and intrauterine conditions, ensure well-balanced diets for infants, provide uniform standards for child care, nutrition, educational attainment, housing, freedom from or better strategies to cope with stressful conditions or traumatic events, and improved access to the appropriate services for each.

References

Acheson D (1998) Independent Enquiry into Inequalities in Health. London: The Stationery Office.
Action on Smoking and Health (2004) Tobacco: Global trends tobacco prevalence and consumption worldwide available on-line at www.ash.org.uk/html/international/html/globaltrends.html.
Barker DJP, Osmond C (1986) Infant mortality, childhood nutrition, and ischaemic heart disease in England and Wales. Lancet i: 1077–81.

Barker DJP, Osmond C, Golding J, Kuh D, Wadsworth MEJ (1989) Growth *in utero*, blood pressure in childhood and adult life, and mortality from cardiovascular disease BMJ 298: 564–7.

Barker DJP, Gluckman PD, Godfrey KM, Harding JE, Owens JA, Robinson JS (1993) Fetal and cardiovascular disease in adult life. Lancet 341: 938–41.

Black D (1980) Inequalities in Health: Report of a Research Working Group. London: DHSS.

Bloemenkamp KW, de Maat MP, Dersjant-Roorda MC, Helmerhorst FM, Kluft C (2002) Genetic polymorphisms modify the response of factor VII to oral contraceptive use: an example of gene-environment interaction. Vasc Pharmacol 39: 131–6.

British Heart Foundation (1999) Joint British Recommendations on Prevention of Coronary Heart Disease in Clinical Practice. Factfile 8/99. London: BHF.

British Heart Foundation (2001) Stopping Smoking – Evidence-based guidance. Factfile 8/2001. London: BHF.

British Heart Foundation (2003) Coronary Heart Disease Statistics Book. British Heart Foundation Statistics Database. Can be purchased on-line at www.bhf.org.uk/publications/description.asp?secondlevel=416&artID=708.

Cade JE, Margetts BM (1991) Relationship between diet and smoking is the diet of smokers different? J Epidemiol. Community Health 45: 270–2.

Capewell S, Beaglehole R, Seddon M, McMurray J (2000) Explanation for the decline in coronary heart disease mortality rates in Auckland, New Zealand, between 1982 and 1993. Circulation 102: 1511–16.

Carroll (1995) The Which Guide to Men's Health. London: Penguin, pp. 173–230.

Department of Health (1992) The Health of the Nation. A strategy for health in England. Cm 1986. London: HMSO.

Department of Health (1998a) Our Healthier Nation. London: The Stationery Office (also on-line at www.archive.official-documents.co.uk/document/doh/ohnation/title.htm).

Department of Health (1998b) Smoking Kills: A White Paper on Tobacco. Cm 4177. London: The Stationery Office.

Department of Health (1999) Saving Lives: Our healthier nation. Cm 4386. London: The Stationery Office.

Department of Health (2000) The National Standard Framework for Coronary Heart Disease. London: HMSO.

Department of Health (2001) House of Commons Select Committee on Health Second Report on Public Health. Cm 5242. London: DoH.

Department of Health (2004) Winning the War on Heart Disease. DH 2004, 35312 1p 5k Mar04 (CWP). London: HMSO.

Department of Health and Social Security (1976) Prevention and Health: Everybody's business. A reassessment of public and personal health. London: HMSO.

Downie RS, Fyfe C, Tannahil A (1991) Health Promotion: Models and values. Oxford: Oxford University Press.

Editorial (2004) Health advice: I'd rather ask my mum. Community Practit 77: 203.

Family Heart Study Group (1994) Randomised controlled trial evaluation cardiovascular screening and intervention in general practice; principle results of British family heart study. BMJ 308: 313–20.

Floud R, Wachter K, Gregory A (1990) Height, Health and History. Nutritional status in the United Kingdom, 1750–1980. Cambridge: Cambridge University Press.

Forsdahl A (1977) Are poor living conditions in childhood and adolescence an important risk factor for arteriosclerotic heart disease? Br J Prevent Social Med 31: 91–5.

Forsdahl A (1978) Living conditions in childhood and subsequent development of risk factors for arteriosclerotic heart disease. 1974–75. J Epidemiol Commun Health 32: 34–7.

Hippisley-Cox J, Pringle M (2001) General practice workload implications of the national service framework for coronary heart disease: cross sectional survey. BMJ 323: 269–70.

Kannel WB (1987) Common ECG electrocardiographic markers for subsequent clinical coronary events. Circulation 75(suppl II): II-25–II-27.

Kannel WB (1988) Contributions of the Framingham Study to the conquest of coronary artery disease. Am J Cardiol 15: 1109–12.

Kannel WB (1991) Epidemiology of essential hypertension: the Framingham experience. Proc R Coll Physns Edinb 21: 273–87.

Kannel WB, Dawber TR, Kagan A, Revotskie L, Stokes J III (1961) Factors of risk in the development of coronary heart disease: six-year follow-up experience. Ann Intern Med 55: 33–50 (www.nhlbi.nih.gov/about/framingham/index.html).

Krantz DS, Manuck SB (1984) Acute psychophysiologic reactivity and risk of cardiovascular disease: A review and methodological critique. Psychol Bull 96: 535–64.

Krantz DS, Raisen SE (1988) Environmental stress, reactivity and ischaemic heart disease. Br J Med Psychol 61: 3–16.

Lalonde M (1974) New Perspective on the Health of Canadians. Working Document presented by Minister of National Health and Welfare in Ottawa, April 1974 (www.phac-aspc.gc.ca/ph-sp/phdd/pdf/perspective.pdf).

Landsbergis P, Klumbiene J (2003) Coronary heart disease mortality in Russia and Eastern Europe. Am J Public Health 93: 1793.

Law MR, Wald NJ (1994) An ecological study of serum cholesterol and ischaemic heart disease between 1950 and 1990. Eur J Clin Nutr 48: 305–25.

Law MR, Wald NJ, Thompson SG (1994) By how much and how quickly does reduction in serum cholesterol concentration lower risk of ischaemic heart disease? BMJ 308: 367–72.

Lupton D (1997) Foucault and the medicalisation critique. In: Peterson A, Bunton R (eds), Foucault: Health and medicine. London: Routledge.

McKeown T (1976) The Role of Medicine: Dream, mirage, or nemesis. London: Nuffield Provincial Hospital Trust.

McPherson K, Britton A, Causer L, National HF (2002) Coronary heart disease: estimating the impact of changes in risk factors. London: The Stationery Office.

Marmot MG, Rose G, Shipley M, Hamilton PJS (1978) Employment grade and coronary heart disease in British civil servants. J Epidemiol Community Health 32: 244–9.

Marmot MG, Shipley MJ, Rose G (1984) Inequalities in death-specific explanations of a general pattern. Lancet i: 1003–6.

Marmot MG, Smith GD, Stansfeld S et al. (1991) Health inequalities among British civil servants: the Whitehall II study. Lancet 337: 1397–3.

Marshall T (2000) Exploring a fiscal food policy: the case of diet and ischaemic heart disease. BMJ 320: 301–5.

Meade TW, Ruddock V, Stirling Y, Chakrabarti R, Miller GJ (1993) Fibrinolytic activity, clotting factors, and long-term incidence of ischaemic heart disease. in the Northwick Park Heart Study. Lancet 342: 1076–9.

Morris JN, Everitt MG, Pollard R et al. (1980) Vigorous exercise in leisure-time: protection against coronary heart disease. Lancet ii: 1207–10.

Morris JN, Clayton DG, Everitt MG et al. (1990) Exercise in leisure time: coronary attack and death rates. Br Heart J 63: 325–34.

National Statistics (2002) Living In Britain. London: HMSO.

Puska P, Salonen JT, Nissinen A et al. (1983) Change in risk factors for coronary heart disease during 10 years of a community intervention programme (North Karelia project). BMJ (Clin Res Ed) 287: 1840–4.

Rose G (1981) The strategy of prevention: lessons from cardiovascular disease. BMJ 1: 1847–51.

Rotter JB (1966) Generalized expectancies for internal versus external control of reinforcements. Psychol Monograph 80.

Scragg R, Jackson R, Holdaway IM, Lim T, Beaglehole R (1990) Myocardial infarction is inversely associated with plasma 25-hydroxyvitamin D$_3$ levels: a community based study. Int J Epidemiol 19: 559–63.

Seedhouse D (2001) Health the Foundations for Achievement, 2nd edn. London: Wiley.

Sigfusson H, Sigvaldson L, Steingrimsdottir I et al. 1(991) Decline in ischaemic heart disease in Iceland and change in risk factor levels. BMJ 302: 1371–5.

Stout RW, Crawford V (1991) Seasonal variations in fibrinogen concentrations among elderly people. Lancet 338: 9–13.

Tones K, Tilford S, Robinson Y (1991) Health Education, Effectiveness and Efficiency. London: Chapman & Hall.

WHO (1986) Ottawa Charter of Health Promotion. International Conference on Health Promotion, Ottawa, Canada.

WHO (1991) Sundsvall Statement on Supporting Environments (www.who.int/hpr/NPH/docs/sundsvall_statement.pdf).

WHO (2004) Tobacco Free Initiative, Tobacco and Poverty: A Vicious Circle. Tobacco Control. WHO Tobacco Control Papers. Geneva: WHO (http://repositories.cdlib.org/context/tc/article/1149/type/pdf/viewcontent/).

Wonderling D, Langham S, Buxton M, Normand C, McDermott C (1996) What can be concluded from the Oxcheck and British Family Heart Studies: commentary on cost-effectiveness analyses. BMJ 312: 1274–8.

Wood D (2002) Guidelines and global risk: a European perspective. Eur Heart J 4(suppl F): F12–18.

Wood DA, Kinmonth AL, Davies D et al. (1994) Randomised controlled trial evaluating cardiovascular screening and intervention in general practice: principal results of British family heart study. Family Heart Study Group. BMJ 308: 313–20.

CHAPTER THREE

Chest pain assessment in the pre-admission setting

ANDREA SAYCELL

History and development of rapid access chest pain clinics

Coronary heart disease (CHD) continues to be the most common cause of death in the UK (British Heart Foundation 2003). The most frequent manifestation of this condition is termed 'angina pectoris' with an estimated 1.4 million people living with angina in the UK (Department of Health or DoH 2000) and around 20 000 people developing angina for the first time every year.

In the late 1990s it was argued that health-care provision for patients with CHD in the UK was inequitable (Payne and Saul 1997). An attempt to remedy this inequity was made in the year 2000 with the publication of the National Service Framework (NSF) for Coronary Heart Disease (DoH 2000). This government document identified and set a number of standards of care that all patients with CHD should expect to receive throughout England and Wales. It highlighted the need for early assessment and rapid diagnosis of patients with coronary disease. Early recognition of signs and symptoms of CHD was seen as paramount to providing prompt, efficient and up-to-date intervention and treatment.

Chapter 4 of that document outlines clearly these aims, treatments and standards of care required in order to provide a service to meet the needs of this client group. Standard 8 is specifically related to the early diagnosis and treatment of angina (DoH 2000, p. 2):

> People with symptoms of angina or suspected angina should receive appropriate investigation and treatment to relieve their pain and reduce their risk of future coronary events.

To achieve this standard, immediate priorities and goals were established which laid down the foundations of rapid access chest pain clinics, including setting out a maximum time that patients should have to wait before an assessment is made:

> By April 2001, there should be 50 rapid access chest pain clinics, to help people who develop new symptoms that their GP thinks might be due to angina, which can be assessed by a specialist within 2 weeks of referral.
>
> DoH (2000, p. 34)

> There should be 100 rapid access chest pain clinics by April 2002 and a nationwide roll-out thereafter.
>
> DoH (2000, p. 36)

Currently the number of rapid access clinics has far exceeded the government target. Within the setting of the rapid access chest pain clinic (RACPC), the aim is to diagnose patients with coronary artery disease swiftly and provide the necessary treatments to optimize their condition and prevent future risk using an evidence-based approach.

What is angina?

Angina is a symptom, not a diagnosis, often experienced as central chest pain or discomfort precipitated by exertion or emotion and relieved by rest, usually reflecting periods of myocardial ischaemia. Myocardial ischaemia occurs when the coronary blood supply is insufficient to maintain myocardial tissue O_2 tension. This in turn leads to an imbalance between O_2 supply and demand, causing myocardial ischaemia and angina.

The amount of O_2 required by the myocardium is dependent primarily on heart rate. As heart rate increases, coronary perfusion is reduced as a result of the decrease in duration of diastole (coronary arteries fill during diastole) and O_2 demand increases as a result of an increase in the workload of the heart, potentially leading to ischaemia.

The major determining factor in the control of myocardial supply is coronary blood flow and so a narrowing within the lumen of a coronary artery can cause critical restriction to the supply of O_2.

Angina is brought on by an increase in O_2 demand that cannot be met by the supply; therefore any factor that increases heart rate can induce symptoms. The most common causes are:

- Exertion: particularly inclines and stairs
- Emotion: especially anger and stress
- Temperature change

- Windy weather
- A large meal: cardiac output rises by 20%; angina can occur within 30 minutes of a meal and is termed 'postprandial angina'.

If someone's angina is unchanging or progressing slowly it can be described as 'stable'. Stable angina is thought to be caused by a gradual occlusion of coronary arteries. A patient with stable angina will often say: 'I'm okay walking on the flat but when I walk uphill I have to stop and rest.' If, however, the severity of angina is increasing rapidly, or if angina is experienced at rest or on minimal exertion or at night, then it can be described as 'unstable'. Typically a patient will say: 'It wakes me up in the middle of the night.' Unstable angina is a medical emergency and the patient requires immediate hospitalization.

There are several tools that help with the grading of the severity of angina and these are useful to determine treatment options; the Canadian Cardiovascular Society provides the grading in the box.

Canadian Cardiovascular Society classification of angina

Class I	Ordinary physical activity does not cause angina
Class II	Angina causes slight limitation of day-to-day activities
Class III	Symptoms cause marked limitation of ordinary activity
Class IV	Symptoms occur when undertaking any physical activity or at rest

It has been shown that there is a close correlation between symptoms and prognosis; even without any further evidence provided by exercise tolerance testing, etc., the prognosis can be calculated. Patients with mild or moderate angina (class I or II) have a better prognosis than those with a severe angina (class III or IV) whose prognosis is poorer (Jain et al. 2003).

Patients attending an RACPC will have an uncertain diagnosis; their chest pain may be cardiac or non-cardiac in origin and so careful assessment is paramount.

Specialist assessment of chest pain

Chest pain is one of the most common reasons for consultation in primary care, accounts for around 30% of emergency medical admissions and is the main reason for referral to cardiology outpatient clinics (Bass and Mayou 2002).

There are many causes of chest pain (see box), with as many as 50% of patients who attend the cardiology clinic having non-cardiac pain (Mayou et al. 1994). Therefore it is necessary to have the ability and skills required to differentiate between non-cardiac and cardiac chest pain. An early diagnosis is of equal value to the patient, whether or not it is cardiac, and the reassurance and explanation of a non-cardiac diagnosis should be regarded as equally important to the practitioner. Newby et al. (1998) found that a firm diagnosis and reassurance of patients with recent onset of non-cardiac chest pain reduce their potential anxiety, morbidity and re-attendance, and also allow inappropriate anti-anginal medication to be discontinued.

The accurate identification of patients with ischaemic heart disease is of course of greatest concern, because around 30% of patients presenting with recent-onset angina have a significant cardiac event within 1–2 years (Ghandi et al. 1995). It is therefore apparent that an early diagnosis, followed by appropriate treatment and interventions, is paramount to the well-being of these patient groups. The consequences of an accurate diagnosis are significant to the patient and the family, specialist practitioner and NHS.

Within the setting of the RACPC, a diagnosis of CHD and informing patients that they have 'angina' is a fundamental issue, allowing the initiation of appropriate drug therapy and identifying patients who are at risk of future 'cardiac events'. It is not the environment to diagnose and treat patients who present with acute coronary syndrome, because this group of patients need swift hospitalization and emergency treatment.

Common causes of non-cardiac chest pain

Musculoskeletal problems: arthritis, costochondritis
Gastric disorders: mainly gastro-oesophageal reflux disease
Referred pain from thoracic spine
Psychological: panic attacks, depression
Pulmonary: pleuritic pain, chest infection

To help with the fundamental question 'Is it cardiac?', perhaps it is more appropriate to ask: 'Does it sound cardiac?' Typical angina usually presents as 'tightness' or 'heaviness' in the chest, precipitated by exertion and relieved by rest. It is often accompanied by breathlessness and further discomfort may be felt in the arms, jaw and neck. The relationship to exertion is the key factor; pain that is not precipitated or affected by exercise is rarely angina. Pain at rest, without other extrinsic factors such as stress, is also highly unlikely to be angina. The American Heart Association provides a classification of chest pain based on clinical characteristics. To rationalize chest pain it must encompass certain components in order to categorize it into typical angina, atypical angina or non-cardiac chest pain:

- Typical/definite angina consists of the following: substernal chest discomfort with characteristic qualities and duration, which is provoked by exertion or emotional stress and relieved by rest or nitroglycerin.
- Atypical/probable angina meets two of these characteristics.

- Non-cardiac chest pain meets one or fewer of the typical angina characteristics.

For those patients who fall into the atypical/probable or non-cardiac categories, the application of a coronary risk factor profile may be of help. Indeed its application to those patients with typical angina symptoms may assist the practitioner to swing the balance even further. Chest discomfort is more likely to represent coronary artery disease when there are also two or more existing risk factors present (Pryor et al. 1983). The risk factors of prevalence are:

- smoking
- hypertension
- diabetes
- hypercholesterolaemia
- family history of premature CHD
- the presence of other vascular disease.

History taking

To establish the presence of CHD risk, it is vital for the nurse to be skilled in the art of communication and able to use these skills to complete a thorough patient assessment. This often takes the form of what the doctor terms 'history taking'. During this interview particular emphasis is placed on pain assessment (for a more detailed account of pain assessment, see Chapter 7). This information is collected together with an assessment of the individual's CHD risk factors. Once completed the assessment should provide a foundation upon which to balance the diagnosis. Investigations also hold valuable information but only when considered together with the assessment as a whole. It is only when all of these factors are put together, rather like a jigsaw puzzle, that a more accurate picture can be formed.

To obtain a good history from a patient, the practitioner requires 'a list' of key questions; a mixture of open-ended and closed questions usually allows and facilitates discussion. During this time body language, attitude and facial expressions can be observed and accounted. It is important to remember that the patient is allowed to give his or her own account; however, this is not always easy.

- Patients may give answers that they think you want to hear or that they think are the correct response.
- Some patients may be vague in their responses requiring more discussion.
- Some patients may not answer the question that they were asked.
- Relatives can also be helpful but be aware that the opposite can also be true.

Pain assessment

Where is the pain?

A classic example of this is when, rather than use words to convey thoughts, a patient may 'rub' over the area with the hand or fist, showing an approximate area in the chest rather than a localized area. A patient who can directly point to a specific location is not usually describing cardiac pain.

However, an important point to remember is that discomfort may be experienced in the usual sites of radiation and not at all in the chest.

What does the pain feel like?

From my experience patients will often dispute that they are feeling any pain. If this is the case it is usually advisable to continue the assessment using the same words that the patient has used, i.e. ache, discomfort, indigestion, tightness.

When does the patient experience the pain?

'I'm fine walking on the flat but start to feel my chest start to ache when I walk uphill' is again a characteristic sign of ischaemic pain.

Others would include worsening in cold weather and during emotional stress.

How long does the pain stay?

Typical angina pain can last for up to about 20 minutes; pain that is constant, without relief and lasting for several hours or more, is unlikely to be cardiac in origin. Also pain that is fleeting and lasts for seconds only is highly unlikely to be cardiac. Not many patients 'time' their pain but they are usually able to give an approximation – 'about 5 minutes'.

It is important to note that chest pain that lasts longer than 15 minutes and is unresponsive to sublingual nitrates may be attributed to myocardial infarction.

Does the pain go anywhere else?

Many people are aware of cardiac pain going into the left arm, but remain unaware of the other usual sites of radiation. Discomfort usually perceived as an ache can be felt in one or both arms, or in the back, shoulders, neck or jaw.

What makes the pain go away?

The most typical response is rest; the patient who finds walking uphill difficult will say that he or she has to stop and rest before continuing. Occasionally patients take relatives' medication, such as glyceryl trinitrate (GTN) spray, and will have found this to be beneficial (although taking other people's medication should be discouraged).

Does the patient experience any other symptoms?

Table 3.1 highlights the signs and symptoms that many patients demonstrate on first presentation and serves as a useful reminder when taking a patient's history.

Table 3.1 Symptoms experienced by patients

Symptom characteristic	Typical	Atypical
Site	Central, left sided	Localized, 'pinpoint' – patient is able to point to exact location
Nature	Tightness, burning pressure, heaviness, ache, 'indigestion'	Sharp, stabbing
Radiation	Arms, neck, back, jaw	–
Duration	Usually < 20 min	Seconds or alternatively hours
Precipitating factors	Exertion requiring increased effort	Comes on at rest
Associated symptoms	Stress	No precipitating factors, occurs at any time
	Post eating	Deep inspiration, coughing
	Breathlessness, sweating, clamminess	–
Relieving factors	Rest, GTN spray	Analgesia, antacids, change of position, etc.

Shortness of breath related to exertion may be either an associated symptom or the only indication of an underlying problem. Other problems include feeling generally unwell and tired. The assessment of the patient's symptoms should be the foundation on which to build, using this information to help answer the question: 'Does it sound cardiac?'

The link between whether symptoms appear to be cardiac from the nature of the symptoms themselves and the presence of CHD is, however, stronger in men than in women (Melin et al. 1985) because women are known to suffer atypical presentations. As stated previously, the likelihood of chest pain being angina is increased when there is the presence of cardiovascular risks.

The assessment of cardiovascular risks forms an integral part of the overall assessment. An increasing number of risk factors associated with typical, cardiac-sounding chest pain increases the probability that symptoms are cardiac in origin. It is also true that, for those patients whose symptoms are not typically cardiac sounding, the presence of numerous risk factors increases the possibility of a cardiac diagnosis.

Exercise tolerance testing

The NSF for Coronary Heart Disease (DoH 2000a) sets standards for the investigation and treatment of stable angina. The exercise tolerance test forms an integral part of this assessment process. It can provide valuable information to confirm exercise-induced ischaemia and an indication of prognosis. A patient presenting with cardiac-sounding chest pain who has not had a myocardial infarction will usually have a normal resting ECG if it is carried out when the patient is pain free. However, a normal resting ECG does not exclude the presence of coronary artery disease. Around 30% of patients with a history of angina and severe three-vessel disease will display a normal ECG at rest and be free of symptoms (Hill and Timmis 2002). It is therefore important to note the significance of obtaining an ECG while the patient has pain. The ECG waveforms can (but not always) be altered while the patient is experiencing chest pain. With this in mind the exercise tolerance test is designed to produce symptoms and to determine functional and ECG response to graded stress.

Not all patients are suitable to perform an exercise tolerance test and the British Cardiac Society describes the contraindications to stress testing within their protocol for cardiac physiologist-managed exercise stress testing published in 2003. It is imperative that the following conditions are excluded before conducting a test:

• aortic stenosis
• hypotension (systolic < 90 mmHg)
• hypertension (systolic > 180 mmHg, diastolic > 100 mmHg)

- left bundle-branch block
- severe angina/rest angina
- acute myocarditis/percarditis
- dissecting aneurysm.

There are a number of different ways of conducting an exercise tolerance test, the most common being the treadmill exercise test conducted within a standard protocol and with continuous ECG and blood pressure monitoring. The most common protocol within the UK is the Bruce protocol (Table 3.2). It consists of graded levels of exercise, which build up in incremental 3-minute stages, increasing in both speed and incline.

Table 3.2 The Bruce protocol

Stage	1	2	3	4	5
Speed in km/h (m.p.h.)	2.7 (1.7)	4.0 (2.5)	5.5 (3.4)	6.8 (4.2)	8.0 (5)
Gradient (%)	10	12	14	16	18
METs	4.6	7.0	10.2	13.5	17.2

Each of the stages equates to a certain metabolic value (MET); this is a calculation of the amount of O_2 consumed per minute at certain levels of workload: 1 MET is the amount of O_2 consumed per minute by an average individual at rest; to carry out the activities of daily living at least 5 METs are required.

Measurable values that are achieved during exercise, such as maximum heart rate, blood pressure recordings, METs, ST-segment depression, exercise and recovery time are important components of the test.

Maximum heart rate

This is a simple calculation and by subtracting the patient's age from 220 the predicted maximum (80%) is obtained in beats per minute, e.g. if patient's age is 54, the maximum heart rate is 166 beats/min. This is useful because it not only provides guidance to end the test, but can also indicate the severity of heart disease. Patients who have severe disease will usually either fail to attain the predicted target heart rate or reach it at a low level of workload (Lancer et al. 1999). However, another reason for reaching maximum heart rate early in the test may be a poor level of fitness.

Blood pressure measurements

In particular falls in systolic blood pressure (≥ 10 mmHg) in response to exercise indicate that the heart is not pumping effectively (left ventricular dysfunction) and frequently signifies the presence of severe coronary artery disease and associated extensive myocardial ischaemia (Sanmarko et al. 1980). The failure of the systolic blood pressure to rise during exercise also suggests severe disease.

Exercise tolerance

The inability to exercise on a standard Bruce protocol and achieve > 7 METs is of significance, because this indicates a poor exercise tolerance related to an increased likelihood and risk of coronary events. Moreover, a patient who is able to demonstrate a good exercise tolerance, achieving > 10 METs, has a good prognosis even when the presence of CHD is established (Roger et al. 1998).

ST-segment changes

ST-segment changes of significance are mostly demonstrated in leads I and V3–6 (Travel 2001); however, from experience notable changes are often additionally seen in leads II, III and aVF. The standard criteria for a significant change in the ST segment are evidence of a horizontal or downsloping depression of > 2 mm. There is also a correlation between the severity of disease and the amount of ST-segment depression, taking into consideration the number of leads affected and the depth of ST depression (Hill and Timmis 2002).

The response to exercise is not the only piece of valuable information; the recovery stage is of equal significance and the information that it can provide should be of equal concern. In around 11% of patients with an abnormal test, ST changes occur during recovery (that were not apparent during exercise) and are equally as important and significant as changes seen in exercise (Martin and McConahay 1972).

ECG changes provide valuable and measurable evidence; however, this information is helpful only when patient response is taken into account. Significant information is gained from basic observations of respiratory rate, signs of fatigue, pain and distress.

It is therefore important to remember that, although careful study of the ECG is required during exercise (and recovery), close observation of the patient is paramount. Many patients will not disclose relevant information, thinking it is of no significance or the result of fear and anxiety. For some patients a simple 'Are you OK?' will prompt a response; for others a more direct approach is required. From experience, the question, 'Have you got chest pain?' has been needed when significant ST changes are clearly apparent on their ECG.

Exercise time

The amount of exercise a patient can tolerate not only reflects their general fitness but is also a prediction of the heart's ability to cope with exercise. An exercise time of 9–12 min is usually regarded as satisfactory.

Conversely, a high probability of coronary artery disease is suggested when an early positive response is shown within 6 minutes of exercise (Hill and Timmis 2002).

Prognostic value of the exercise tolerance test

The exercise tolerance test is useful to estimate the future risk of cardiac events, by providing prognostic information, and to indicate the severity and location of myocardial ischaemia. There are many useful scoring tools to help provide prognostic information, among which is the most recognized, the Duke Treadmill Score (Mark et al. 1991). It was designed to provide survival estimates based on the results from the exercise test, including amount of ST-segment depression, chest pain and exercise duration.

Equation of score

Treadmill score = Duration of exercise in minutes (using the Bruce protocol)
− 5 × Maximal ST deviation in mm
− 4 × Treadmill angina index

Treadmill angina index:
0 = no angina
1 = non-limiting angina
2 = limiting angina

High risk = Treadmill score < −10
   79% 4-year survival rate
   5.25% annual mortality rate

Moderate risk = Treadmill score −10 to +4
   95% 4-year survival rate
   1.25% annual mortality rate

Low risk = Treadmill score ≥ +5
   99% 4-year survival rate
   0.25% annual mortality rate

For example, a patient who exercises for 6 minutes with ST-segment depression of 2 mm and associated limiting angina would have a treadmill score of −12 and therefore be considered at moderate risk: $6 - (5 \times 2) - (4 \times 2) = -12$

High-risk patients have the poorest prognosis and generally should undergo coronary angiography, because many will have severe CHD. Low-risk patients have the best prognosis and are unlikely to benefit from further intervention.

Exercise tolerance testing (Figure 3.1), when assessed objectively, is a reliable predictor of risk. Even without the application of a scoring system, good prognosis can generally be predicted when the exercise test is well performed (Dargie 1993). Therefore, if patients complete a time that is comparable to their age and it does not precipitate symptoms or symptoms become apparent only at the end of a good exercise time this can be considered a well-performed test. Conversely, it has also been shown that greater degrees of ST segment depression generally correlate with more extensive disease (Merck 2000).

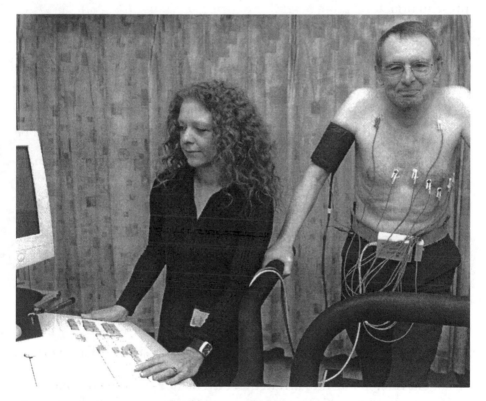

Figure 3.1 Patient on a treadmill.

After a cardiac diagnosis, risk reduction and the provision of advice and support are equally important to appropriate intervention and pharmacological management.

Lifestyle management

Modification of the lifestyle of a patient with CHD should not only be directed at the individual; it has been proved far more effective and beneficial when the patient's family are included (Pyke et al. 1997).

The patient who has been diagnosed with CHD needs to understand the importance of reducing risk factors and in doing so reducing risk of future events. Risk factors will differ according to the individual but, by modifying and reducing them, there will be an improvement in outcome in patients with angina (de Bono 1999). The specialist chest pain nurse will take time to identify the patient's risk profile and use evidence-based care (identified in Chapters 2 and 12) to facilitate the patient's lifestyle change where necessary.

The following section is a brief overview of the referral criteria and the patient journey through the RACPC; it concludes with a real case presentation.

Referral criteria for RACPC

- Patients who have suffered chest pain in the previous 24–48 h.
- Patients with established CHD with worsening symptoms may be referred, although it may be appropriate to access the 2-week cardiology clinic.
- Patients in whom CHD is extremely unlikely (women < 40 and men < 30 years) should not be referred except in exceptional circumstances.
- Patients suspected of having acute MI should be referred to the A&E department in the usual way.

The rapid access chest pain service is designed to provide swift and accurate diagnosis of patients with recent-onset chest pain of clinical concern. Where possible patients will be given an appointment on the day of referral.

Pathway of patients attending RACPC

- Patient presents at GP surgery with chest pain, possibly cardiac in origin.
- GP faxes patient details to RACPC.
- Patient is telephoned to arrange a convenient appointment time.
- Most (approximately 90%) are seen on the day of referral.
- Patient attends clinic.
- Assessment, including patient history, relevant risk factors, current medications and suitability for exercise tolerance test (ETT).
- Patient undergoes ETT.

- Blood testing if applicable, based on findings in clinic:
  - full blood count
  - urea and electrolytes
  - troponin T
  - lipid profile
  - thyroid function test.
- Diagnosis based on findings.
- Patient informed of probable diagnosis and treatment plan:
  - non cardiac: referred back to GP, patient is reassured that symptoms are non-cardiac
  - cardiac at low risk: medical therapy and cardiologist or GP review to assess
  - cardiac at medium risk: medical therapy and referral for coronary angiogram.
  - cardiac at high risk: medical therapy and referral for urgent coronary angiogram and direct admission to hospital.

Referrals for further investigations are made where necessary, such as:

- chest radiograph
- 24-hour blood pressure or ECG monitoring
- echocardiogram.

Information about the diagnosis is given, i.e. angina, medical therapies, interventions, such as coronary angiogram, are explained and appropriate lifestyle advice given along with a 24-hour helpline card. The GP is informed of probable diagnosis and treatment plan via fax after the patient's appointment.

Conclusion

There are about 0.5 million attendances to A&E departments every year in the NHS as a result of acute chest pain. It has been suggested that the care that these patients receive is poor and this is emphasized by the inappropriate discharge of patients with acute coronary syndrome and unnecessary admissions to hospital of patients with benign non-cardiac chest pain (Goodacre 2000). By improving access to cardiology services the implementation of an RACPC allows an early diagnosis and risk stratification of patients with coronary artery disease.

For those patients with non-cardiac chest pain unnecessary admissions may be avoided. This, in itself, has major benefits for the patient: first, because the stress associated with being admitted to hospital is avoided and, second, through reassurance that their symptoms are not cardiac in origin. Potentially this can reduce anxiety, morbidity and re-attendance of patients with non-cardiac chest pain, and allows inappropriate medical therapy to be discontinued.

Newby et al. (1998) would agree. In a study of rapid access chest pain services in the UK it was shown that the management of this group of patients has improved and hospital admission rates were reduced. Admissions with non-cardiac chest pain were reduced by 21% and, conversely, 42% of patients referred overall were diagnosed with coronary artery disease.

It would appear that there is a steady accumulation of evidence to support the work of RACPCs and, although evidence of reduced costs, admissions, etc. is evident, perhaps more importantly it provides an improved and effective patient experience.

Case study

The following account details the journey of an actual patient who attended an RACPC after referral by her GP. The patient's name has been changed in order to protect confidential patient information in accordance with the Nursing and Midwifery Council (NMC 2002).

Mrs Booth attended her GP surgery on Monday morning, following episodes of chest pain and shortness of breath on exertion over the weekend. After her appointment she was referred to an RACPC and given an appointment for that afternoon.

On arrival at the clinic a history was obtained, along with details of risk factors and assessment of chest pain.

She was a 64-year-old woman, previously fit and well who enjoyed an active social life, line dancing, walking and bowls, and who had never previously experienced exertional difficulties.

She described a central chest tightness and shortness of breath which presented when she was out walking the dog; it lasted about 5 minutes and she presumed that it was because the dog was 'pulling' on the lead. Later in the day it returned when she was coming home from the shop (uphill). Again it was perceived as a tightness in the middle of her chest, accompanied by shortness of breath and an 'ache in her jaw'. She experienced a further three episodes, all related to exertion which were relieved by sitting down and resting.

Past medical history:

Hypertension treated with atenolol 50 mg once daily
No known drug allergies

Risk factors for CHD:

Family history, sister had myocardial infarction at 53 years of age
Non-smoker (lifelong)
Lipid profile unknown
Resting ECG revealed normal sinus rhythm, 88 beats/min
Blood pressure was slightly elevated at 162/92 mmHg
Heart sounds normal.

She completed an exercise tolerance test (Bruce protocol), reporting chest tightness and shortness of breath at 4 minutes and 13 seconds of exercise; corresponding ST segment changes were seen on ECG in the form of horizontal ST depression of 2.4 mm. The exercise test was therefore terminated. During recovery the ST changes worsened, becoming downsloping, and lasted for a further 6 min despite O_2 therapy and sublingual GTN.

This woman was admitted to the cardiology ward and referred for urgent coronary angiography, which was performed on the following day.

Further reading

Hampton JR (1997) The ECG in Practice, 3rd edn. Edinburgh: Churchill Livingstone.
Ford MJ, Munro JF (2000) Introduction to Clinical Examination, 7th edn. Edinburgh: Churchill Livingstone.
Purcell H, Kaddoura S (eds) (2001) Angina: A systematic guide to investigation and treatment. St Louis, MO: Mosby.

References

Bass C, Mayou R (2002) ABC of psychological medicine. Chest pain. BMJ 325: 588–91.
British Heart Foundation (2003) Coronary Heart Disease Statistics Database (www.heartstats.org).
Dargie HJ (1993) Guidelines for cardiac exercise testing. Eur Heart J 14: 969–88.
de Bono D (1999) Investigation and management of stable angina: revised guidelines 1998. Heart 81: 546–55.
Department of Health (2000) The National Service Framework for Coronary Heart Disease. London: HMSO.

Ghandi MM, Lampe FC, Wood DA (1995) Incidence, clinical characteristics, and short term prognosis of angina pectoris. Br Heart J 73: 193–8.

Goodacre SW (2000) Should we establish chest pain observation units in the UK? A systematic review and critical evaluation of the literature. J Accid Emerg Med 17: 1–6.

Hill J, Timmis A (2002) ABC of clinical electrocardiography: Exercise tolerance testing. BMJ 324: 1084–7.

Jain A, Wadehra V, Timmis AD (2003) Management of stable angina. Postgrad Med J 79: 332–6.

Kennedy RL, Burton AM, Fraser HS et al. (1995) Review of triage, diagnosis and readmission rates in patients with acute chest pain. Heart 73: 107 (abstract).

Lancer MS, Francis GS, Okin PM (1999) Impaired chronotropic response to exercise stress testing as a predictor of mortality. JAMA 282: 524–9.

Mark DB, Shaw L, Harrel FE (1991) Prognostic value of a treadmill exercise score in outpatients with suspected coronary artery disease. N Engl J Med 325: 849–53.

Martin CM, McConahay DR (1972) Maximal treadmill exercise electrocardiography: correlations with coronary arteriography and cardiac haemodynamics. Circulation 46: 956–62.

Mayou R, Bryant B, Forfar C (1994) Non-cardiac chest pain and benign palpitations in the cardiac clinic. Br Heart J 72: 548–53.

Melin JA, Wijns W, Van Butsele RJ (1985) Alternative diagnostic strategies for coronary heart disease in women. Circulation 71: 535–42.

Merck Manual (2000) www.merck.com.

Newby DE, Fox KA, Flint LL, Boon NA (1998) A 'same day' direct access chest pain clinic: improved management and reduced hospitalisation. Q J Med 333–7.

Nursing and Midwifery Council (2002) Code of Professional Conduct: Standards for conduct, performance and ethics. London: NMC.

Payne N, Saul C (1997) Variations in the use of cardiology services in a health authority: Comparison of coronary artery revascularisation rates with prevalence of angina and coronary mortality. BMJ 314: 257–61.

Pryor DB, Harrell FE, Lee KL, Califf RM, Rosati RA (1983) Estimating the likelihood of significant coronary artery disease. Am J Med 75: 771–80.

Pyke SD, Wood DA, Kinmonth AL, Thompson SG (1997) Change in coronary risk and coronary risk factor levels in couples following lifestyle intervention Arch Family Med 6: 354–60.

Roger V, Jacobsen S, Pellikka P et al. (1998) Prognostic value of treadmill exercise testing. Circulation 98: 2836–41.

Sanmarco ME, Pontius S, Selvester RH (1980) Abnormal blood pressure response and marked ischaemic ST-segment depression as predictors of severe coronary artery disease. Circulation 61: 572–8.

Travel ME (2001) Stress testing in cardiac evaluation-current concepts with emphasis on the ECG. Chest 70: 545–7.

CHAPTER FOUR

Care of the patient with acute coronary syndrome in the accident and emergency department

DEBRA VICKERS AND IAN JONES

The term 'acute coronary syndrome' has recently been adopted to encompass the spectrum of clinical manifestations of acute coronary artery disease (Fox 2000), from acute ST-elevation myocardial infarction (MI) through non-ST-elevation MI to unstable angina. The use of the term 'non-ST-elevation MI' replaces the more traditional terms of 'non-Q-wave MI' or 'subendocardial MI' (Jones 2003). Unstable angina occupies the beginning of this spectrum, causing disability and risk that are greater than for stable angina but less than for non-ST-elevation MI (Braunwald et al. 1994). Studies in the 1990s found that the risk of death or non-fatal MI complicating unstable angina ranges from 8% to 16% at 1-month follow-up (Bertrand et al. 2000). Although non-ST-elevation MI was thought for many years to have a similar prognosis to unstable angina, some studies indicate that the prognosis for this group is similar to ST-elevation MI (Aguire et al. 1995).

It is now apparent that the acute coronary syndromes share a common anatomical substrate (Bertrand et al. 2000). As stated in Chapter 1, they occur as a result of the rupture or erosion of an atheromatous plaque (Forrester 2000). However, unfortunately plaque formation is neither linear nor predictable; new high-grade lesions have been noted in arterial segments that had recently been within normal limits (Theroux and Fuster 1998). Small plaque disruption, localized thrombus formation and subsequent repair of the fibrous plaque most probably cause this unpredictable progression. However, the patient may be symptom free during the whole process.

Symptoms of acute coronary syndromes

As a result of the common underlying pathology and disease process discussed in an earlier chapter, the presenting symptoms are often identical
regardless of the subsequent diagnosis. During the acute phase of this syndrome patients will often present with chest pain. Typical cardiac chest
pain is often described as central crushing chest pain radiating down the
left arm and/or up into the jaw. The pain, if thought to be caused by an
acute coronary syndrome, usually lasts in excess of 20 min, and is unre-
lieved by nitrate therapy. The discomfort is not sharp or highly localized
and may be associated with dyspnoea, nausea and/or vomiting (European
Society of Cardiology/American College of Cardiology 2000) and as a
result of autonomic dysfunction the patient may be sweaty, cold and clammy (Quinn et al. 2002). However, atypical presentations of acute coronary
syndromes are not uncommon. They are often observed in young and elderly people, women and patients with diabetes (Bertrand et al. 2000).
Atypical presentations can include stabbing pain, epigastric pain, pleuritic pain and dyspnoea (Lee et al. 1985).

Diagnosis of acute coronary syndromes

Diagnosis of an acute coronary syndrome can be made either prospec-
tively or retrospectively (Jones 2003). The criteria adopted to aid
diagnosis of acute MI include either elevation of certain enzymes or
pathological findings (European Society of Cardiology/American College
of Cardiology Committee 2000).

The first criterion is a typical rise and gradual fall of troponin, or a
more rapid rise and fall (subfraction of creatine kinase or CK-MB) of additional biochemical markers of myocardial necrosis, with at least one of the
following:

- ischaemic symptoms, e.g. chest pain
- development of pathological Q waves on the ECG
- ECG changes indicative of ischaemia (ST-segment elevation or depression)
- coronary artery intervention.

Although these criteria are helpful in diagnosing MI retrospectively,
they are of little use in the acute phase of the illness. Unfortunately, the
biochemical markers that have been identified can be within normal limits for several hours after an MI and therefore of limited use. The
practitioner relies on a good history and the ECG.

The diagnosis of unstable angina is essentially a clinical one, made on
the basis of clinical history and ECG (Unstable Coronary Artery Disease

Council 1998). A normal ECG does not exclude unstable angina but the following all support the diagnosis:

- ST-segment depression > 0.5 mm
- transient ST-segment elevation > 1 mm
- T-wave inversion.

Non-ST-elevation MI is diagnosed retrospectively, as is MI occurring without the subsequent Q-wave development on the 12-lead ECG (Maynard et al. 2000).

Treatment options for acute coronary syndromes

Patients with unstable angina are at high risk of MI and death (Hamm et al. 1992). Hyde et al. (1999) argue that as little as 0.5 mm ST elevation can reduce overall survival rate. Yet despite the optimal treatment benefits for acute ST-elevation MI being clear (Ryan et al. 1999), as discussed below the management options for unstable angina and non-ST-elevation MI patients remain in doubt (Maynard 2000).

The general principles for treatment of acute coronary syndromes are as follows (Califf 2000):

- Open the artery and keep it open.
- Perfuse the myocardium and prevent electrical accidents.
- Enhance the recovery of function.
- Enhance healing.
- Prevent recurrence.
- Practise according to the evidence available.

In essence the patient will require treatment that may include pharmacological, interventional and nursing therapies during the acute phase of the illness in order to address all aggravating factors (Jones 2003).

Unfortunately the means by which these aims are to be achieved for unstable angina/non-ST-elevation MI are rather more complex than that of ST-elevation MI. In the latter the gold standard is the dissolution of a persistent thrombus by the use of thrombolytic therapy (International Study of Infarct Survival or ISIS II 1988). However, more recently evidence has emerged to suggest that primary percutaneous coronary intervention is more beneficial than in-hospital thrombolysis, although the feasibility and capability of providing 24-hour angioplasty services within the UK are unknown at this time. Some tertiary cardiac centres are able to offer this service to their local population and others have extended their service to offer primary angioplasty to their near neighbours, but, while it is anticipated that these kind of services will expand, they remain the exception rather than the rule, so thrombolysis remains the most commonly used treatment. Unfortunately, thromblysis has been shown to be ineffective (Thrombolysis in Myocardial Infarction or TIMI IIIB Investigators 1994), and in some cases harmful, when given to patients without ST elevation (Boden et al. 1998). Therefore the patient with unstable angina is categorized into order of risk. These categories are important for the choice of pharmacological and interventional treatment because the relationship between risks and outcome have been defined in clinical trials (Fox 2000). These risk groups have been developed following the study of a number of databases and the outcomes of patients within these databases. Some drugs are available to all patients regardless of categorization, e.g. aspirin, whereas other drugs such as glycoprotein GPIIb/IIIa inhibitors may be prescribed only to the more high-risk groups. A number of risk stratification formulae are available from the aforementioned databases and share common themes, including age, severity of ST depression, elevated troponins, heart failure, prior coronary heart disease (CHD) and diabetes. Risk status requires regular review because patients' conditions change or their risk status changes in light of new information such as cardiac enzyme levels (Fox 2000). One such risk stratification formula is that devised by the European Society of Cardiology/American College of Cardiology (2000) (Figure 4.1), which provides a simple and easy-to-follow flow diagram for patients presenting with acute coronary syndromes.

Another widely used risk stratification formula is taken from the findings of the Global registry of Acute Coronary Event (Grainger et al. 2003). This observational study was designed to develop a simple means of assessing mortality risk in patients with acute coronary syndrome. A number of variables are required to formulate the calculations including ST segment deviation, creatinine levels, age, blood pressure and heart rate among others. All the variables required are easily obtainable in clinical practice and, once collated, the tool is able to provide the clinician with the patient's percentage risk of in-hospital death. Such a tool could be invaluable in cardiac triage.

Investigations

Electrocardiograph (ECG)
Urea and electrolytes (Us&Es)
Full blood count
Glucose
Troponin levels
Lipid breakdown

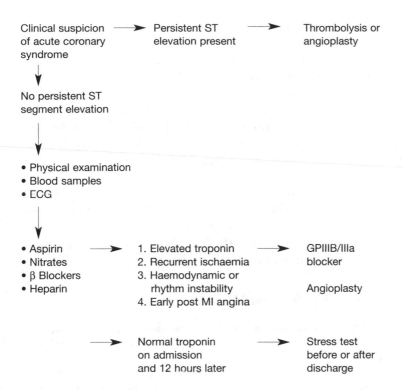

Figure 4.1 Flow diagram of people presenting with acute coronary syndromes. (From Bertrand et al. 2000.)

Emergency nursing care

A more detailed overview of nursing care is provided in Chapter 7. Patients presenting with a possible acute coronary syndrome should be assessed as soon as possible by an appropriately trained member of staff. The initial assessment should be rapid, and aimed at establishing a diagnosis, assessing the haemodynamic state and determining suitability for thrombolysis. Comprehensive history taking and examination should be deferred until the patient has received appropriate emergency care.

Emergency care consists of relief of pain, breathlessness and anxiety, and administration of thrombolytic therapy and aspirin as early as possible. The following interventions are priorities:

- Establish venous access.
- Institute rhythm monitoring to aid rapid detection and treatment of cardiac arrhythmias.
- Provide adequate analgesia: intravenous opiates are indicated to provide rapid relief of pain. Uncontrolled pain and anxiety are associated with

sympathetic activation, with resulting detrimental effects on cardiac performance, O_2 consumption and the arrhythmia threshold. Intramuscular injections should be avoided because they are associated with unpredictable absorption, may cause a haematoma if the patient is subsequently thrombolysed and can affect cardiac enzyme estimations. The choice of agent is diamorphine 2.5–5 mg by slow intravenous injection, followed by metoclopramide 10 mg as an antiemetic. The dose should be repeated every 5 min until adequate analgesia is achieved. Respiratory depression produced by diamorphine can, if necessary, be rapidly reversed by naloxone.

• Provide supplemental O_2: hypoxia is common in patients with acute MI and may increase myocardial necrosis or have adverse metabolic effects. Supplemental O_2 will optimize O_2 delivery and limit ischaemia.
• Start treatment with aspirin, and with thrombolysis if indicated after rapid assessment of clinical features and exclusion criteria.

Thrombolysis in acute ST-elevation MI

Doesn't thou love life? Then do not squander time, for that is the stuff of life.

Benjamin Franklin

Some 240 000 people have an acute MI (AMI) in England and Wales each year; of these up to 50% will die within 30 days of the event. Over half the deaths occur before medical assistance arrives or the patient reaches hospital. The onset of symptoms is usually sudden and the highest risk of death is within the first hour of experiencing symptoms – around one-third of deaths occur within the first hour (National Institute for Clinical Evidence or NICE 2002). Intravenous thrombolytic therapy is an established treatment for AMI. It is estimated by the NICE (2002) that about 50 000 patients receive thrombolysis in England and Wales each year. However, evidence suggests that thrombolysis continues to be underused.

The importance of early administration of thrombolytic treatment to eligible patients with AMI is highlighted in the UK in the National Service Framework (NSF) for Coronary Heart Disease (Department of Health or DoH 2000a) and *The NHS Plan* (DoH 2000b).

Thrombolytic therapy has been an established treatment for MI for over two decades. The benefits of prompt treatment have been well documented in large randomized trials (Fibrinolytic Therapy Trialists' Collaborative Group 1994, Boersma et al. 1996). A benefit in the mortality rate has been shown to be maintained for at least 10 years after treatment with streptokinase (Baigent et al. 1998).

A clear message from the trials is that the benefits associated with thrombolysis are inversely proportional to the delay in starting treatment

(Boersma et al. 1996). In patients seen within the first few hours of symptom onset, each minute of delay is reportedly associated with 11 days of life lost – thus every half an hour of delay is equated to a year of life lost (Rawles 1997). Treatment within an hour of onset of symptoms is associated with a 50% reduction in mortality rate. It has been subsequently recommended that, in terms of its potential for saving lives, action to initiate thrombolytic therapy in eligible patients should be afforded urgency similar to that given to the management of cardiac arrest (Cannon et al. 1994).

The NSF for CHD (DoH 2000a) set standards for improved prevention, diagnosis, treatment and rehabilitation of patients with CHD. Standards 5, 6 and 7 specifically address the management of patients with suspected MI.

Standard 5

People with symptoms of a possible heart attack should receive help from an individual equipped with and appropriately trained in the use of a defibrillator within 8 min of calling for help, to maximize the benefits of resuscitation should it be necessary.

Standard 6

People thought to be having a heart attack should be assessed professionally and, if indicated, receive aspirin. Thrombolysis should be given within 60 min of calling for professional help. Of eligible patients 75% should receive thrombolysis within 30 min of hospital arrival by April 2002, and within 20 min of hospital arrival by April 2003.

Standard 7

NHS trusts should put in place agreed protocols/systems of care so that people admitted to hospital with proven heart attack are appropriately assessed and offered treatments of proven clinical and cost-effectiveness to reduce their risk of disability and death.

Working towards and achieving the aims proposed in the NSF for CHD (DoH 2000a) has led to much organizational adaptation, as well as changes in the way patients thought to be experiencing AMI are treated. Organizational strategies that have evolved to suit local circumstances include the following:

- Policies for direct admission to a coronary care unit (CCU) assessment by a GP (Burns 1989).
- Pre-hospital thrombolysis (GREAT Group – Rawles 1997, Quinn et al. 2002a).
- Direct admission to CCU after assessment by ambulance personnel, including 12-lead ECG interpretation (Bannerjee and Rhodes 1998).

- Acute chest pain specialist nurses based in the accident and emergency (A&E) department (Pyatt et al. 1999, Wilmhurst et al. 2000).
- Thrombolysis coordinator facilitating treatment by an A&E team (Gamon et al. 2002).
- Nurse-initiated thrombolysis in a CCU (Caunt 1996, Smallwood 2000b).

Whichever strategy or model is employed – depending on local circumstances – every effort should be made to streamline pre-hospital and in-hospital procedures, which should be the subject of regular audit. The NSF for CHD targets of 20-min 'door–needle' time, and 60-min overall 'call–needle' time for patients meeting criteria for thrombolysis, with no exclusion criteria at the time of presentation, should be achievable.

Inclusion criteria

Thrombolysis should be considered for all patients presenting with 12 h of onset of chest pain who have ST-segment elevation or new left bundle-branch block (LBBB) on their ECG. Aspirin or an alternative anti-platelet agent should be given alongside or before thrombolysis in all circumstances. There is no evidence of benefit from the administration of thrombolysis to patients with normal ECGs or ST-segment depression at presentation. In these circumstances the ECG should be repeated at regular (15-min) intervals or continuous ST-segment monitoring instituted. If the criteria for thrombolysis are not fulfilled in a patient presenting with prolonged cardiac chest pain and ST-segment depression, management should be along the lines given in Chapter 7 for the management of acute coronary syndrome.

Patients suitable for thrombolysis are selected on the basis of the following criteria:

- Presentation within 12 h of the onset of ischaemic cardiac chest pain in a patient with:
  - ST-segment elevation of at least 1 mm in two or more limb leads
  - ST-segment elevation of at least 2 mm in two adjacent chest leads
  - new, or presumed to be new, LBBB
  - true posterior MI.
- Absence of contraindications.

Clinical features

The pain associated with AMI is typically retrosternal, crushing and severe. Pain often radiates to the arms, back or neck, and is often accompanied by nausea, sweating and vomiting, related to increased autonomic activation and the release of toxins from injured myocardial cells. The pain associated with AMI is usually sudden in onset and not usually affected by respiration, movement or changes in posture. The pain may also by atypical, i.e. sited in the epigastrum, neck, arms or back, or unusual in character. In inferior infarction, particularly, the pain may mimic dyspepsia. In some patients (particularly those with diabetes and who are elderly), the pain may be minimal or even absent, with predominant symptoms consisting of nausea, vomiting, dyspnoea and syncope. In some patients AMI occurs without any symptoms, and is often recognized only retrospectively by the presence of abnormalities of the electrocardiogram (ECG). For each individual patient, the pain from a cardiac event may vary in intensity and radiation, but is broadly similar in character, on each occasion. Ask the patient to compare the pain with any earlier, proven ischaemic events – if the patient feels that the pain is similar – and then even atypical presentations are probably the result of cardiac ischaemia.

As several conditions can produce similar clinical features and even ECG changes to those presented in MI, it is important that they can be correlated with the clinical presentation to produce a reasonable diagnosis. It is for this reason that taking an accurate clinical history is paramount. Essential baseline questions that should be asked of any patient with chest pain should include:

- When did the pain begin (recently, minutes or hours)?
- Where do you feel it (chest)?
- When did it start?
- Did it spread anywhere (arms, neck, back)?
- How would you describe the pain (crushing, stabbing)?
- Has the pain been constant, or does it come and go?
- Does it feel like any discomfort or pain that you have had in the past (especially patients with pre-existing heart disease)?
- Is there anything that seems to aggravate or alleviate the pain (exercise, rest, deep inspiration)?
- Did you break out in a sweat, have nausea or vomiting, or become short of breath?

This list is not exhaustive, but the answers to these questions should be considered the minimum information necessary for an adequate history of chest pain.

ECG changes (Figure 4.2)

The following are typical changes of AMI.

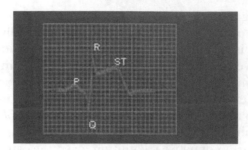

Figure 4.2 ECG changes indicating acute myocardial infarction (AMI). Reproduced with kind permission of Boehringer Ingelheim.

ST-segment elevation in the leads overlying the area of infarction

This usually occurs in the early stages of infarction and may exhibit quite a dramatic change. ST-segment elevation is often upward and concave, although it can appear convex or horizontal. ST-segment elevation is not unique to AMI, and therefore is not confirmatory evidence unless the other clinical features of AMI are present. Basic requirements of ST changes for diagnosis are: elevation of at least 1 mm in two or more limb leads (I, II, III, AVR, AVL or AVF) or at least two or more chest leads (VI–V6). Some ST-segment elevation may be seen in leads VI and V2 normally; however, if there is also elevation in V3 the cause is unlikely to be physiological.

Pathological Q waves in the leads overlying the area of infarction

Q waves are usually associated with full-thickness AMI, develop within a few hours of the infarct and persist long term. Associated with the development of the Q wave is a reduction of the R-wave amplitude in affected leads. As Q waves are a relatively late change, they are not useful for the diagnosis of AMI in the emergency setting, in the case of a patient who has presented to emergency care early after symptom onset.

T-wave inversion in the leads overlying the area of infarction

The T wave is the most unstable feature of the ECG tracing and changes occur very frequently under normal circumstances, limiting their diagnostic value. However, T-wave inversion develops as the ST-segment elevation subsides, and usually resolves over 7–14 days. An early sign of AMI might be the development of tall, peaked T waves in the area overlying the infarction.

Bundle-branch block

Is the pattern produced when either the right bundle or the entire left bundle fails to conduct an impulse normally? The ventricle on the side of the failed bundle branch must be depolarized by the spread of a wave of depolarization through ventricular muscle from the unaffected side. This is obviously a much slower process and usually the QRS duration is prolonged to at least 0.12 s (for a right bundle-branch block or RBBB) and 0.14 s (for LBBB).

Sequence of changes in evolving AMI (Figure 4.3)

- The ECG changes that occur as a result of AMI do not all occur at the same time. There is a progression of changes correlating to the progression of the infarction.
- Within minutes of the clinical onset of infarction, there are no changes in the QRS complexes; therefore there is no definitive evidence of infarction. However, there is ST-segment elevation providing evidence of myocardial damage.
- The next stage is the development of a pathological Q wave and the loss of an R wave. These changes occur at variable times and so can occur within minutes or can be delayed. Development of a Q wave is the only proof of infarction (although Q waves may be present in lead III in the absence of infarction but disappear on inspiration).

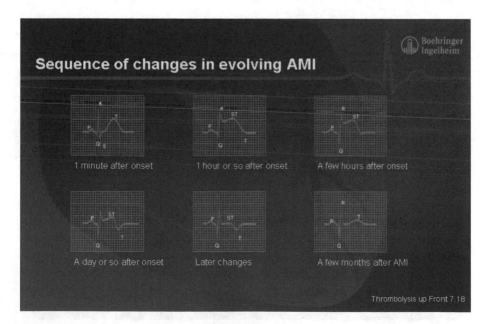

Figure 4.3 The evolving sequence of ECG changes. Reproduced with kind permission of Boehringer Ingelheim.

- As the Q wave forms, the ST-segment elevation is reduced and after about 1 week the ST changes tend to revert to normal, although the reduction in R-wave voltage and the abnormal Q waves usually persist.
- The late change is the inversion of the T wave and, in a non-ST-elevation MI (NSTEMI), this T-wave change may be the only sign of infarction.
- Months after the MI the T waves may gradually revert to normal, but the abnormal Q waves and reduced voltage R waves persist.
- In terms of diagnosing AMI in time to make thrombolysis a life-saving possibility, the main change to look for on the ECG is ST-segment elevation.

Location of infarction and its relationship to the ECG (Figure 4.4)

Different leads on the 12-lead ECG look at different aspects of the heart, and so infarctions can be located by noting the changes that occur in different leads. Using these we can define where the changes will be seen for infarctions in different locations.

Anterior infarction

This usually occurs as a result of the occlusion of the left anterior descending coronary artery, causing infarction of the anterior wall of the

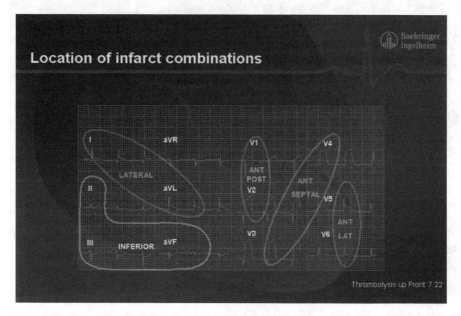

Figure 4.4 Location of infarct and its relationship to the ECG. Reproduced with kind permission of Boehringer Ingelheim.

left ventricle and the intraventricular septum. It may result in pump failure caused by loss of myocardium, ventricular septal defect, aneurysm or rupture and arrhythmias, and an increased risk of early death.

ST-segment elevation in leads I, aVL and V2–V6, with ST-segment depression in II, III and aVF, are indicative of an extensive anterior infarction.

ST-segment elevation in leads V2–V4 indicates a septal infarction, usually associated with more distal occlusion of a well-collateralized left anterior descending artery or one of its branches. These patients usually sustain a smaller infarct, with a lower risk of complications and a better prognosis.

ST-segment elevation in leads I, AVL, V5 and V6 indicates lateral infarction, caused by occlusion of the circumflex artery or the diagonal branch of the left anterior descending artery. These patients usually sustain a relatively limited infarct with a lower risk of complications and a better prognosis.

Inferior infarction

This may occur as a result of occlusion of the right circumflex coronary arteries causing infarction of the inferior surface of the left ventricle, although damage may occur to the right ventricle and the intraventricular septum.

ST-segment elevation in leads II, III and AVF, and often ST depression in leads I and AVL, and the precordial leads, indicate inferior infarction. Patients with inferior infarction have a relatively low incidence of heart failure and tachyarrhythmias, but an increased incidence of bradyarrhythmias (caused by damage to the AV node). Patients with inferior infarction generally have a good prognosis, although those with very extensive infarction (indicated by changes in the inferior, lateral and posterior leads) are a high-risk subgroup. Hypotension in patients with inferior infarction may be the result of right ventricular involvement (ST elevation in V3R and V4R); these patients respond well to intravenous fluids and have a good prognosis, unlike patients with hypotension caused by excessive left ventricular impairment.

Posterior infarction

This is difficult to diagnose, but may be indicated by tall R waves in V1–V3 associated with ST-segment depression in those leads, in a patient with a history of ischaemic chest pain. An ECG recording of leads V7, V8 and V9 should be obtained; ST elevation in these leads would indicate the need to proceed with thrombolytic therapy.

Some patients will undoubtedly present with a history highly suggestive of cardiac ischaemia, but with a normal or equivocal ECG. The ECG should be repeated at regular (every 15-min) intervals, or continuous cardiac monitoring started. These patients should be admitted to hospital, especially if the symptoms are new because they may have an acute coronary syndrome or an evolving infarct. Care and investigations should consist of those described for the care of the patient with acute coronary syndrome in Chapter 7.

Exclusion criteria for thrombolysis

There are risks associated with thrombolytic therapy, the most important of which is haemorrhagic stroke. This affects 0.5–1.5% of patients and is associated with high mortality and long-term disability in survivors. The risk of haemorrhagic stroke after thrombolysis increases with age and increasing blood pressure (Simoons et al. 1993).

The list of exclusion criteria continues to evolve, varies somewhat in detail from hospital to hospital, and in general decreases as our experience with thrombolytic therapy increases. Many contraindications are now regarded as relative, rather than absolute, and must be interpreted within the clinical context. The patient must be conscious and coherent. Criteria include the following:

- History of stroke with residual neurological defect
- Pregnancy
- Any immediate major bleeding risk
- Active peptic ulceration, oesophageal varices or recent (within 6 months) gastrointestinal haemorrhage (dyspepsia alone is not a contraindication)
- Sustained hypertension: systolic > 200 mmHg and/or diastolic > 110 mmHg
- Surgery, major trauma or head injury within the previous month
- Prolonged or traumatic cardiopulmonary resuscitation
- Recent internal bleeding from any site
- Known coagulation disorder, including uncontrolled anticoagulation therapy
- Menstruation (very low risk)
- Diabetic retinopathy (should be considered a very relative contraindication, because the risk of intraocular bleeding is small, and the potential benefit of thrombolysis in patients with diabetes far outweighs this risk).

Balancing the risk against the benefits of thrombolytic therapy is a very important decision when presented with a suspected AMI. Some contraindications rule out patients immediately because the risk is too great. However, with relative contraindications the risks and benefits must be weighed carefully. Providers of the care need to assess how much harm they may do for the benefit that thrombolysis will achieve.

If there is any doubt about the appropriateness or otherwise of administering thrombolysis, a senior colleague should be consulted without delay. If the risks of thrombolysis outweigh the perceived benefits, the urgent referral for percutaneous coronary intervention (PCI) should be considered at the earliest opportunity.

Differential diagnosis

The classic symptoms of MI are chest pain, breathlessness, nausea and vomiting, dizziness or fainting, palpitations and sweating. As these symptoms can be similar to those of other conditions, some of which may also present with ST-segment elevation on the ECG, it is important to distinguish between these conditions and MI to try to provide a definite diagnosis.

Conditions that may present with similar symptoms to MI are angina, dissecting aortic aneurysm, pericarditis, oesophageal pain, musculoskeletal pain, pulmonary embolism or pneumothorax, and (rarely) skin conditions.

Angina

Pain of an MI is described as a tightness or crushing pain, although its severity varies widely. The pain occurs typically in the chest, but often radiates to the left arm. The pain is not sudden; it usually builds up rapidly to constant severity lasting several hours. The pain may fluctuate as a result of the formation and breaking away of thrombi, or coronary artery spasm. Angina presents with the same symptoms as MI, but the pain is less severe, and is often precipitated by and occurs during exertion. A diagnosis of angina rather than MI is likely if the pain is resolved within 20 min, or if the pain is relieved by nitrates. The ECG will show ST-segment depression or T-wave inversion in the affected leads rather than ST-segment elevation.

Dissecting aortic aneurysm

This occurs when a tear occurs in the inner wall of the aorta, as a result of hypertension and associated atherosclerosis. The pain of aortic dissection is severe and of sudden onset. This condition may be associated with hypertension, aortic regurgitation, neurological signs, widened mediastinum and pulse deficits. The pain is usually severe precordial or epigastric searing, or tearing pain leading to the neck, abdomen, legs or back of the chest between the scapulae. The pain is totally abrupt in onset and at its worst in the first second. The site of the pain may change as the aneurysm expands.

Pericarditis

This is an inflammation of the pericardium and the associated pain is very similar to that of an MI. However, the pain of pericarditis is accentuated by inspiration and relieved by leaning the patient forwards. It is commonly seen after an infarction, or in a young adult with acute postviral pericarditis. A pericardial rub is common. ST-segment changes are common early features, although the segment is concave upwards and may sometimes be seen globally across the ECG.

Oesophageal or upper gastrointestinal pain

Dyspeptic pain arising from the upper gastrointestinal tract is usually burning in nature, may have a clear relationship to posture or food, and is often relieved by antacids. Oesophageal pain may, however, be very similar to the pain of cardiac ischaemia. If the pain is unrelated to food, further cardiological investigation may be necessary to obtain a correct diagnosis. Pain caused by ischaemia of the inferior surface of the heart often mimics dyspepsia.

Musculoskeletal pain

Musculoskeletal pain from the chest wall (e.g. costochondritis) may also mimic that of an AMI. It is usually unilateral, localized and sharp and exacerbated by movement or local pressure. There may be a history of trauma.

The pleura in pneumonia, pulmonary embolism or pneumothorax

Pain arising from the pleura is unilateral, sharp and stabbing, and worse on inspiration. There may be associated signs of pneumonia, pulmonary embolus or deep vein thrombosis. Most patients who have a pulmonary embolus have no ECG changes apart from a tachycardia or atrial fibrillation. Spontaneous pneumothorax is a strong possibility in patients with chronic obstructive pulmonary disease, who present with chest pain and dyspnoea in the absence of ECG evidence of MI. A chest radiograph is vital to rule out the presence of air in the pleural space.

Acute skin conditions

These can (rarely) cause chest pain. The unilateral pain of shingles precedes the rash, and may present in a similar fashion to MI.

Consent to treatment

The clinician providing treatment is responsible for ensuring that the patient has given valid consent before treatment begins, although the consultant responsible for the patient's care will remain ultimately responsible for the quality of medical care provided (DoH 2001).

There is a debate to be had, however, about the validity of consent obtained from patients with acute MI and related conditions during the acute phase of illness (Kucia and Horowitz 2000, Sugarman 2000, Agard et al. 2001).

Choice of thrombolytic agent

In the UK, four thrombolytic agents are currently licensed to treat AMI (Table 4.1). There is a long history of use of one agent, streptokinase, whereas the other three, alteplase, reteplase and tenecteplase, are newer.

Streptokinase

Streptokinase can be used up to 12 hours after the onset of AMI symptoms and is administered as an intravenous infusion over a period of an hour.

Administration of streptokinase is often associated with hypotension, infrequently with allergic reactions and, rarely, anaphylaxis. Patients treated with streptokinase develop anti-streptococcal antibodies, which can inactivate the drug if subsequent treatment is needed. Consequently patients must be treated with streptokinase only once.

Table 4.1 Thrombolytic drugs currently used in the UK

Drug	Bolus/Infusion	Considerations/disadvantages
Streptokinase	Infusion	Infusion; associated with hypotension/allergy
Alteplase	Infusion	Infusion
Reteplase	Bolus	Two doses required
Tenecteplase	Bolus	Weight-adjusted dose

Alteplase

Alteplase (recombinant human tissue plasminogen activator or rtPA) can be delivered as a standard or accelerated regimen. The accelerated regimen, which is most commonly used, is indicated up to 6 h after onset of symptoms of AMI and is delivered by an intravenous bolus injection, followed by two intravenous infusions – the first given over 30 min and the second over 60 min. The standard regimen is indicated between 6 and 12 h after symptom onset and requires a bolus injection followed by five infusions over 3 h. Unlike streptokinase, alteplase does not stimulate the production of antibodies and so can be used repeatedly if indicated.

An infusion of heparin must follow alteplase (5000-unit bolus and 1000 units/h infusion, for at least 48 h).

Reteplase

Reteplase can be given up to 12 h after onset of symptoms of AMI. It is given as two intravenous bolus injections, exactly 30 min apart. Each bolus should be given slowly over 2 min. Like alteplase, it can be used repeatedly if indicated. Reteplase should also be followed by heparin (regimen as for alteplase), beginning after the second bolus dose.

Tenecteplase

Tenecteplase is indicated up to 6 h after the onset of symptoms of AMI. It is administered as a single, weight-adjusted, intravenous bolus injection given over 5–10 s. Again this is followed by heparin (regimen as for alteplase).

Managing the complications of thrombolysis

Cerebrovascular event

The most significant complication of thrombolysis is intracerebral haemorrhage. If there is any evidence of a stroke, thrombolysis should be stopped (if an infusion is the thrombolytic used), along with any intravenous anticoagulant therapy. Specialist medical advice (haematologist) should immediately be sought about reversal of the thrombolytic agent. Computed tomography (CT) and neurological opinion will help to determine the mechanism of the stroke and guide therapy.

Haemorrhage

Minor bleeding at venepuncture sites is relatively common, and rarely requires any specific therapy other than direct compression of the site. Gingival bleeding can be treated with saline mouthwashes and reassurance. If a major bleed occurs, the thrombolytic infusion (if used) should be stopped, along with any intravenous anticoagulant therapy. Reversal of the thrombolytic agent should be considered urgently, after urgent referral to senior cardiology and haematology colleagues.

Arrhythmias

Arrhythmias are a common complication of MI and should be treated in the normal manner according to advanced life support guidelines. Reperfusion arrhythmias such as accelerated or slow idioventricular rhythm may occur – these are usually benign and do not require treatment.

Hypotension

Hypotensive reactions can occur with any thrombolytic agent, but are common with streptokinase. Alteplase, reteplase and tenecteplase rarely cause hypotension. If the hypotension is accompanied by bradycardia this should be treated with atropine. If symptomatic hypotension occurs, any treatment should be stopped (in the case of infusion). Hypotension will usually resolve after streptokinase has been discontinued for 5 or 10 min, particularly if the patient is laid flat or tilted head down. Steptokinase may be recommenced if the blood pressure normalizes. If recurrent hypotension occurs after streptokinase infusion, use of an alternative thrombolytic agent should be urgently considered. Volume replacement may be indicated if the hypotension is the result of haemorrhage. In the case of severe persistent hypotension, fluids and ionotropes may be administered cautiously if necessary.

Allergy

Allergic reactions are most likely to occur when using streptokinase, and are the result of the effect of pre-existing anti-streptococcal antibodies. Alteplase, reteplase and tenecteplase rarely cause allergic reactions. Mild urticarial reactions are the most common allergic response, and should be treated with 200 mg hydrocortisone and 10 mg chlorpheniramine intravenously. If a more severe reaction with bronchospasm occurs, 250–500 μg of intramuscular adrenaline (epinephrine) should be administered, along with nebulized bronchodilators. Major anaphylaxis is very rare.

Failed re-perfusion

Achievement of successful re-perfusion is associated with infarct artery patency, restoration of rapid anterograde blood flow into a patent microcirculation and resolution of chest pain. In a significant number of patients re-perfusion therapy fails. Failure of re-perfusion is associated with continuing chest pain, extensive infarction, electrical and haemodynamic instability, mechanical complications and a poor prognosis. In the International Joint Efficacy Comparison of Thrombolytics (INJECT) Trial (Schroder et al. 1995), those with no ST-segment resolution had a 17.5% hospital mortality rate, those with partial resolution a 4.3% mortality rate and those with total resolution a 2.5% mortality rate.

There are few accurate markers of successful reperfusion. Probably the best are the prompt resolution of chest pain and reduction in ST-segment elevation (Sutton et al. 2000). A more quantitative correlate of re-perfusion may be gained from cardiac enzyme release (i.e. troponin T or I, creatine kinase myoglobin or CK-MB); however, as a result of the frequency of measurement required over a short time period after thrombolysis, this is an impractical solution.

Patients should therefore have a 12-lead ECG recorded at 60–90 min (or according to local protocol) after commencing thrombolysis. Patients with clinical evidence of failure to re-perfuse (e.g. continuing pain, persisting or sometimes worsening ST-segment elevation), particularly in the presence of haemodynamic instability, have a poor prognosis. Management strategies include:

- 'rescue' thrombolysis (note that streptokinase should not be given more than once)
- 'rescue' PCI.

These patients should be discussed with a cardiologist or senior colleague at the earliest opportunity, and the strategy chosen will depend on clinical factors and the level of locally available (tertiary centre) expertise. In haemodynamically stable patients who have had only a small infarct, the risks associated with PCI or repeat thrombolysis may in fact outweigh the potential benefits. However, patients who have had a large infarct, with marked ST-segment elevation, ongoing pain and haemodynamic instability, where failure to re-perfuse is established within the first 4 h of the infarct, a 'rescue' procedure stands a better chance of re-establishing adequate re-perfusion, salvaging myocardium and improving prognosis.

Conclusion

Early treatment saves lives. Treatment within the 'golden hour' from onset of symptoms is associated with at 50% reduction in mortality from AMI. Patients presenting with STEMI within 12 h of onset of symptoms, with no contraindications, should receive thrombolysis within 20 min of hospital arrival, and within 60 min of 'call for help'.

After a provisional diagnosis of AMI, emergency care consists of relief of pain, and breathlessness and anxiety, and then administration of thrombolytic therapy and aspirin as soon as possible.

The decision to administer thrombolytic therapy in the presence of STEMI should be taken by a suitably trained and competent practitioner, who must carefully weigh up the benefits of thrombolysis against the possible risk of harm to the patient. Failure to re-perfuse or re-occlude after thrombolysis may be associated with poor prognosis. These patients should be discussed with a senior colleague urgently with a view to PCI or rescue thrombolysis.

References

Agard J, Hermeren G, Herlitz J (2001) Patients' experiences of interventional trials on the treatment of myocardial infarction: is it time to adjust the informed consent procedure to the patients capacity? Heart 86: 632–7.

Aguire FV, Younis LL, Chaitman BR et al. (1995) Early and 1 year clinical outcome of patients evolving non-Q wave and Q wave MI after thrombolysis: results from the TIMI II study. Circulation 91: 2541–8.

Baigent C, Collins R, Appleby P, Parish S, Sleight P, Peto R (1998) ISIS-2: 10 year survival among patients with suspected acute myocardial infarction in randomised comparison of intravenous streptokinase, oral aspirin, both or neither BMJ 316: 1337–43.

Bannerjee S, Rhodes WE (1998) Fast-tracking of myocardial infarction by paramedics. J R Coll Physns Lond 32: 36–40.

Bertrand ME, Simoons ML, Fox KAA et al. (2000) Management of acute coronary syndromes: acute coronary syndromes without persistent ST segment elevation. Recommendations of the Task Force of the European Society of Cardiology. Eur Heart J 21: 1406–32.

Boden WE, O Rourke RA, Crawford MH et al. (1998) Outcomes in patients with acute non Q wave myocardial infarction randomly assigned to an invasive as compared with a conservative management strategy. Veteran Affairs non Q wave infarction Strategies in Hospital (VANQWISH) trials investigators. N Engl J Med 338: 1785–92.

Boersma E, Maas A, CP, Deckers JW, Simoons M (1996) Early thrombolytic treatment in acute myocardial infarction: Reappraisal of the golden hour. Lancet 348: 771–4.

Braunwald E, Jones RH, Mark DB et al. (1994) diagnosing and managing unstable angina Circulation 90: 613–22.

Burns JMA (1989) Impact of a policy of direct admission to a Coronary Care Unit on the use of thrombolytic treatment. Br Heart J 61: 322–34.

Califf RM (2000) Evidence to practice in acute coronary syndromes. Am J Cardiol 86(12b): 1M–3M.

Cannon C P, Antman FM, Walls R, Braunwald E (1994) Time as an adjunctive agent to thrombolytic therapy. J Thrombos Thrombolys 1: 27–34.

Caunt J (1996) The advanced nurse practitioner in CCU. Care Crit Ill 12: 136–9.

Department of Health (2000a) The National Service Framework for Coronary Heart Disease. London: HMSO.

Department of Health (2000b) The NHS Plan – A plan for investment, a plan for reform. London: HMSO.

Department of Health (2001) Reference Guide to Consent for Examination or Treatment. London: HMSO.

European Society of Cardiology and American College of Cardiology (2000) Myocardial infarction redefined: A consensus document of the Joint European Society of Cardiology/American College of Cardiology Committee for the Redefinition of Myocardial Infarction. Eur Heart J 21:1502–13.

Fibrinolytic Therapy Trialists' (FTT) Collaborative Group (1994) Indications for thrombolytic therapy in suspected acute myocardial infarction. Collaborative overview of early mortality and major morbidity results from all randomised trials of more than 1000 patients. Lancet 343: 311–22.

Forrester J (2000) Role of plaque rupture in acute coronary syndromes. Am J Cardiol 86(suppl): 15J–23J.

Fox KAA (2000) Acute coronary syndromes: presentation – clinical spectrum and management. Heart 84: 93–100.

Gamon R, Driscoll P, Cooper A, Barnes P, Parr B (2002) Can Emergency Department-initiated thrombolysis supported by a Thrombolysis Co-ordinator reduce treatment times. Care Crit Ill 18: 104–6 .

Ghuran A, Uren N, Nolan J (2003) Emergency Cardiology: An evidence based guide to acute cardiac patients. London: Arnold.

Grainger CB, Goldberg RJ, Dabbous O et al. for the global Registry of Acute Coronary Events Investigators (2003) Predictors of hospital mortality in the global Registry of Acute Coronary Events. Arch Intern Med 163: 2345–53.

Hamm CW, Ravkilde J, Gerhardt W et al. (1992) The prognostic value of serum Troponin T in unstable angina. N Engl J Med 327: 146–50.

Hyde TA, French JK, Wong CK, Straznicky IT, Whitlock RML, White HD (1999) Four-year survival of patients with acute coronary syndromes without ST-Segment Elevation and prognostic significance of 0.5mm ST-segment depression. Am J Cardiol 84: 379–85.

International Study of Infarct Survival II Collaborative Group (1988) Randomised controlled trial of streptokinase, oral aspirin, both, or neither among 17 187 cases of suspected acute myocardial infarction (ISIS 2). Lancet ii: 349–60.

Jones I (2003) Acute coronary syndromes: Identification and patient care. Professional Nurse 18: 289–92.

Kucia AM, Horowitz JD (2000) Is informed consent to clinical trials an 'upside selective' process in acute coronary syndromes? Am Heart J 139: 94–7.

Lee T, Cook F, Erb R (1985) Acute chest pain in the emergency room. Arch Intern Med 145: 65–9.

Maynard SJ, Scott J, Riddell W, Adgey AAJ (2000) Management of acute coronary syndromes. BMJ 321: 220–3.

National Institute for Clinical Excellence (2002) Drugs for Early Thrombolysis in the Treatment of Myocardial Infarction. London: HMSO.

Nolan J, Greenwood J, Mackintosh A (1998) Cardiac Emergencies: A pocket guide. Oxford: Butterworth Heinemann.

Pyatt J, Hughes C, Mullins P, Saltiss S. (1999) The effect of an acute chest pain nurse specialist on the delivery time of thrombolytic therapy in AMI. Br J Cardiol 6: 499–507.

Quasim A, Malpass K, O'Gorman D, Heber ME (2002) Safety and efficacy of nurse initiated thrombolysis in patients with acute myocardial infarction. BMJ 324: 1328–31.

Quinn T, Butters A, Todd I (2002a) Implementing paramedic thrombolysis – and overview. Accident Emergency Nursing 10: 189–96.

Quinn T, Webster R, Hatchett R (2002b) Coronary heart disease: Angina and acute myocardial infarction. In: Cardiac Nursing, A Comprehensive Guide. London: Churchill Livingstone.

Rawles J (1997) Quantification of the benefit of earlier thrombolytic therapy: 5 year results of the Grampian region early antistreplase trial (GREAT). J Am Coll Cardiol 30: 1181–6.

Ryan TJ, Antman EM, Brooks NH et al. (1999) update: ACC/AHA guideline for the management of patients with acute myocardial infarction. A report of the American College of Cardiology/American Heart Association task force on practice guidelines (Committee on the management of Acute Myocardial Infarction). J Am Coll Cardiol 34: 890–911.

Schroder R, Wegscheider K, Schroder K, Dissmann R, Meyer-Sabellek W (1995) Extent of early ST segment elevation resolution: a strong predictor of outcome in patients with acute myocardial infarction and a sensitive measure to compare thrombolytic regimens. A substudy of the International Joint Efficacy Comparison of Thrombolytics (INJECT) trial. J Am Coll Cardiol 26: 1657–64.

Simoons ML, Maggioni AP, Knatterud G et al. (1993) Individual risk assessment for intercranial haemorrhage during thrombolytic therapy. Lancet 342: 1523–8.

Smallwood A (2000a) Medical consultants' attitudes towards nurse assessment and initiation of thrombolysis prior to medical screening. Nursing Crit Care 5(1): 15–21.

Smallwood A (2000b) Nurse-initiated thrombolysis in coronary care. Nursing Standard 15(2): 38–40.

Sugarman J (2000) Is the emperor really wearing new clothes? Informed Consent for Acute Coronary Syndromes. Am Heart J 140: 2–3.

Sutton AGC, Campbell PG, Price DJA et al. (2000) Failure of thrombolysis by streptokinase: detection with a simple electrocardiographic method. Heart 84: 149–56.

Theroux P, Fuster V (1998) Acute coronary syndromes: Unstable angina and non Q wave myocardial infarction. Circulation 97: 1195–206.

TIMI IIIB Investigators (1994) Effects of tissue plasminogen activator and a comparison of early invasive and conservative strategies in unstable angina and non-Q wave myocardial infarction: results of the TIMI IIIB trial. Thrombolysis in myocardial ischemia. Circulation 89: 1545–56.

Unstable Coronary Artery Disease Council (1998) Managing Unstable Coronary Artery Disease: A practical guide. London: Open Line.

Wilmhurst P, Purchase A, Webb C, Jowett C, Quinn T (2000) Improving door to needle times with nurse initiated thrombolysis. Heart 84: 262–6.

CHAPTER FIVE

Drugs affecting the cardiovascular system

IAN JONES AND ELIZABETH LAWSON

When caring for cardiac patients, it is imperative that the health professional has an understanding of the various drug regimens that patients are prescribed, and is able to detect and counter the side effects that these drugs may cause. This chapter provides an overview of the common classes of drugs used in cardiac care.

β Blockers

β Blockers (atenolol, bisoprolol, propranolol, metoprolol) are now widely accepted as a first-line secondary prevention treatment in coronary heart disease and the mainstay of anti-hypertensive treatment. They have been shown to reduce sudden deaths, re-infarction rates after myocardial infarction (MI) and total mortality (Yusef et al. 1988). The extent of mortality reduction is estimated to be 12/1000 patients treated per year (Freemantle et al. 1999). The benefits of these drugs are thought to be related to their ability to reduce the heart rate by blocking the β-adrenoreceptors in the heart (receptors are also found in the liver, blood vessels, bronchi and pancreas). This blockade reduces the effects of stimulant catecholamines such as adrenaline (epinephrine). They also reduce the level of catecholamines in the circulation and decrease myocardial O_2 demand, resulting in a reduction in myocardial contractility, heart rate and blood pressure, thereby reducing cardiac workload (Verheught 1999). Renin release will also be inhibited as sympathetic nerves stimulate the juxtaglomerular cells to release it.

β Blockers may also reduce the size of an MI and/or control angina in patients with acute coronary syndromes (Yusef et al. 1988), and should be prescribed for all patients with an acute coronary syndrome (ACS) unless contraindicated (British Cardiac Society 2000). Some β blockers have also been found to be effective in the management of chronic heart failure. A more detailed account of its therapeutic effects in this group of patients is provided in Chapter 13.

Side effects

The side effects of β blockers are bradycardia and bronchospasm; patients with diabetes may experience hypoglycaemia, fatigue, cold peripheries and erectile dysfunction.

As a result of the presence of β cells in the lungs, β blockers can cause bronchospasm. Some β blockers are termed 'cardioselective' and are more capable of influencing the β_1 cells present in the heart, as opposed to the β_2 cells that are present in the lungs. However, it should be noted that even cardioselective β blockers (metoprolol, atenolol) are not without risk. Some β blockers are water soluble and some fat soluble. Atenolol is water soluble, so it is less likely to cross the blood–brain barrier and give rise to nightmares and sleep disturbances.

Calcium channel blockers

Calcium (Ca^{2+}) channel blockers (verapamil, diltiazem, amlodopine, nifedipine), although often considered as one class, can be subdivided into three further groups:

* dihydropyridines
* phenylalkylamines
* benzthiazepines.

Dihydropyridines have been shown to have a detrimental effect (SPRINT 1988). However, the DAVIT II (1990) study showed a beneficial effect of prescribing verapamil, a phenylalkylamine in post-MI patients without heart failure. Therefore, the British Cardiac Society (2000) argue that certain calcium channel blockers may be prescribed to control heart rate when β blockers are contraindicated, or as an additional therapy where symptoms persist despite treatment with nitrates and β blockers.

All calcium channel blockers reduce the Ca^{2+} flow through cardiac cell membranes, including myocardial, vascular and conductive cells. By preventing the opening of Ca^{2+} channels, there is a reduced movement of Ca^{2+} into myocardial and smooth muscle cells. Consequently, this results in a reduction of myocardial contractility and a relaxation of vascular smooth muscle. The inhibition of contraction in the blood vessels increases the vascular diameter of the blood vessels, resulting in a reduction of the blood pressure. By reducing the amount of Ca^{2+} inside the cardiac myocytes, the contraction rate (heart rate) is reduced, ensuring an overall reduction in myocardial O_2 demand. However, when discussing Ca^{2+} channel blockers, it is imperative to note that despite having similar pharmacological actions the effects of individual drugs are varied.

Verapamil produces a greater effect on the conduction system, in particular the atrioventricular (AV) node, so reducing heart rate. Benzthiazepines are used predominantly for angina as a result of their vasodilatory effect, but they may be used for hypertension; dihydropyridines are used predominantly for hypertension as a result of its vasodilatory and negative inotropic effects. Any discussion needs to ensure that the evidence for individual agents within this class are highlighted separately and placed within their particular context.

Side effects

The side effects of Ca^{2+} channel blockers are bradycardia, heart block, hypotension, headaches malaise, gynaecomastia, gum hyperplasia, nausea and vomiting, and palpitations.

Angiotensin-converting enzyme inhibitors

Angiotensin-converting enzyme (ACE) inhibitors (captopril, enalapril, fosinopril, lisinopril, quinapril) are now used quite readily in cardiac care. It was not so long ago that patients needing ACE inhibition were admitted to hospital to be monitored while receiving their first dose of the drugs. Thankfully, those days are now behind us and ACE inhibitors are often started in primary care.

Although ACE inhibitors are often used for hypertension, there is also a wealth of evidence to support the use of these drugs in secondary prevention and heart failure. The ISIS 4 (1995) study provided moderate reductions in mortality for patients after an MI. However, the AIREX (Hall et al. 1997) and Trace (Køber et al. 1995) studies, which focused on post-MI patients with left ventricular dysfunction, showed dramatic improvements, thereby ensuring that ACE inhibitors would form part of secondary prevention protocols. In heart failure studies the evidence is also overwhelming. In both mild-to-moderate (V-HeFT-II – Cohn et al. 1991) and severe chronic heart failure (CONSENSUS I 1987), the drugs provide an impressive mortality reduction, so much so that the National Institute for Clinical Excellence (NICE 2003) now recommend that all patients with symptomatic left ventricular systolic dysfunction receive ACE inhibition.

Remember that renin is released from the juxtaglomerular cells of the kidney.

The drugs work by influencing the renin–aldosterone system within the renal system. Renin converts the protein angiotensinogen into the shorter protein angiotensin I, a decapeptide that is subsequently converted to a shorter protein – an octapeptide angiotensin II – by ACE. Angiotensin II binds to angiotensin II receptors found on vascular smooth muscle, increasing the intracellular concentration of calcium leading to vasoconstriction primarily of arterioles. This vasoconstriction is strongest in the skin, the kidneys and the splanchnic (abdominal) region:

Angiotensin I + ACE = Angiotensin II.

Inhibition of the renin–angiotensin–aldosterone system may be through either reducing the rate and amount of angiotensin II produced or blocking the angiotensin II receptors. ACE inhibitors act as the name suggests, inhibiting the activity of ACE. When the drug binds to the active site of the enzyme the rate of production and the amount of angiotensin II in the blood are significantly reduced. This has a number of effects:

* Reduction in the calcium availability to the arterioles, promoting vasodilatation.
* Reduction in the stimulation of the adrenal cortex to secrete aldosterone, reducing sodium and fluid retention.

The overall result is a reduction in the blood pressure. This outcome is beneficial in its own right and is often the only outcome required in hypertensive patients, but it is even more important for patients with heart failure. In heart failure the patient frequently develops a reduction in cardiac output as a result of the inability of the left ventricle to pump adequately. As this is undesirable the body compensates by activating the renin–aldosterone system. These compensatory mechanisms aim to maintain cardiac output, blood pressure and peripheral perfusion. However, sustained activation of these compensatory mechanisms leads to progression of left ventricular systolic dysfunction and worsening heart failure (Exner and Schron 2001). A more detailed review of the evidence for this group of drugs in heart failure is provided in Chapter 13.

Side effects

* The side effects of ACE inhibitors include dry cough, hypotension, maculopapular rash and eosinophilia, which is immune system generated.
* By limiting the production and secretion of aldosterone, potassium excretion could be reduced, resulting in hyperkalaemia.
* By decreasing the renal vasoconstriction urine production may be reduced resulting in an elevation of urea and creatinine values.

ACE inhibitors must not be used in pregnancy because the inhibition of angiotensin II production and the possible increased production of prostaglandins appear to affect the developing child adversely.

Angiotensin II receptor inhibitors

These drugs (losartan and valsartan) have similar effects to ACE inhibitors in reducing blood pressure, but this is achieved by blocking the angiotensin II receptor sites.

Side effects

The side effects include the following:

* The major advantage of this type of drug is that it achieves the reduction in blood pressure in a similar way to the ACE inhibitor drugs, but is not associated with the cough.
* Hypotension.
* Hyperkalaemia.

Diuretics

Diuretics affect the renal system by increasing the flow of urine. The aim of most diuretics is to increase the excretion of sodium chloride in the urine by interfering with the reabsorption of sodium chloride. They are commonly used to manage hypertension primarily because they increase urine output and reduce blood volume, which improves cardiac output and reduces blood pressure. They can also relieve oedema caused by cardiac failure. Different diuretic agents act at different sites of the nephron, which impacts on the effectiveness of the response.

Thiazides

Thiazides (bendrofluazide, chlorthalidone) are moderately effective diuretics. They act on the early segment of the distal convoluted tubule of the nephron and inhibit sodium (Na^+) reabsorption by blocking the transport mechanism. Potassium loss using these diuretic agents particularly at high doses is significant and can be severe.

Side effects

Side effects include postural hypotension, hyponatraemia, hypokalaemia, hyperuricaemia, hyperglycaemia and allergic reactions.

Furosemide (frusemide, Lasix)

Furosemide is termed a loop diuretic because it has its effect at the loop of Henle of the nephron. Loop diuretics are filtered via the glomerulus into the nephron and are potent diuretic agents. Furosemide inhibits the transport mechanism in the ascending loop of Henle so that sodium chloride is not reabsorbed and remains in the filtrate. By inhibiting this reabsorption, sodium chloride remains in the filtrate, attracts water to it and increases the amount of urine output (diuresis). Loop diuretics also have some vasodilatory effect, which will reduce blood pressure but importantly will increase the glomerular filtration rate, so increasing urine production. Intravenous furosemide is extremely effective in treating acute pulmonary oedema. The effects are almost instantaneous.

Side effects

- Hypovolaemia caused by overzealous administration.
- Hypotension caused by a reduction in fluid volume.
- Hypokalaemia: increased urine production increases the secretion of potassium and a reduction in the fluid volume of the blood stimulates aldosterone secretion, which increases potassium excretion. This is very important if using digoxin concurrently.

Potassium-sparing diuretics

This class of diuretic (spironolactone and amiloride) tends to be regarded as a weaker and less powerful diuretic. The K$^+$-sparing diuretics act on the later segment of the nephron and can play a significant role in producing diuresis and avoiding K$^+$ supplementation.

There are two major classes of potassium-sparing diuretics: aldosterone antagonists and Na$^+$ channel inhibitors.

These diuretic agents have their effect on the distal convoluted tubule of the nephron. Spironolactone acts as an inhibitor of aldosterone by occupying the aldosterone receptor. By blocking the action of aldosterone sodium chloride is excreted, followed by water, which increases urine output although K$^+$ is conserved and hence the term 'potassium sparing'. Amiloride is not an aldosterone antagonist but it inhibits the transport of sodium from the tubular lumen back into the blood by blocking the Na$^+$ channels. Consequently, sodium chloride is again not reabsorbed into the body but remains in the filtrate with its concomitant water. K$^+$ then remains in the body.

Side effects

Hyponatraemia, hyperkalaemia and hypotension have been reported.

Cardiac glycosides

Digoxin is a leaf extract from the plant *Digitalis lanata* (Grecian foxglove). It is commonly prescribed for the treatment of congestive cardiac failure or atrial fibrillation.

Remember that at rest the cells of the heart have a high concentration of K^+, a low concentration of Na^+ and a low concentration of Ca^{2+} inside the cell. On contraction the Na^+ and Ca^{2+} concentrations rise and the K^+ concentration lowers. To re-establish the resting concentrations of these electrolytes requires a Na^+/K^+ pump to become activated. This pump will drive Na^+ back out of the cells again and return the K^+ intracellularly.

The first effect of digoxin is to inhibit the Na^+/K^+ pump. This produces cardiac myocytes with an increased intracellular concentration of Na^+ and a reduction in K^+ that will reduce the heart rate by slowing the conduction at the sinoatrial (SA) and AV nodes (negative chronotropic effect).

The second effect of digoxin results from the increased intracellular concentration of Na^+, which limits the outward movement of Ca^{2+}. This increases the Ca^{2+} available within the cardiac myocytes, increasing the power of contraction (positive inotropic effect). This effect has been debated for many years with the result that digoxin is in and out of vogue for patients who have left ventricular impairment. The Digitalis Investigation Group (1997) found that, although the use of digoxin for these patients did not reduce overall mortality, it was able to reduce the rate of readmission.

Side effects

Digoxin has a *very narrow* therapeutic range (the differences between the therapeutically effective dose and the toxic dose are small).

Toxicity can arise from hypokalaemia (caution with diuretic choice and management), which results because digoxin competes to occupy the K^+ site on the Na^+/K^+ pump. When K^+ availability is low (hypokalaemia) the digoxin is far more effective on the pump, which enhances its effect.

Digoxin toxicity can lead to hyperkalaemia because a lot of K^+ is extruded. This will have a detrimental effect on the nerve supply to the heart suppressing the activity of the SA node and the AV node, resulting in AV block. Arrhythmias may also occur as a result of the excessive elevation of intracellular Ca^+ (tachyarrhythmia).

Common extra-cardiac side effects include: nausea, vomiting, abdominal pain and diarrhoea.

Lipid-lowering drugs

Remember that atherosclerotic plaques have a very complex structure, but mainly they have a fatty core. The arteries become narrowed as a result of the presence of the plaques. Lipids are necessary for a number of bodily processes, including formation of myelin, cell membranes and steroid hormone synthesis.

Lipoproteins are graded by their density. The least dense particles, very-low-density lipoproteins (VLDLs), are not usually associated with atherosclerosis but low-density-lipoprotein (LDL) particles appear to penetrate damaged arterial walls easily. There is a strong positive correlation between LDLs (cholesterol) and coronary vascular disease.

Statins

There are now a number of studies that have produced overwhelming evidence that lipid-lowering therapy in CHD patients significantly reduces mortality and morbidity (Scandinavian Simvastatin Survival Study Group 1994 [4S Study], Sacks et al. 1996 [CARE], LIPID Study Group 1998). These studies have included patients either after an MI or with stable angina and cholesterol levels ranging from 4 to 7 mmol. The overall reduction in mortality rate in these studies ranges from 9% to 30%. The higher reduction was noted in the 4S Study, which recruited higher-risk patients; conversely the smallest reduction was noted in the CARE study, which recruited lower-risk post-MI patients. The studies discussed have provided an amazing insight into post-ST-elevation MI management and ensured that statin treatment is included in all secondary prevention protocols. The Myocardial Ischaemia Reduction with Aggressive Cholesterol Lowering (MIRACL) trial (Schwartz et al. 2001) has gone one step further by proving the effectiveness of statin therapy in patients with unstable angina and non-ST-elevation MI. Therefore, it should now be accepted that statin therapy is a major contributor to long-term mortality reduction in all acute coronary syndromes.

Originally statin therapy was introduced on the assumption that reducing cholesterol levels would reduce the prevalence of cholesterol-rich atheromatous plaques. However, evidence has been accumulating that intense cholesterol lowering with statins favourably influences a multitude of factors relevant to the pathophysiology of recurrent events in acute coronary syndromes (Waters and Hsue 2001), including the following:

- Statins are less effective at lowering triglyceride levels but do reduce their availability.
- There is improvement in vascular endothelial function through an increase in nitric oxide formation.
- Modification of the inflammatory processes is involved in plaque formation by reducing the number of white blood cells found in plaques.
- Reduction in smooth muscle cell proliferation is commonly associated with plaque formation.

The drugs work by reducing the hepatic production of cholesterol, which reduces the amount of cholesterol in the blood that can participate in plaque formation. In the liver, an essential process in the formation of cholesterol is the conversion of 3-hydroxy-3-methylglutaryl coenzyme A (HMG-CoA) into mevalonic acid, after which a sequence of chemical processes creates cholesterol. This process is enhanced by the action of a hepatic enzyme HMG-CoA reductase, which is inhibited by statins. Consequently, the production of cholesterol in the liver is reduced.

Side effects

Statins are generally well tolerated but a number of the following precautions are necessary:

- Caution needed if patient has existing liver disease.
- Grapefruit juice inhibits the metabolism of statins so avoid co-administration.
- Statins should not be given to pregnant women, because cholesterol is vital to the developing fetus.
- Myalgia (muscle pain) should be reported; it is experienced when statins are taken with fibrates.

In addition the following side effects have been reported:

- Headache
- Nausea
- Vomiting and diarrhoea
- Hypersensitivity reactions.

Fibrates

Fibrates (bezafibrate, ciprofibrate and fenofibrate) lower the hepatic production of VLDLs, essentially triglyceride, but they have some effect on lessening the level of cholesterol.

Side effects

Fibrates are generally are well tolerated but the following side effects can occur:

- Nausea and diarrhoea.
- Myositis which can result in acute renal failure. It is particularly associated with concomitant use of HMG-CoA (statins).
- Fibrates are not suitable for use in individuals with renal impairment because there is reduced excretion.

Nitrates

Few studies have evaluated the efficacy of using nitrates (glyceryl trinitrate or GTN, Glytrin Spray, Transiderm-Nitro and oral isosorbide mononitrate) for patients with acute coronary syndromes, yet many cardiologists consider intravenous nitrates to be the most effective way of relieving chest pain and signs of ischaemia (Abrams 2000). In fact about two-thirds of hospitalized patients with acute coronary syndromes receive intravenous nitrates (Abrams 2000). Nitrates are potent vasodilators, which act by releasing NO (nitrous oxide) into vascular tissue. NO activates an intracellular enzyme called guanylyl cyclase which can decrease the amount of Ca^{2+} inside muscle cells; this is how the dilatation is achieved and the main effect of GTN is predominantly vascular dilatation, which decreases the preload by reducing venous return. Through a reduction in the venous return the cardiac workload is reduced and so is the cardiac O_2 requirement. Second, the nitrates dilate the large coronary arteries; however, it is proposed that it is unclear whether this is effective in relieving ischaemia and preventing infarction in patients with acute coronary syndromes (Verheught, 1999), although this therapeutic effect should not be discounted

Nitrate therapy can be administered orally, intravenously or via the submucosal route. The preparations consist of nitroglycerin, isosorbide dinitrate and isosorbide mononitrate. As a result of their similarity in pharmacology, the agents are chosen depending on their duration of action and the formulation available (Sanghani and Filer 2000). In the acute phase administration tends to preclude the oral route because of the inability to titrate therapy according to changes in the patient's condition. Common side effects include hypotension and headaches. The latter, although not life threatening, can have deleterious effects on the patient's experience. The former is of major importance and intravenous nitrates would need to be reduced if the patient showed any signs of hypotension. It is worth noting at this point that the patient may have been previously hypertensive and therefore a normal blood pressure while receiving nitrate therapy may be grossly abnormal for that individual. Symptom awareness as well as blood pressure monitoring is vital when caring for such a patient.

There has been a long-held belief within coronary care nursing that the administration of intravenous nitrates can have a detrimental effect on the use of intravenous heparin. However, on searching the literature it is unclear whether this interaction actually exists. It can be argued that the introduction of low-molecular-weight heparin may actually make the argument redundant. One major issue affecting the use of nitrate therapy that needs to be explored is the concept of nitrate tolerance. It is accepted that prolonged use of nitrates should include a nitrate-free period. Some studies have shown that during nitrate tolerance the body becomes more sensitive to catecholamines, thus increasing vasoconstriction and worsening the clinical picture (Caramori et al. 1998).

Side effects

Side effects include dizziness resulting from reduction in vascular pressure, throbbing headaches after cerebral blood vessel dilatation and flushing of the skin.

Side effects after intravenous administration include nausea, hypotension, palpitations and abdominal pain. These are usually associated with a too rapid administration.

GTN is contraindicated where there is underlying hypotension and hypovolaemia, aortic stenosis and a previous history of hypersensitivity reactions to nitrate-based products.

Potassium channel activators

The K^+ channel activators have similar properties to those of nitrates and may be indicated (unlicensed indication) in the treatment of refractory unstable angina in addition to nitrates, β blockers or Ca^{2+} channel blockers where symptoms persist (British Cardiac Society 2000). In the Cesar 2 study (Patel et al. 1999), nicorandil was shown to be a safe and effective anti-ischaemic agent, but it was found to have no effect on mortality or non-fatal MI.

Side effects

Side effects include nausea and vomiting, hypotension, flushing, hepatic disturbance and oral ulceration.

Anti-thrombotics

As discussed earlier, when an atheromatous plaque ruptures a highly thrombogenic surface is exposed. Factor VIIa and tissue factor VIIa complex promote the generation of factor Xa (Ardissino et al. 1997). The resultant effect is the production of large quantities of thrombin, as well as activation of platelets (Weitz 1995). These platelets adhere to the site of injury attracting additional platelets and blood cells and, if left intact, a fibrin-rich mesh encapsulates this material to form a resistant thrombus. A number of drugs are now available that act at various points of the

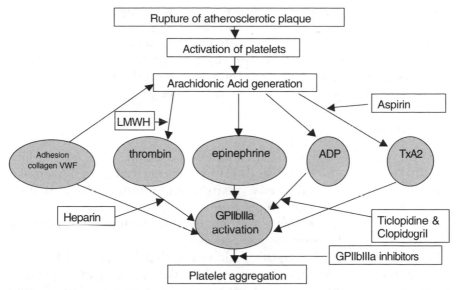

Figure 5.1 The platelet aggregation process after atherosclerotic plaque rupture and pharmacological actions. AA, amino acid; GPIIb/IIIa, glycoprotein IIb/IIIa; MWH, low-molecular-weight heparin; TxA$_2$, thromboxane A$_2$; vWF, von Willebrand's factor. Reproduced with kind permission of Lilly.

coagulation process in order to provide an anti-thrombotic effect. To understand the modes of action of these drugs it is imperative first to understand the coagulation process (Figure 5.1).

Thrombolytic agents

Numerous studies have established thrombolysis as a significant and effective strategy in the management of MI in both the short and the long term (ISIS II 1982, GUSTO 1993, Fibrinolytic Therapy Trialists (FTT) Collaborative Group 1994) if given within 12 h of the onset of pain. Speed of administration is associated with a successful outcome, which is achieved by rapid assessment and diagnosis (Boersma et al. 1996), so much so that the National Service Framework (NSF) for Coronary Heart Disease (DoH 2000) recommends that 75% of eligible patients should be thrombolysed within 20 min of hospital arrival (door to needle)

Thrombolysis involves the dissolution of the clot by the conversion of plasminogen to plasmin to dissolve the fibrin mesh surrounding the thrombus. Successful dissolution of the clot will lead to re-establishment of the blood flow, preserving the cardiac muscle.

There are currently a number of thrombolytic agents available in the UK that work in similar ways and with the appropriate evidence base to support their use. In reality the choice of individual agent tends therefore to be based on cost or personal preference. The newer bolus agents such as reteplase and tenecteplase obviously have the advantage of not requiring an initial infusion. This approach is particularly attractive to thrombolysis by paramedics. More information on the dosages and clinical usage of thrombolysis is available in Chapter 7.

Streptokinase

This drug was one of the first agents to be used and was shown to have beneficial effects in the ISIS II study (1982). It is derived from β-haemolytic streptococci and administered as an intravenous infusion because it is a protein. Streptokinase binds to plasminogen which undergoes a structural conformational change that allows it to dissolve the fibrin mesh. It is the least expensive of the thrombolytic agents.

The disadvantage of using streptokinase is that it depletes fibrinogen and is potentially allergenic to the patient; the patient can respond by producing antibodies to streptokinase which, on repeated administration, can be rendered ineffective. The indicators of an allergic reaction include rash, fever and flushing.

Current recommendations suggest avoiding reusage of streptokinase to prevent ineffective treatment and delayed benefit in the light of developing non-allergenic thrombolytic agents.

Recombinant tissue-type plasminogen activators

These drugs (alteplase, reteplase, tenecteplase) are the most recent additions to the series of thrombolytic drugs. Alteplase (tissue-type plasminogen activator or tPA) has in the recent past been used sparingly because of its cost. Many units have adopted the GUSTO I (1993) findings and used alteplase for patients with anterior MI and streptokinase for inferior MI. However, the introduction of a single-bolus thrombolytic with equal effects to that of alteplase (ASSENT 2 1999) has appealed to most clinicians.

In addition, these agents are hypoallergenic compared with streptokinase and consequently can be re administered with no immune response. All are administered intravenously, have a marked affinity for thrombi and are active in the dissolution of the clot. They are markedly more expensive than streptokinase.

Side effects

The potential for thrombolytic agents to potentiate serious bleeding is the major adverse effect. Bleeding may be from the site of administration, but it may occur in alternative sites including cerebral haemorrhage. A sudden drop in blood pressure shortly after commencing streptokinase is not uncommon.

Contraindications

For contraindications, see page 112.

Aspirin

Aspirin is regarded as a first-line antiplatelet agent. It is easily available and inexpensive. Several studies have shown a significant risk reduction of acute MI or death for patients who received aspirin at the time of their acute event (Theroux et al. 1993). Despite these studies being carried out in the very early stages of the thrombolytic era and at a time when interventional cardiology was less well established in the UK, a meta-analysis by the Antiplatelets Trialists' Collaboration in 1994, and updated in 2002, supported these findings. Unless specific contraindications exist, aspirin is recommended for all patients at high risk of having another vascular event (Antiplatelet Trialists' Collaboration 1994). Aspirin should also be regarded as a first-line treatment for secondary prevention in CHD.

Aspirin acts on the cyclo-oxygenase pathway of platelet activation and aggregation and blocks thromboxane production (Abrams 2000). In doing so it reduces the aggregating properties of the platelets (Sanghani and Filer 2000). Thromboxane contributes to the adhesiveness of platelets and activation of other platelets to enlarge the plug. Aspirin reduces the production of thromboxane by platelets, therefore making them 'less sticky'. The effect of aspirin on platelets is irreversible and lasts for the lifespan of the platelets affected (Hepinstall 2000). However, platelet aggregation can be stimulated by other means (Sanghani and Filer 2000), as illustrated in figure 5.1, and therefore it is regarded as a relatively weak platelet inhibitor especially when compared with glycoprotein GPIIb/IIIa inhibitors (Abrams 2000). Aspirin is well absorbed orally and generally well tolerated (Sanghani and Filer 2000). However, aspirin inhibits cyclo-oxygenase enzymes located not only on platelets but also in the gastric mucosa, which may result in peptic ulceration. Suggested dosages of aspirin are an initial dose of 300 mg followed by a maintenance daily dose of 75–100 mg (Antiplatelet Trialists' Collaboration 2002). Large doses of aspirin are associated with a number of side effects and toxic effects, including salicylate poisoning.

Side effects

Side effects include haemorrhage, gastrointestinal disturbance and broncho-spasm.

Clopidogrel

Clopidogrel belongs to the thienopyridine family of anti-platelet agents. These drugs irreversibly inhibit platelet aggregation induced by the release of ADP, thereby reducing ischaemic events (CAPRIE Steering Committee 1996). In the past clopidogrel was only used for post-MI patients who had a true aspirin allergy. The CURE study (Clopidogrel in Unstable Angina to prevent Recurrent Events Trial Investigators 2001) provided evidence over a 12-month period that the relative risk of MI, stroke or cardiovascular death was reduced by an additional 20% when patients with unstable angina/non-ST-elevation MI were given clopidogrel in addition to standard therapy, compared with those given standard therapy alone. However, the risk of bleeding is increased among patients who received clopidogrel. These findings have been immediately acted upon by the American College of Cardiology and the American Heart Association, which have recommended that clopidogrel should be prescribed in addition to aspirin when patients present with unstable angina or non-ST-elevation MI (cited in Braunwald et al. 2002). The European Society of Cardiologists is currently reviewing the situation.

Side effects

Side effects include gastrointestinal disturbance, bleeding disorders, nausea, vomiting, headache, dizziness, leukopenia and decreased platelets.

Heparin

Heparin is a mainstay of therapy for hospitalized patients with acute coronary syndromes (Abrams 2000). It acts indirectly as an anticoagulant by binding with anti-thrombin III and increasing its ability to destroy circulating thrombin; this results in the inactivation of a number of clotting factors including thrombin and factors IX, X, XI and XII. Heparin cannot be absorbed by the gastrointestinal tract because of its size and charge, so it is given only by injection, either subcutaneously or intravenously.

Although unfractionated heparin inhibits both thrombin and factor Xa with the same effectiveness, low-molecular-weight heparin (LMWH) has a greater effect on factor Xa, thereby inhibiting thrombin and clotting times to a lesser extent (Manhapra and Borzak 2000, Holdright 2001). Several studies of LMWH combined with aspirin have shown them to be as safe and efficient or superior as unfractionated heparin (FRISC-1 1996, Cohen et al. 1997). However, the benefits of prescribing LMWH are not exclusive to the therapeutic effects. LMWH possesses a longer half-life than unfractionated heparin, which allows for subcutaneous administration. The ease of subcutaneous administration, the fact that clotting time does not need to be monitored, and the fact that it would appear to have a comparable anticoagulant effect (Wallentin 2000) when compared with unfractionated heparin all ensure that, from a clinical perspective, LMWH is more favourable. The one disadvantage of LMWH is the purchasing cost when compared with unfractionated heparin, although when comparing these therapies it is vital to include the costs of additional expenditure, such as blood tests, increased nursing time, disposable equipment such as syringes, infusion lines, etc., which are required when administering unfractionated heparin. One such cost analysis was carried out in a small study by Fox and Bosanquet (1998), who found that a cost saving of £23 per patient could be achieved when reverting to LMWH. However, the study itself was quite small and definitive costings were regarded as unrealistic. Later, the principal findings were supported by O'Brien et al. (2000), who found that a decreased risk of subsequent clinical events also resulted in cost savings.

Side effects

Bleeding may result from excessive anticoagulation, so laboratory analysis of clotting studies are essential for unfractionated heparin. Weight estimation is also vital for LMWH to avoid over-anticoagulation.

As heparin is easily and quickly eliminated from the body, discontinuation of administration should be sufficient if bleeding should occur. However, the antidote to heparin is protamine sulphate, which could be given.

Glycoprotein IIb/IIIa inhibitors

Platelets generally circulate around the body as smooth inactive cells. When blood vessels are damaged glycoprotein receptors located on platelets are activated by von Willebrand's factor. Platelets are then activated and change their shape. This change of shape leads to the expression of the glycoprotein (GP)IIb/IIIa receptors on the surface of the platelets. These altered receptors can now bind to fibrinogen, which is an essential stage of their activation. This phase is followed by the activation of cyclo-oxygenase and thromboxane formation, mentioned earlier.

Aspirin, as stated previously, is a relatively weak anti-platelet agent because it blocks only one of the many signal pathways that lead to platelet aggregation. Similarly heparin, as an indirect inhibitor of thrombin, blocks only one of the many stimuli that promote platelet aggregation (Almony et al. 1996). Activation of the platelet GPIIb/IIIa receptor is the final common pathway leading to platelet aggregation (Boersma et al. 2002). Therefore inhibition of the receptor site has been seen as a major breakthrough. As a result of these potential benefits, there have been a number of trials that have investigated the use of the GPIIb/IIIa inhibitors in patients with unstable angina or non-ST-elevation MI (GUSTO-IV-ACS Investigators 2001).

Boersma et al. (2002) carried out a meta-analysis of all major randomized clinical trials of GPIIb/IIIa inhibitors used in acute coronary syndromes (ACSs). They found that GPIIb/IIIa inhibitors reduce the occurrence of death or MI in patients with ACS not routinely scheduled for early revascularization. They also found evidence that event reduction was greatest in patients at high risk of thrombotic complications. Troponin levels were recorded in only one of the six trials analysed, but in a subgroup analysis troponin-positive patients were found to benefit most from this type of treatment. The treatment effect also seemed larger in those with ST-segment depression than in those without, but the difference did not reach significance. These aforementioned studies and subsequent meta-analysis have ensured that GPIIb/IIIa inhibition is now regarded as a feasible therapeutic option.

Recent guidelines published by the British Cardiac Society (2000) and the National Institute for Clinical Excellence (NICE 2002) recommend that certain GPIIb/IIIa inhibitors should be prescribed for up to 96 h for high-risk patients with unstable angina or non-ST-elevation MI. Patients with recurrent and refractory unstable angina despite treatment should also be prescribed GPIIb/IIIa inhibitors (CAPTURE 1997) and heparin continued until they undergo coronary angiography and possible myocardial revascularization (British Cardiac Society et al. 2000, NICE 2002).

There are a number of different GPIIb/IIIa inhibitors. Two are currently licensed in the UK for intravenous use in medical treatment: tirofiban (Aggrastat) and eptifibatide (Integrilin). Abciximab (ReoPro) is licensed in the UK for intravenous use as an adjuvant to percutaneous coronary intervention (PCI) and stabilization of refractory unstable angina before PCI. Oral use of GPIIb/IIIa inhibitors is currently not licensed in the UK.

Glycoprotein IIb/IIIa inhibitors sites can be blocked by those drugs that inhibit the binding of fibrinogen and reduce the coagulation process.

Side effects

Again bleeding is a potential danger of administering these agents. Consequently they should not be given to patients who have undergone recent surgery or trauma, or those who have an existing clotting disorder.

Patients can also experience nausea and vomiting, fever, pain and allergic reactions.

Diamorphine

Arguably intravenous diamorphine is the most widely used drug in acute cardiac care. It is seen as the ideal analgesic for cardiac patients. Not only is it an opiate offering all the analgesic powers of opiate medication, but it also seems to provide an anxiolytic or calming effect. The drowsy state that patients often find themselves in after administration of an opiate can be seen as a positive effect when considering the harmful effects of acute anxiety and the associated physiological response of increased catecholamine production. Diamorphine is also able to produce a vasodilatory effect, thus reducing preload and myocardial O_2 demand.

The drug itself works centrally as an analgesic, but it can have an adverse effect on the respiratory and vomiting centre in the brain. Therefore, when giving intravenous diamorphine (2.5–5 mg) the health professional should observe for a reduction in the patient's respiratory rate and administer 400 µg naloxone, if required, to reverse the effects of the drug. However, the fear of these effects should not mean that patients with ischaemic pain do not receive adequate analgesia.

In addition an intravenous antiemetic should be administered prophylactically. In practice 10 mg of intravenous metoclopramide is often the drug of choice as a result of the limitations of other antiemetic drugs, e.g. stemetil can be given only orally or via the intramuscular route, and cyclizine causes the unwanted effect of vasoconstriction.

Side effects

Side effects include nausea and vomiting, constipation, drowsiness, respiratory depression and hypotension.

Anti-arrhythmia therapy

There are a number of ways of classifying drugs that produce an anti-arrhythmia effect. The more contemporary classifications are based on the area of the heart that is targeted rather than the pharmacology of the drug, and these drugs are listed in the box but are are described in more detail in the *British National Formulary*.

Drugs that affect supraventricular arrhythmia alone

Adenosine
Digoxin
Verapamil
β Blockers

Drugs that affect ventricular arrhythmia alone

Lidocaine (lignocaine)
Mexiletine
Phenytoin

Drugs that affect supraventricular and ventricular arrhythmia

Amiodarone
β Blockers
Disopyramide
Flecainide
Procainamide
Propafenone
Quinadine

The more traditional classification is the Vaughan Williams classification of anti-arrhythmics (1970), which is the classification chosen for this text. However, it is worth remembering that these drugs only suppress the arrhythmia and are not able to cure the problem. In fact, in some cases the drugs themselves are found to be the cause of additional arrhythmia. Alternative strategies should be considered when anti-arrhythmic therapy is prescribed. If the arrhythmia is induced by ischaemia, then revascularization may be an option, or in other cases referral to an electrophysiologist should be considered for radiofrequency ablation or an implantable defibrillator.

Vaughan Williams separated anti-arrhythmia drugs into categories based on their pharmacology. The classification was based on four different types of drugs, most of which are still in use today in some way, shape or form. It is inappropriate to discuss each individual drug available in an introductory text, so the mechanisms of drug actions are described in their historical groupings:

- Membrane-stabilizing agents, e.g. lidocaine, flecainide
- β Blockers, e.g. sotalol, esmolol
- Drugs increasing refractory period, e.g. amiodarone
- Calcium antagonists, e.g. verapamil.

Membrane-stabilizing agents

This category can be further subdivided into three groups: class 1a, 1b and 1c. However, the basic pharmacology behind the use of this group of drugs (remembering back to the action potential where Na^+ enters the cell rapidly and K^+ exits the cell) is that they interfere with the rapid Na^+ transfer by stabilization of the cell membrane and slow cardiac conduction.

β Blockers

This group of drugs, which has been discussed in more detail earlier in the chapter, inhibits arrhythmia by blocking the receptor site to which catecholamines such as adrenaline (epinephrine) link. The result is not only reduced heart rate but also reduced risk of all arrhythmias.

Drugs prolonging repolarization

During each heart beat there are times when each cell is susceptible to an additional stimulus and times when they are unable to be stimulated regardless of how strong the stimulus may be; this period of stability is called the refractory period. This group of drugs works by prolonging the refractory period and is therefore useful for all arrhythmias.

Calcium channel blockers

Calcium antagonists are discussed in more detail earlier in the chapter but their anti-arrhythmia effect is based on their ability to slow the inward transfer of Ca^{2+} into the cardiac cell, thus prolonging phases 2 and 3 of the action potential. This is particularly important within the AV node and therefore some Ca^{2+} channel blockers are very effective in treating supraventricular arrhythmia.

Inotropes

An inotrope is so called because it increases the contractility of the cardiac cell or force of contraction. The most commonly used inotrope in the UK is dobutamine because it is able to produce an inotropic effect while providing additional vasodilatation without producing a chronotropic effect (increased heart rate). This drug is given intravenously, ideally via a central line, to improve the blood pressure of patients in low-output states such as cardiogenic shock. It is a derivative of isoprenaline and works by stimulating β cells to contract more forcibly.

Side effects

The side effects are arrhythmia and tachycardia.

A number of additional drugs are frequently used to support the life of patients with cardiac conditions such as atropine, adrenaline (epinephrine), magnesium sulphate and lidocaine (lignocaine). A review of these drugs is undertaken in Chapter 6.

References

Abrams J (2000) Medical therapy of unstable angina and non-Q wave myocardial infarction. A Symposium: Acute coronary syndromes. Am J Cardiol 86: 28J–33J.

Almony GT, Lefkovits J, Topol EJ (1996) Anti-platelet and anti-coagulant use after myocardial infarction. Clin Cardiol 19: 357–65.

Antiplatelets Trialists' Collaboration (1994) Collaborative overview of randomised trials of antiplatelet therapy – I: Prevention of death, myocardial infarction, and stroke by prolonged antiplatelet therapy in various categories of patients. BMJ 308: 81–106.

Antiplatelets Trialists Collaboration (2002) Collaborative meta-analysis of randomised trials of antiplatelet therapy for prevention of death, myocardial infarction and stroke in high risk patients. BMJ 324: 71–86.

Ardissino D, Merlini PA, Ariens R, Coppola R, Branucci E, Manucci PM (1997) Tissue factor antigen and activity in human coronary atherosclerotic plaques. Lancet 349: 769–71.

ASSENT-2 Investigators (1999) Single bolus tenectaplase compared with front-loaded alteplase in acute myocardial infarction: the ASSENT-2 double blind randomised trial. Lancet 354: 716–22.

Boersma E, Maas ACP, Deckers JW, Simoons ML (1996) Early thrombolytic treatment in acute myocardial infarction: Reappraisal of the golden hour. Lancet 348: 771–4.

Boersma E, Harrington RA, Moliterno DJ et al. (2002) Platelet glycoprotein IIb/IIIa inhibitors in acute coronary syndromes: a meta-analysis of all major randomised clinical trials. Lancet 359: 9302.

Braunwald E, Antman EM, Beasley JW et al. (2002) Guideline update for the management of patients with unstable angina and non-ST segment elevation myocardial infarction. A report of the American College of Cardiology/American Heart Association Task Force on Practice Guidelines (Committee on the management of patients with unstable angina). J Am Coll Cardiol 40: 1366–74.

British Cardiac Society Guidelines and Medical Practice Committee and Royal College of Physicians Clinical Effectiveness and Evaluation Unit (2000) Guideline for the management of patients with acute coronary syndromes without persistent ECG ST segment elevation. Heart 85: 133–42.

CAPRIE Steering Committee (1996) A randomised, blinded, trial of clopidogrel versus aspirin in patients at risk of ischaemic events (CAPRIE). Lancet 348: 1329–39.

CAPTURE (1997) Randomised placebo-controlled trial of abciximab before and during coronary intervention in refractory unstable angina: the CAPTURE study. Lancet 349: 1429–35.

Caramori PA, Adelman AG, Azevodo ER, Newton GE, Parker AB, Parker JD (1998) Therapy with niroglycerin increases coronary vasoconstriction in response to acetylcholine. J Am Coll Cardiol 32: 1969–84.

Clopidogrel in Unstable Angina to prevent Recurrent Events (CURE) Trial Investigators (2001) Effects of clopidogrel in addition to aspirin in patients with acute coronary syndrome without ST-segment elevation. N Engl J Med 345: 494–502.

Cohen M, Demmers C, Gurfinkel EP et al. for the ESSENCE Study Group (1997) A comparison of low molecular weight heparin with unfractionated heparin for unstable coronary artery disease. N Engl J Med 337: 447–52.

Cohn JN, Johnson G, Ziesche S et al. (1991) A comparison of enalapril with hydralazinc-isosorbide dinitrate in the treatment of chronic congestive heart failure. N Engl J Med 325: 303–10.

CONSENSUS Trial Study Group (1987) Effects of enalapril on mortality in severe congestive cardiac failure: results of the Cooperative North Scandinavian Enalapril Survival Study (CONSENSUS). N Engl J Med 316: 1429–35.

Danish Study Group on Verapamil in Myocardial Infarction (DAVIT II) (1990) Danish Verapamil infarction Trial II. Am J Cardiol 66: 779–85.

Department of Health (2000) The National Service Framework for Coronary Heart Disease. London: HMSO.

Digitalis Intervention Group (1997) The effect of digoxin on mortality and morbidity in patients with heart failure. N Engl J Med 336: 525–33.

Exner DV, Schron EB (2001) Impact of pharmacologic therapy on health related quality of life in heart failure: findings from clinical trials. In: Moser D, Riegel B (eds), Improving Outcomes in Heart Failure: An interdisciplinary approach. Aspen, MA: Jones & Bartlett.

Fibrinolytic Therapy Trialists' (FTT) Collaborative Group (1994) Indications for thrombolytic therapy in suspected acute myocardial infarction. Collaborative overview of early mortality and major morbidity results from all randomised trials of more than 1000 patients. Lancet 343: 311–22.

Fox KAA, Bosanquet N (1998) Assessing the UK cost implications of the use of low molecular weight heparin in unstable coronary artery disease. Br J Cardiol 5: 92–104.

Freemantle N, Cleland J, Young P, Mason J, Harrison J (1999) Beta blockade after myocardial infarction: Systematic review and meta regression analysis. BMJ 318: 1730–7.

FRISC Study Group (1996) Fragmin during instability in coronary artery disease. Lancet 347: 561–8.

GUSTO Angiographic Investigators (1993) The effects of tissue plasminogen activator, streptokinase or both on coronary artery patency, ventricular function and survival after acute myocardial infarction. N Engl J Med 329: 1615–22.

GUSTO-IV-ACS Investigators (2001) Effect of glycoprotein IIb/IIIa receptor blocker abciximab on outcome in patients with acute coronary syndrome without early coronary revascularization: the GUSTO IV-ACS randomized trial. Lancet 357: 1915–24.

Hall AS, Murray GD, Ball SG (1997) Follow up of patients randomly allocated ramipril or placebo for heart failure after myocardial infarction. Acute infarction Ramipril Efficacy eXtension study. Lancet 349: 1493–7.

Hepinstall S (2000) The importance of platelet aggregation in coronary heart disease. Br J Cardiol 7: 27–30.

Holdright DR (2001) Dalteparin sodium (Fragmin) in the management of acute coronary syndromes. Br J Cardiol 8: 147–60.

International Study of Infarct Survival II (ISIS 2) Collaborative Group (1982) Randomised controlled trial of streptokinase, oral aspirin, both, or neither among 17187 cases of suspected acute myocardial infarction. Lancet ii: 349–60.

International Study of Infarct Survival IV Collaborative Group (1995) Fourth international study of infarct survival. Lancet 345: 669–85.

Køber L, Torp-Pederson C, Carlson JR et al. (1995) A clinical trial of the angiotensin converting enzyme inhibitor trandolapril in patients with left ventricular dysfunction after MI. N Engl J Med 33: 1670–6.

LIPID Study Group (1998) Prevention of cardiovascular events and death with pravastatin in patients with coronary heart disease and a broad range of initial cholesterol levels. The Long-term Intervention with Pravastatin in Ischaemic Disease (LIPID) Study Group. N Engl J Med 339: 1349–57.

Manhapra A, Borzak S (2000) Treatment possibilities for unstable angina. BMJ 321: 1269–75.

National Institute for Clinical Excellence (2002) Guidance on the use of glycoprotein IIb/IIIa inhibitors in the treatment of acute coronary syndromes: NICE Technology Appraisal Guidance No. 12. London: NICE.

National Institute for Clinical Evidence (2003) Management of chronic heart failure in primary and secondary care (www.nice.org.uk).

O'Brien BJ, Willan A, Blackhouse G, Goeree R, Cohen C, Goodman S (2000) Will the use of low molecular weight heparin in patients with acute coronary syndromes save costs in Canada? Am Heart J 139: 423–9.

Patel J, Purcell HJ, Fox KM, on behalf of the Clinical European Studies in Angina and Revascularisation (CESAR) Study Group (1999) Cardioprotection by opening of the KATP channel in unstable angina. Is this a clinical manifestation of myocardial preconditioning? Results of a randomised study with nicorandil. Eur Heart J 20: 51–7.

Sacks FM, Pfeffer MA, Moye LA et al. (1996) The CARE study. Efficacy of pravastatin on coronary events after myocardial infarction in patients with average cholesterol levels. Five year follow up of patients with starting cholesterol < 6.2mmol/l treated with pravastatin. N Engl J Med 335: 1001–9.

Sanghani P, Filer L (2000) The Pharmacological Management of the Cardiac Patient in Cardiac Nursing: A comprehensive guide. London: Churchill Livingstone.

Scandinavian Simvastatin Survival Study Group (1994) Randomised trial of cholesterol lowering in 4444 patients with coronary heart disease: the Scandinavian Simvastatin Survival Study (4S). Lancet 344: 1383–9.

Schwartz GG, Olsson AG, Ezekowitz MD et al. (2001) Effects of atorvastatin on early recurrent ischaemic events in acute coronary syndrome: The Myocardial Ischaemia Reduction with Aggressive Cholesterol Lowering (MIRACL) study. JAMA 285: 1711–18.

SPRINT Study Group (1988) Secondary Prevention Re-Infarction Israeli Nifedipine Trial. Eur Heart J 9: 354–64.

Theroux P, Waters D, Qui S et al. (1993) Aspirin versus heparin to prevent myocardial infarction during the acute phase of unstable angina. Circulation 88: 2045–8.

Vaughan Williams EM (1970) Classification of anti arrhythmic drugs. In: Sandhoe E, Flensted Jensen E, Losen KH (eds), Symposium on Cardiac Arrhythmias. Sodertalje, Sweden: AB Astra, p. 49.

Verheught FWA (1999) Acute coronary syndromes: drug treatments. Lancet 353(suppl II): 2023.

Wallentin L (2000) Efficacy of low molecular weight heparin in acute coronary syndromes. Am Heart J 139: S29–32.

Waters DD, Hsue PY (2001) What is the role of intensive cholesterol lowering in the treatment of acute coronary syndromes? Am J Cardiol 88: 7J–16J.

Weitz JI (1995) Activation of blood coagulation by plaque rupture: mechanisms and prevention. Am J Cardiol 75: 23–5.

Yusef S, Witte J, Friedman L (1988) An overview of results of randomised trials in heart disease: unstable angina, heart failure, primary prevention with aspirin and risk factor modifications. JAMA 260: 2259–63.

CHAPTER SIX
Resuscitation

DENIS PARKINSON

The aim of this chapter is to introduce the concepts surrounding resuscitation with a focus on simplicity and ease of use. It is not intended to be an all-embracing text and there is an expectation that the reader would use it as a starting point on the path to gaining knowledge and experience in this area.

Any nurse involved with the care of the cardiac patient needs to be familiar with all aspects of resuscitation because of the nature of their work. This includes technical skills, ethical issues and post-resuscitation care, to name but a few examples. This text aims to present these issues in a logical and, above all, accessible way. Cardiac patients are at risk of cardiac arrest and their nurses should be in a position to deal with this complication should it arise.

Simply put, a cardiac arrest can be defined as the failure of the heart to pump sufficient blood to maintain cerebral perfusion. Circulatory arrest indicates complete, or virtually complete, cessation of blood flow to vital organs. This occurs immediately following cardiac arrest or if cardiac massage is interrupted during cardiopulmonary resuscitation (Gilston 1987).

Cardiopulmonary arrest may occur because of a primary airway, breathing or circulatory problem or a secondary problem relating to a disease process. The cardiovascular and respiratory systems often interact, e.g. severe illness may increase O_2 consumption.

The most common cause of cardiac arrest is myocardial infarction (MI) (Thompson and Webster 1992), which is usually the result of a fissuring or ruptured atheromatous plaque causing thrombosis within a coronary artery. MI can occur without any previous symptoms. Over 50% of patients who die after acute coronary occlusion will do so within the first hour (Myerburg et al. 1993). This is commonly the result of cardiac rhythm problems, more specifically ventricular fibrillation (VF). The risk of VF after MI is highest at the onset of symptoms and reduces as time passes.

There are two other rhythms associated with cardiac arrest: asystole and pulseless electrical activity (PEA). Both are associated with cessation of circulation. When the heart fails to maintain the cerebral circulation for about 4 min, the brain can become irreversibly damaged (Thompson and Webster 1992).

Brain death usually occurs because of failure of oxygenation of brain cells. This will result from a failure in ventilation or a compromise of the heart's ability to pump blood to the brain tissues. The brain has no secondary stores of oxygen that can be used, hence the short time to damage occurring.

Rapid diagnosis and treatment of cardiac arrest are essential. As has been mentioned already there is a high mortality after cardiopulmonary arrest so, if patients can be identified before the arrest, and the arrest prevented, more lives can be saved. In hospitals, almost 80% of patients who suffer cardiac arrest will have had some deterioration in clinical signs in the hours preceding the event (Schein et al. 1990). The most common symptoms are breathing problems, an increase in heart rate and a fall in cardiac output. Therefore there is a vital role for nurses to play in detecting these signs earlier in a patient's journey. Nurses should be aware and constantly observing their patients for signs of hypotension, confusion, restlessness, lethargy or a deteriorating level of consciousness. All can be predictors of impending cardiopulmonary arrest.

Breathing problems can be indicated by shortness of breath, an increase in respiratory rate and a fall in O_2 saturation. A fall in cardiac output could be indicated if a patient becomes cold, clammy or cyanosed. Their pulse could weaken and their urine output may fall to less than 30 ml/h.

The management of cardiac arrest by the nurse requires rapid decision-making and actions based on several of these key points. The chance of restoring adequate heart rhythm and successfully resuscitating the patient rapidly reduces over time. Where nursing staff have access to resuscitation equipment and can defibrillate on their own initiative, e.g. on coronary care units (CCUs), the successful resuscitation rate can approach 75% (Mackintosh et al. 1979). Also external cardiac massage, as performed in resuscitation, produces only a limited cardiac output. All of these circumstances point to the need for prompt action.

Recognition of impending and actual cardiac arrest is an essential skill for a nurse to develop and can be dealt with in a systematic way, linking to airway, breathing and circulation in turn.

Airway assessment is vital. A conscious patient will complain of difficulty in breathing or could be choking. It may also be noisy. With silent breathing complete airway obstruction may be present. A nurse should approach this situation using the techniques described in the Resuscitation Council's basic life support (BLS) algorithm (Resuscitation Council UK 2005). Access to advanced life support techniques should also be available.

In summary, then, cardiorespiratory arrest can follow airway obstruction, breathing inadequacy or cardiac dysfunction. Hospitalized patients who have a cardiorespiratory arrest usually display warning signs and symptoms in the hours preceding the arrest. The nurse has a role in identifying early signs of deterioration and this can lead to the prevention of the arrest. Nursing responsibilities can include being able to recognize a cardiorespiratory arrest accurately, i.e. an abrupt loss of consciousness, absent major pulses and absent respirations. A nurse should be able to commence resuscitation and summon help appropriately. There is a responsibility to maintain patient dignity throughout the procedure and beyond, and there may be an opportunity to support colleagues who are less experienced and, as expertise grows, to act as role model. The patient's family will also require a high level of support. Nurses must remain up to date with current practice and have an understanding of ethical issues that may arise.

The following sections of this chapter describe some of the techniques with which nurses should familiarize themselves. The guiding protocol for advanced resuscitation is used to provide a context for use. This is followed by an introduction to post-arrest care and some ethical issues.

Basic life support

Resuscitation Council UK guidelines

There are specific guidelines for the application of BLS techniques and nurses should be competent in using them (Resuscitation Council UK 2005). Even though this text is aimed at nurses working within a cardiac environment, it must be stressed that despite being in a clinical setting safety of the area must still be checked. Under no circumstances should resuscitation present an unnecessary risk to the team.

The aim of BLS is to maintain an adequate circulation and ventilation until action can be taken to correct the underlying cause of the arrest. Irreversible brain damage often occurs after about 4 min. It is clear then that any delay in starting BLS could have a profound effect on the outcome for the patient. Patients who have VF have a much greater chance of survival but this is linked to access to defibrillation, which is addressed later in the chapter.

There are some elements within the BLS protocol that can be adapted within a health-care setting to be more efficient in terms of both time and use of expertise. However, it may be helpful to review the layperson's protocol and then address these issues at the end. After all, it is conceivable that these techniques may be used by any health-care professional in a public setting, where there may be limited access to help or equipment.

There are three aims of resuscitation: first, protection of the brain by restoring its flow of oxygenated blood with cardiac massage and artificial ventilation; second, restoration of an adequate spontaneous cardiac output; and, third, correct post-arrest care.

The definitive sign of cardiac arrest is the absence of the carotid or other large artery pulse. Although this is not taught in laypeople's BLS it is essential for health-care staff.

Restoration of an oxygenated blood supply to the brain involves external cardiac massage and artificial ventilation. However, in some cases this achieves less than 5% of normal flow. Faced with a possible cardiac arrest the following sequence should be followed:

- The safety of rescuer and patient should be ensured and the patient should be checked for a response using a gentle shake of the shoulders and a question: 'Are you alright?'
- If there is a response or movement leave the patient in the position in which he or she was found unless it is unsafe to do so.
- Check the patient's condition and summon help if needed.
- Reassess regularly.

Airway

Patients should be placed on their backs and the airway opened by placing your hand on the forehead and tilting their head back gently. Any visible obstruction should be removed from the patient's mouth. Dentures should be removed if loose and left in place if well fitting. Using your fingertips under the point of the patient's chin, lift the chin which will have the effect of opening the airway.

Breathing and Circulation

A diagnosis of cardiac arrest can be made if a victim is unresponsive and not breathing normally (Resuscitation Council UK 2005).

Keeping the airway open, look, listen and feel for breathing. Look for chest movements. Listen at the patient's mouth for breath sounds. Feel for air on your cheek. This should be done for no more than 10 seconds in total.

If the patient is breathing normally he or she should be placed in the recovery position. His or her continued breathing should be checked and help should be summoned. If the patient is not breathing or the breathing is inadequate, help should be requested. It may be necessary to leave the patient to summon help.

If the patient is not breathing chest compressions should be started. Chest compressions or external cardiac massage can provide only a limited cardiac output. Cerebral blood flow is only 3–15% of normal and cardiac output about 20–25% of normal. It is therefore important that the technique used should be as efficient as possible (Redmond 1986).

Place the heel of one hand in the centre of the victim's chest and place the heel of your other hand on top of the first hand. Interlock the fingers of your hands and ensure that pressure is not applied over the ribs. Do not apply any pressure over the upper abdomen or the bottom end of the bony sternum. Position yourself vertically above the patient's chest and, with your arms straight, press down the sternum 4-5 cm.

After each compression pressure on the chest should be released without removing the hands from the sternum. The rate should be about 100 compressions per minute.

After 30 compressions rescue breaths should be given. The airway should be opened using the head-tilt and chin-lift manoeuvre. To carry out this procedure pinch the soft part of the patient's nose closed with your index finger and thumb. Maintain chin lift with the other hand and open the mouth slightly. Take a normal breath and place your lips around the patient's mouth, ensuring a good seal (in hospital this will rarely be

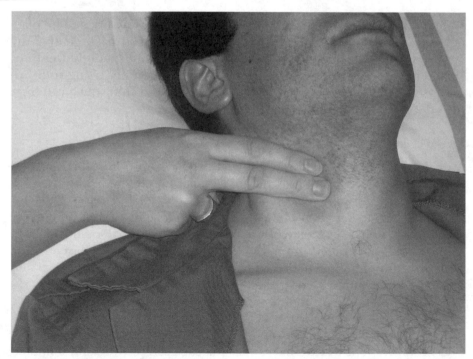

Figure 6.1 Carotid pulse being checked.

necessary because of pocket masks which allow "no contact" rescue breathing to take place).

Watch the chest and blow steadily into the mouth for about 1 s to make the chest rise as in normal breathing. Keeping the airway open, remove your mouth and watch for the chest to fall as the air is expelled. Repeat this sequence to deliver a second breath. Do not attempt more than 2 breaths each time before returning to chest compressions. Continue with chest compressions and rescue breaths at a ratio of 30:2. Resuscitation should continue until qualified help arrives and takes over, the patient starts breathing normally or you become exhausted.

Immediate life support

As hospital settings allow access to equipment and expert personnel there are some modifications that can be applied. In a clinical area, if health-care professionals see a patient apparently collapsed they should shout for help first and then assess for a response with 'shake and shout'. As more staff may be available some of the techniques can be performed simultaneously. It is possible to check for a pulse at the same time as checking breathing and if one or both are absent then the cardiac arrest team should be called. If a patient has a pulse and is breathing then further assessment is warranted. O_2, ECG monitoring and venous access should be instigated. It is essential that access to a defibrillator is not delayed.

A Guedel airway should be inserted and O_2 administered as soon as possible (Figures 6.2 and 6.3). Bag–valve–mask equipment (Figure 6.4) can be used if the professional is competent with such equipment. The ultimate in airway management is the use of an endotracheal tube (Figure 6.5). The passage of this tube into the bronchus is termed 'intubation' and should be carried out only by a skilled practitioner because of the risk of laryngeal damage. Once the airway is secured with a cuffed tracheal tube, compressions should not be interrupted for ventilation. Breaths can be delivered asynchronously at a rate of 12/min.

It is essential that, as soon as there is access to a defibrillator, monitoring leads should be applied to assess the cardiac rhythm and allow rapid defibrillation if indicated. Appropriate drugs should be made available to the cardiac arrest team.

Defibrillation

A nurse working with cardiac patients is in a prime position to contribute to an increased survival rate. One of the key factors contributing to reduced mortality in cardiac care is quick and easy access to safe and appropriate defibrillation. A nurse should know what is meant by defibrillation, when it is indicated and how to deliver a shock safely. Many

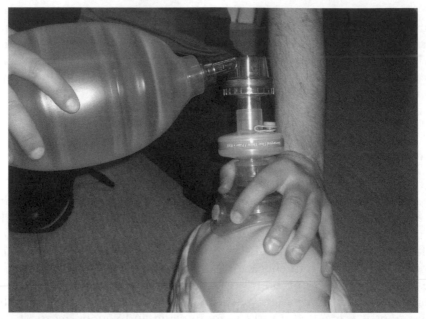

Figure 6.2 Manikin being ventilated.

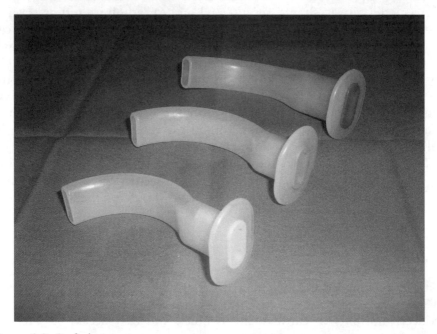

Figure 6.3 Oral airways.

clinical areas will have their own programmes of staff development, which should be aimed at achieving competence in this technique.

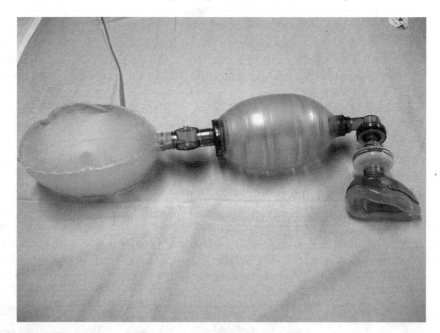

Figure 6.4 Bag and mask.

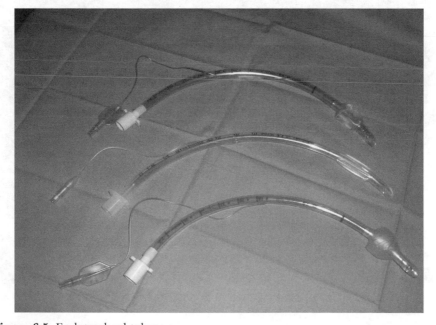

Figure 6.5 Endotracheal tubes.

The main indications for defibrillation are VF and pulseless ventricular tachycardia (VT). If a patient develops either of these conditions, cardiac output stops and cerebral damage can occur within 3 min. The need for rapid defibrillation is apparent. BLS is appropriate as a holding measure if there is a delay in obtaining equipment, but early defibrillation is vital to maximize the potential to restore a life-sustaining rhythm. Success is greater when the delay between the arrest and defibrillation is shorter.

To achieve the change from VF/VT to a normal rhythm, an electrical current is delivered to the myocardium externally in order to depolarize the cardiac muscle. This allows the normal pacemaker within the heart to take over control again. The shock is delivered through electrodes placed on the patient's chest (Figure 6.6).

The ideal electrode position is one that allows maximum current flow through the myocardium. The most common approach is where one electrode is placed to the right of the upper sternum below the clavicle and the second is placed level with the fifth left intercostal space in the anterior axillary line (leads V5–V6 on the ECG). The electrodes are marked positive and negative but in actual fact they can be used in either position.

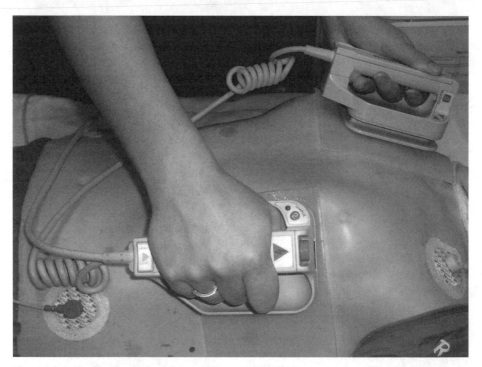

Figure 6.6 Defibrillator paddles on chest of manikin.

If defibrillation is unsuccessful in this position, an alternative position that could be adopted would be to apply one electrode to the left of the lower sternal border and the second just inferior to the left scapula. This is known as the anterior/posterior position. To achieve this position the patient must be rolled to the right, which can interfere with chest compressions so it is not the position of first choice.

Safety to the cardiac arrest team and the patient is vital. Electricity is dangerous and there are several basic safety principles of which a nurse must be aware. Wet surroundings or clothes can be dangerous. Therefore, it may be necessary to dry the patient's chest. A form of electrocution can occur if any member of the team is in physical contact with the patient during defibrillation.

The electrodes should never come into contact with each other. The person delivering the shock must shout 'stand clear' and visually check the area surrounding the patient to ensure that no one is touching the patient, bed or equipment. Any high-flow O_2 should also be removed to prevent arcing of the current, which could be an explosive combination with a major risk of fire.

Some clinical areas dealing with cardiac patients will use a manual defibrillator that needs the electrodes to be manually charged by the operator as opposed to an automated machine. This should be done only on the patient's chest and not in the air. The electrodes should not be held by the operator in the same hand. As a result of the need for rapid sequential shocks, the paddles can be held on the chest between shocks and if necessary the current setting can be altered by another member of the team. The electrodes should not be placed over medicinal patches such as transdermal glyceryl trinitrate (GTN), ECG electrodes or monitoring wires.

When using a manual machine the operator determines the need for a shock and so detailed knowledge of cardiac rhythms is essential for its appropriate use. The energy of the shock is set manually, the operator charges the defibrillator and the shock is manually administered. There is a universal advanced life support algorithm that indicates when defibrillation is appropriate (Figure 6.7).

In addition to life-saving defibrillation these machines can also be used to deliver synchronized shocks or cardioversion in the treatment of other cardiac rhythms such as atrial fibrillation or VT when a pulse is present. In these instances the shock must be synchronized to occur on the R wave rather than the T wave of the ECG. This reduces the risk of the operator inducing VF. Such machines usually have a switch allowing this synchronization to be performed but a visual confirmation by the operator is essential. Also when the shock is delivered, to facilitate the correct delivery time, there may be a slight delay from discharge to delivery. The electrodes must be kept

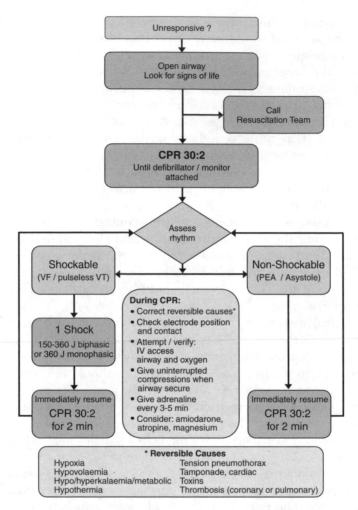

Figure 6.7 Universal advanced life support (ALS) algorithm. BLS, basic life support; CPR, cardiopulmonary resuscitation; VF, ventricular fibrillation; VT, ventricular tachycardia. The algorithm for advance life support guidelines (2005) is published with kind permission of the Resuscitation Council UK.

firmly in place at this stage. It is essential that any member of staff be familiar with the operation of any equipment within the clinical area. The time to determine correct operation is not during an emergency procedure. Ideally, cardioversion should be carried out only in a specialist clinical area.

It is not uncommon for patients with a cardiac history to have an implanted cardiac pacemaker and there are some safety issues associated with this eventuality. The current may travel along the pacemaker wire, causing burns at the point of contact with the myocardium. The electrodes should therefore be placed at least 12–15 cm from the pacemaker to minimize this risk. If the resuscitation is successful, the pacemaker threshold should be checked regularly for several months to ensure no long-term damage.

Drugs

The management of cardiac patients has a large pharmacological basis and the same is true of the management of patient's undergoing cardiac arrest. It is not possible to examine every drug that may be used in this situation, but there is a need to have some knowledge of the common drugs that a nurse may encounter when dealing with a cardiac arrest. An awareness of special precautions and contraindications is also essential.

There are only a few drugs that are used in the immediate stages of a cardiac arrest and the evidence for their use is fairly limited.

Oxygen

If available, high-concentration O_2 should be given to all patients undergoing cardiac arrest. After the restoration of a spontaneous circulation, a sufficient quantity of O_2 should be administered to maintain O_2 saturation > 95%.

Adrenaline (epinephrine)

This is the first drug used in cardiac arrest of any cause. It is indicated after each 3-5 min of resuscitation. An initial 1 mg intravenous dose should be administered. If intravenous access is delayed or not possible 2-3 mg diluted into a volume of 10 ml sterile water may be given via the tracheal tube. Higher doses are not indicated for patients with refractory cardiac arrest.

The dose of adrenaline used in cardiac arrest produces vasoconstriction. This warranted effect increases systemic vascular resistance during cardiopulmonary resuscitation (CPR), resulting in an increase in cerebral and coronary perfusion. However, if the heart is beating the drug stimulates an increase in heart rate and the force of contraction. This is potentially harmful because myocardial O_2 demand is increased, which can worsen ischaemia. In addition another potential problem is that adrenaline causes the myocardium to become more excitable, which in turn can lead to the stimulation of unwanted cardiac rhythms. Potentially the drug could lead to a recurrence of VF (Raehl 1987, Resuscitation Council UK 2000, Jowett and Thompson 2003).

Atropine

This drug is indicated in cardiac arrests caused by asystole or PEA with a rate < 60 min. The recommended dose in this situation is 3 mg i.v. in a single dose. Atropine is also used in the treatment of bradycardias and different doses apply in these situations.

Atropine blocks the effect of the vagus nerve on both the sinoatrial (SA) node and the atrioventricular (AV) node. This effect increases sinus automaticity and improves AV node conduction. As the dose increases side effects become apparent, which could be blurred vision, dry mouth or urinary retention. However, these effects are irrelevant within the context of a cardiac arrest. Pupils can dilate and after resuscitation can contribute to acute confusion.

Interestingly there is little evidence for the use of atropine in asystolic cardiac arrest and the evidence that does exist is mainly anecdotal. The general feeling seems to be that the prognosis for a patient in asystolic arrest would not be made worse by use of the drug.

Amiodarone

This drug is indicated for refractory VF/pulseless VT. A further 150 mg can be given for refractory VF/VT followed by 900mg over 24 hours. An initial dose of 300 mg amiodarone diluted in 5% dextrose to a volume of 20 ml should be considered if there is no response to the first three defibrillatory shocks. The drug can be administered peripherally in an emergency, but ideally should be given via a central line. This is because of the caustic nature of the drug. Amiodarone is also the drug of choice for many arrhythmias outside the arrest situation. Doses will vary in these circumstances according to local protocols.

Amiodarone increases the duration of the action potential in atrial and ventricular myocardium. This prolongs the Q–T interval. Similar to many anti-arrhythmic drugs amiodarone has pro-arrhythmic effects but compared with other drugs the incidence is not as great. Major side effects that can present with the use of amiodarone are hypotension and bradycardia. Although associated with many side effects when taken orally long term, these are irrelevant in an emergency setting.

Note that amiodarone crystallizes if mixed with saline.
Although not forming the main stay of pharmacological treatment in cardiac arrest, the following drugs may be considered in certain situations and so an awareness of their use is indicated:

- Magnesium sulphate can be used for refractory VF if there are low levels of magnesium, and also for tachyarrhythmia in similar circumstances. Magnesium may also be warranted in a particular type of VT called torsades de pointes. Particular attention should be paid to patients who have endured a recent large diuresis induced by diuretics.

This type of fluid loss will often create hypomagnesaemia with subsequent arrhythmias.

- Lidocaine (lignocaine) can be used for refractory VF/pulseless VT in the absence of amiodarone.
- Sodium bicarbonate can be indicated in severe metabolic acidosis or hyperkalaemia. Its use can be problematic and nurses are referred to local protocols.

Finally in this section calcium chloride can be used in PEA caused by hyperkalaemia, hypocalcaemia or an overdose of Ca^{2+} channel-blocking drugs.

There are also many drugs used in the peri-arrest period with which the nurse should be familiar. As a result of limitations of space it is not possible to examine this area in detail but reference to local and national protocols is advised (Resuscitation Council UK 2005).

Advanced life support protocol

The aim of this section is to equip nurses with a logical procedure for the management of cardiac arrest – essentially the synthesis of the various techniques described so far into the UK resuscitation algorithm for the treatment of cardiac arrest.

Heart rhythms associated with cardiac arrest can be split into two groups (Figures 6.8–6.11): VF/pulseless VT and other rhythms, which include asystole and PEA (non-VF/VT). The essential difference in treatment is the need for defibrillation in the VF/VT group. Many other aspects of treatment are the same for all situations.

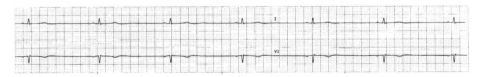

Figure 6.8 An example of pulseless electrical activity.

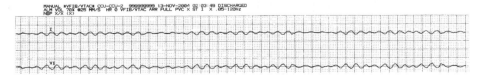

Figure 6.9 Ventricular fibrillation.

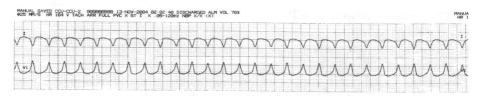

Figure 6.10 Ventricular tachycardia.

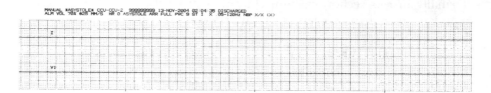

Figure 6.11 Asystole.

Most patients who survive cardiac arrest have been treated for VF/VT so it is essential that the cardiac rhythm is assessed as soon as possible. BLS should be started if there is any delay in obtaining a defibrillator, but this must not hold up the delivery of appropriate shocks.

If an arrest is witnessed or monitored and a defibrillator is not immediately available, a precordial thump should be administered within 30 s. A sharp blow with the closed fist on the patient's sternum may convert VF into a sustaining rhythm. Once the arrest is confirmed and the patient is attached to a defib monitor the rhythm is assessed.

VF/ VT should be treated with a single shock followed with an immediate resumption of compressions and ventilations at a ratio of 30:2. Do not check for a pulse or reassess rhythm. After 2 min check the rhythm and give another shock if indicated. The energy levels to be used are 360J for monophasic defibrillators and 150-360J for biphasic defibrillators. This process should continue if there is no change in the patient's condition. If in doubt as to whether the rhythm is fine VF or asystole do not defibrillate but continue chest compression and ventilation.

If VF/VT persists after a second shock give adrenaline 1mg IV and repeat every 3-5 min if VF/VT persists. If VF/VT persists after 3 shocks give amioderone 300mg by bolus injection.

In non VF/VT defibrillation is not indicated. If asystole is suspected, confirmation should be obtained by checking gain and lead connections to the machine. Increasing the gain increases the size of the rhythm display, allowing the display to be read in more detail.

With a confirmed non VF/VT arrest compressions and ventilations should be performed at the ratio of 30:2. The rhythm should be rechecked after 2 min. If there is no change in the ECG continue. If organised electrical activity is seen check a pulse. If no pulse is present continue. Adrenaline 1 mg should be given IV as soon as access is achieved and then readministered every 3-5 min. In the case of asystole a one off dose of atropine 3 mg is indicated. The individual providing chest compressions should change every 2 min to prevent inefficiency due to tiredness.

During both of these cycles the time in which CPR is administered should be used to carry out other essential care as well. This includes checking electrodes, their position and contact. The airway should be secured and the patient intubated if possible, but this should be performed only by a suitably qualified professional. Once the patient is intubated CPR should consist of compressions at 100/min and respirations at 12/min asynchronously. Oxygen should be administered at a high flow rate and IV access should be secured if not present already. The need for amioderone, atropine/cardiac pacing, sodium bicarbonate and calcium chloride should be considered if appropriate.

The survival of those patients with refractory VF/VT or non VF/VT depends on prompt identification and treatment of a reversible cause and therefore the common causes of cardiac arrest should be considered for each patient and the appropriate intervention performed. There are eight major causes split into two groups of four for ease of recall: the 4 "Hs" and the 4 "Ts".

Hypoxia

Oxygen 100% should be administered and ventilation should be adequate. The chest should be seen to rise and fall and breath sounds should be audible on both sides of the chest.

Hypovolaemia

Pulseless electrical activity can be caused by severe bleeding. Causes may include trauma, gastrointestinal bleeding or a ruptured aortic aneurysm. Appropriate fluids should be administered.

Hyperkalaemia and other metabolic disorders

This could be evident from blood results or the patient's history (e.g. renal failure), and an ECG may provide further information.

Hypothermia

This can affect responses to treatment and a patient can become hypothermic during a prolonged period of resuscitation.

Tension pneumothorax

This can follow central line or pacemaker insertion. Diagnosis must be rapid and decompression performed by needle thoracocentesis followed by chest drain insertion.

Cardiac tamponade

This is difficult to diagnose during a cardiac arrest because symptoms are hidden by the arrest, i.e. hypotension and distended neck veins. The patient's clinical history may suggest this.

Therapeutic or toxic substances

These could be involved, whether or not deliberate. An overdose of calcium channel blockers or tricyclic antidepressants may lead to cardiac arrest.

Thromboembolic or mechanical obstruction

This would include massive pulmonary embolus, and this could potentially be treated with thrombolysis. In cardiac patients myocardial rupture after myocardial infarction is a potential problem.

A nurse should be aware of the sequence of events within the life support protocol and, although not expected to perform beyond the role, an awareness of treatments and potential problems is essential, particularly in the care of cardiac patients.

Post-resuscitation care

Care of the patient is ongoing after a successful resuscitation from a cardiac arrest. It is rare for a patient to recover immediately and there are several areas that will need addressing. It is vital to check level of consciousness with attention to cardiac, renal and cerebral functions. If the patient has had a cardiac arrest on a general ward, transfer to a specialist cardiac unit should be considered.

Care after arrest should be tailored to a patient's individual needs. Some patients may recover immediately with no significant after-effects, some may be unconscious for an extended period of time and some may never regain consciousness.

Any underlying causes of the arrest need to be addressed, as do any problems caused by the arrest itself, e.g. aspiration of stomach contents. Urea and electrolytes need to be adjusted if necessary as does acid–base balance. The level of treatment necessary will vary.

A systematic approach to patient assessment is vital.

Cardiac

From a cardiac perspective, heart rhythm and rate should be closely monitored and a 12-lead ECG is a mandatory investigation. Anti-arrhythmic drugs may be required, e.g. a 24-h infusion of amiodarone. Possibly thrombolysis for a myocardial infarction may be warranted; blood pressure monitoring will be necessary and possibly haemodynamic monitoring. There may be a need for inotropic drugs such as dobutamine to support the blood pressure.

Respiratory

The respiratory system requires O_2 therapy to continue post-arrest and arterial blood gases should be taken. Control of blood levels of CO_2 can decrease cerebral oedema.

Renal

The renal system may also need support after an arrest. This could involve a low-dose infusion of dopamine to stimulate renal function by stimulating renal perfusion (British Medical Society and Royal Pharmaceutical Society of Great Britain 2004) and commonly some strong diuretic such as furosemide (frusemide). Urinary catheterization may be necessary to facilitate accurate hourly urine measurement.

Neurological

Hypoxia during the arrest can lead directly to cerebral damage. Reduction of cerebral oedema and avoidance of hypertension can minimize this outcome. Also avoidance of excessive blood glucose levels will help.

Gastrointestinal

There is a risk of irritation to the gastrointestinal system. During CPR air may have been forced into the stomach. Passing a nasogastric tube can help to alleviate feelings of discomfort. Antacids may help and a light diet should be available when the patient is able to eat. In addition the throat may be painful from airway management during the arrest.

During a cardiac arrest the patient may have been incontinent or soiled as a result of blood loss. Personal hygiene needs should be met including oral care, clean sheets and clothing. The patient may also complain of pain either caused by their underlying condition or resulting from the trauma experienced during the cardiac arrest. Appropriate medication should be administered and position altered.

It may be necessary to transfer a post-arrest patient to another environment and it is essential that this is performed in a safe manner. If this is deemed necessary, all monitoring should continue. All cannulae, drains and catheters should be secured. Suction, O_2 and defibrillation equipment should accompany the patient. The personnel who accompany the patient should be capable of assessing the condition and responding to changes including another cardiac arrest.

There is also a psychological element to the patient's care that should be addressed. Some patients may have limited recall of events and the nurse should be there to answer questions and concerns with openness and sensitivity. Sometimes patients are disoriented and may experience short-term memory problems. Again an approach that supports the patient psychologically is warranted. Some patients may have memories of the event that could be described as near-death experiences and often the opportunity to talk may help. Feelings of fear and anxiety are common. Patients may be worried about the same thing happening again. Honest and realistic answers are needed.

A patient may have been told that he or she has had a myocardial infarction and there are issues around this as well. Experiencing the trauma of a cardiac arrest is difficult enough but patients may have to deal with serious and life-changing events after a successful resuscitation.

There is also an opportunity for the nurse to offer support to the family. Unfortunately some patients do not survive and bereavement support should be managed in a supportive way. Families can be anxious and frightened and they should not be neglected. Information should be given in a sensitive way and if possible in a written form because details can be hard to retain (see Chapter 7). Honesty is vital.

There may be other patients who witnessed the cardiac arrest to varying degrees especially in an environment such as a CCU. Patients may be very aware of their own situations and worried that the same thing may happen to them. Without breaching confidentiality the nurse will have to reassure other patients in the clinical area. This should also be carried out in as sensitive a manner as possible.

Finally it should be mentioned that the staff involved with the management of the cardiac arrest should themselves receive support. Both from a professional and from a psychological perspective staff may need to talk and clarify issues. Even if someone is very experienced and appears to be coping well, the opportunity to debrief should be made available.

Participation in a cardiac arrest can be a valuable learning experience and staff should be encouraged to reflect on it. However, any critique of the events as they occurred should be positive. To apportion blame for any aspects of the event is undesirable and non-productive.

Ethical and wider issues

A generally accepted statement seems to be that CPR should be targeted at patients who will benefit from it. However, this opens the way to several interesting points.

A standard of care has been set up by the European Resuscitation Council, suggesting that it is reasonable to expect all health-care professionals to be able to perform BLS and that arrangements are made to facilitate access to advanced life support measures – in effect, patients have access to resuscitation.

The current state of medicine allows doctors to prolong the life of many patients. Resuscitation has saved many lives and importantly maintained an acceptable quality of life. However, it is at times inappropriate.

Resuscitation is often carried out on patients who are mortally ill whether as a result of cardiac problems, cancer or many other conditions. Resuscitation is not an appropriate treatment for the dying and does little to promote dignity and respect if used inappropriately. Sometimes inappropriate resuscitation may be the result of poor communication within health-care settings and the overriding urge to resuscitate first and then ask questions. This is particularly relevant in cardiac arrests that occur outside the hospital setting. Sometimes it is impossible to know enough about an individual to allow assessment of the appropriateness of CPR. Many hospitals are switching the emphasis away from dealing with arrests as they happen to predicting and avoiding the onset of cardiac arrest and possible inappropriate resuscitation. Resuscitation should really be used only where there is a good likelihood of a satisfactory outcome.

Many institutions address this by the use of 'Do Not Attempt Resuscitation' (DNAR) orders which can be applied to individual patients. There are guidelines in the UK issued jointly by the Resuscitation Council, the British Medical Council and the Royal College of Nursing. All patients should be resuscitated unless there is a specific DNAR order in place.

There are various criteria that can be used in making these decisions. The patient's own wishes or the wishes of the family or close friends can be taken into account, although relatives cannot consent. Final responsibility rests with the consultant responsible for the patient. Knowledge of the short- and long-term prognosis is helpful as is objective knowledge of the patient's quality of life. The effect of resuscitation on the patient and how he or she will cope with it could be considered.

In these situations it should not be seen as failure if a patient dies, providing that it happens with as much peace and dignity as possible. The nurse is in a prime position to facilitate this process. Nurses tend to build relationships with patients and their families that are among the strongest within the health-care team. The nurse should act as an advocate for the patient, ensuring that the patient's wishes and the wishes of the family are taken into account. For a patient to die with dignity, support and compassion can be seen as professionally important as successful resuscitation.

References

British Medical Society and Royal Pharmaceutical Society of Great Britain (2004) British National Formulary 47. London: Pharmaceutical Press.

Gilston A (1987) Cardiopulmonary resuscitation. Med Int 2: 1572–5.

Jowett NI, Thompson DR (2003) Comprehensive Coronary Care, 3rd edn. London: Baillière Tindall.

Mackintosh AF, Crabb ME, Brennan H (1979) Hospital resuscitation from ventricular fibrillation in Brighton. BMJ 1: 511–13.

Myerburg RJ, Kessler KM, Castellanos A (1993) sudden cardiac death: epidemiology, transient risk and intervention assessment Ann Intern Med 119: 1187–97.

Raehl CL (1987) Advances in drug theory of cardiopulmonary arrest. Clin Pharmacy 6: 118–39.

Redmond AD (1986) Post resuscitation care. BMJ 292: 1442–6.

Resuscitation Council UK (2000) Advanced Life Support Provider Manual, 4th edn. London: Resuscitation Council UK.

Resuscitation Council UK (2005) Resuscitation Guidelines 2005. London: Resuscitation Council UK.

Schein RMH, Hazday N, Pena M, Ruben BH, Sprung CL (1990) Clinical antecedents to in-hospital cardiac arrest. Chest 98: 1388–92.

Thompson DR, Webster RA (1992) Caring for the Coronary Patient. London: Butterworth Heinemann.

Vincent R (2003) Resuscitation. Educ Heart 89: 673–80.

CHAPTER SEVEN

Care of the patient with acute coronary syndrome in the CCU

IAN JONES

Historical overview of the coronary care unit

A number of steps have been taken to reduce the mortality from coronary heart disease (CHD), but arguably none is more important than the introduction of the coronary care unit (CCU) (Braunwald 1998). Before the introduction of CCUs, the mortality rate for a patient with an acute myocardial infarction (MI) was around 30%; this was reduced initially to 15% but further reduced to 6% with the introduction of aggressive re-perfusion therapy (Antman and Braunwald 1997). The concept of a unit dedicated to the care of patients with CHD was first proposed by Julian in 1961. Julian's beliefs were possibly based on the emerging evidence that not only was external cardiac massage effective in restoring life (Kouwenhoven et al. 1960) but that Jude et al. (1961) had singled out cardiopulmonary resuscitation (CPR) as being most effective in post-MI patients.

> It became very clear that the potential of cardiopulmonary resuscitation was great but could not be realised because of the inherent delays when patients with myocardial infarction were scattered throughout the hospital.
>
> Julian (2001, p. 622)

It was therefore considered logical to admit all patients suffering from an acute MI to a specialist unit. Julian argued that this type of unit would need to be staffed by personnel who were experienced in the recognition and management of cardiac arrhythmias and arrest. But despite Julian's early observations it was Hughes Day (1962) who was first reported to have used the term 'coronary care unit' when he noted that, despite a mobile crash trolley being used in a 200-bedded hospital, cardiac arrest results remained poor because patients with acute MI were cared for throughout the building. He concluded that this group of patients should be cared for in a specialist CCU. The concept of coronary care was quickly adopted in the USA but much more slowly in Europe. The fact that there had not been any data published that provided conclusive proof that these units were effective in reducing mortality caused a great deal of antagonism in some quarters. Other studies (Mather et al. 1976, Hill et al. 1978) found that there was no benefit from in-hospital treatment. The negative results of these studies influenced the Department of Health not to support the development of CCUs in England and Wales (Julian 2001).

When CCUs were finally opened physicians were responsible for the constant monitoring of the patient's condition, but they soon tired of this role, complaining of inactivity and boredom. A system of specialized care was then conceived, whereby nurses would have the primary responsibility for surveillance as well as emergency treatment. However, the management of cardiac arrest was to form only part of the nurse's role. Julian (1961) also noted that nurses could make a more positive impact if they were taught to recognize and manage cardiac arrhythmias. Meltzer and Kitchell (1961) had shown that nearly half of all deaths from acute MI were caused by arrhythmia and that 80% of all sudden deaths were caused by ventricular fibrillation (VF). Bayes de luna et al. (1989), who identified that ventricular tachycardia (VT) or VF caused 85% of all circulatory collapses, later supported these data. Zoll et al. (1956) had reported that VF could be successfully terminated with external defibrillation. It therefore seemed logical that, if nurses were able to recognize cardiac arrhythmias and defibrillate patients with life-threatening ventricular arrhythmias, the in-hospital mortality rates would reduce. Killip and Kimball (1967) wrote:

> In our opinion, optimal treatment cannot be attained unless certain prerogatives hitherto reserved for the physician are delegated to the nurse.

Therefore the coronary care nursing role was born. However, although the role may have been born out of the need to provide technological input to patients with a high mortality rate, the technical elements of the role should not overshadow the additional fundamental skills required to care for a patient in a CCU.

Nursing care

This chapter concentrates on the care of the patients within the CCU. It assumes that the patient has received some nursing and medical care within the accident and emergency department.

Therapeutic goals

Nursing care for the cardiac patient will differ depending on the patient's condition. For one group of patients the care will centre around two main aims:

- The first priority is to keep the patient alive by preventing complications and allowing the myocardium to heal.

- The second is to facilitate the rehabilitation process.
  The aim of nursing care for the second group of patients will be:
- to allow the patient to die with dignity
- to offer emotional support to the family

This chapter therefore discusses the nursing care required to achieve these goals.

Assessment

Assessment is the foundation on which we build our nursing care and, like any building, adequate time needs to be devoted to ensure that the foundations are solid. Very often in critical care environments, the assessment process will take place in two phases: the first is the emergency phase where the priority is to gain enough information to stabilize the patient or indeed keep him or her alive; the second, in which a more detailed history is taken, is often carried out at a later stage. This is not uncommon and quite acceptable. However, the nurse must ensure that this second phase is completed as soon as practically possible. The assessment process is often the first point of contact between the patient and nurse and it is within this time frame that the beginnings of the therapeutic relationship are formed. Good communication skills are paramount to this process as is the need to empathize with the patient's situation. Proctor et al. (1996) found that patients' perceptions of the CCU play a major part in the recovery process. The admitting nurse can often demystify the complexities of the CCU and improve the patient's understanding of the environment.

Priorities on admission

Before transferring the patient to the CCU the nurse will ensure that the patient is pain free, attached to a cardiac monitor and receiving O_2 therapy, and that intravenous access has been established. On admission to the CCU the patient may be anxious and distressed. The nurse needs to adopt a confident attitude and deal with the patient and relatives in a calm and collected manner. The patient should be transferred on to an appropriate cardiac bed while being monitored. The bed area itself should be large enough for nursing care to be carried out without hindering other patients or indeed restricting the movement of the nurse. Once in bed the patient's vital signs should be recorded, including an ECG, and the results documented. The nurse needs quickly to familiarize her- or himself with the patient's recent treatment and ensure that all appropriate care has been given. The patient's pain should also be reassessed and ongoing treatment administered if warranted. It may be difficult to obtain a detailed history from the patient at this point and it may be more appropriate to obtain only the information necessary to care for the patient over the next few hours. Additional information can be gained at later date.

Mobility

All patients with acute coronary syndrome will need to be placed under enforced bed rest for a minimum of 12 h. Rest is a fundamental part of the myocardial recovery process and although bed-rest periods have been shortened over the last 40 years the principle of resting the heart continues to form part of contemporary nursing care. However, although bed rest is desirable for reduction of myocardial demand, it poses a number of risks in its own right. All patients will need some form of risk assessment to be completed to establish the likelihood of pressure ulcer development; this will need to be repeated at regular intervals. There are a number of tools available to score pressure ulcer risk. However, in an evaluation of pressure ulcer prevention and treatment, McGough (1999) was unable to distinguish between a number of recognized pressure ulcer risk assessment tools, so the choice of assessment tool may be made locally. The risk of pressure ulcer is increased in acute coronary syndromes because of the potential reduction in peripheral perfusion (Bliss 1990, Royal College of Nursing or RCN 2001). In a shocked patient, the peripheries are likely to shut down, reducing blood supply to the peripheral tissues. The nurse will need to maintain regular observation of the skin and advise the patient to alternate the position in bed (RCN 2001).

In addition, the reduction in lower limb movement while in bed can increase the risk of deep vein thrombosis (DVT). The risk may also be increased because of the patient's predisposition to thrombus formation. However, it may be counteracted by the administration of anticoagulants. Heparin is often given to reduce the risk of thrombus formation in acute coronary syndromes. Passive or active limb movement should also be encouraged to reduce the risk of DVT and promote continued muscle usage.

Although ambulation is encouraged for stable patients within 12–24 h, patients who continue to experience pain, arrhythmia or haemodynamic disturbances will require longer periods of bed rest. These effects are symptoms of underlying pathological problems that need ongoing management. One such management is the reduction in myocardial workload. Bed rest appears to achieve this goal.

Most hospitals will use a post-MI mobility plan and, although intended purely for patients after an MI, it is frequently used for patients with unstable angina until MI has been excluded. Such protocols tend to prescribe a gradual increase in exercise on a daily basis. The traditional guidelines have tended to advise bed rest for 12–24 h, followed by the patient being allowed to sit in a chair on the second day and to walk one way to the bathroom on the third day. By the fourth day the patient is allowed to walk to and from the bathroom and on the fifth day should be fully mobile. However, yet again these guidelines are far too mechanistic. A number of variables need to be considered before planning the mobility regimen, including the person's physical condition, response to the cardiac event, underlying co-morbidity and the proximity of the patient's bed to the toilet. An alternative means of planning a mobility regimen for patients is to adopt a perceived exertion scale such as the Borg scale, similar to that used in cardiac rehabilitation programmes. Patients are asked to rate how hard they feel they have worked in an exercise class. In the acute stage the nurse could adopt such a scale and agree goals with patients, allowing them to mobilize within certain limits. This would allow patients to manage their own condition.

Maintaining a safe environment

The patient with an acute coronary syndrome is critically ill and requires a commensurate level of care. A fundamental part of the nursing role is to monitor the patient adequately to detect and hopefully prevent complications. To achieve this goal the nurse needs to have a good understanding of cardiac physiology and therapeutics. The box below lists a number of observations that nurses need to master to care for the patient effectively.

Routine observations

Blood pressure
Rhythm
Respiratory rate
Pain assessment
Temperature
Fluid balance
Venflon site
Signs of haemorrhage (if thrombolysed or receiving anticoagulation
    therapy)
Skin integrity
Psychological state

Cardiac monitoring (an arrhythmia is a symptom, not a diagnosis)
All patients admitted to a CCU should be attached to a cardiac monitor.
To the patient and junior nurse the monitoring system is intimidating, yet
the principles of cardiac monitoring are simple, i.e. to detect abnormal
rhythms. The more advanced machinery will allow a 12-lead tracing which
can subsequently monitor changes in the ST segment, allowing the practitioner to detect evidence of ischaemia or infarction. However, most
CCUs continue to use 3- or 5-lead systems, so 12-lead monitoring is
beyond their scope and nurses will need to rely on the principles of monitoring. Marriott (1988) identifies four key principles:

1. Use lead with maximal information.
2. Ensure maximal mechanical convenience.
3. One lead is not enough.
4. Know when to use other leads.

A monitoring lead that satisfactorily fulfils most of these requirements
is the modified chest lead (MCL) 1. The positive electrode is placed in the
V1 position. The negative electrode is placed on the left shoulder and the
neutral is placed on the right shoulder (Figure 7.1).

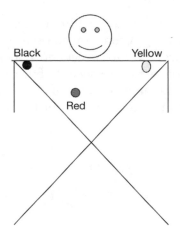

Figure 7.1 The modified chest lead (MCL).

The benefits of this lead placement, as opposed to the more traditional lead II placement, is that MCL1 provides a much greater analysis of the
P wave, along with an ability to distinguish between right and left bundle-
branch block and right and left ventricular ectopics (Marriott 1988). In
the absence of 12-lead ECG monitoring, MCL1 remains the most effective
and least intrusive means of monitoring cardiac rhythm. However, it should

be noted that, although the data produced by a monitor (if interpreted correctly) can improve the likelihood of a correct decision, the monitoring system itself is merely a tool to assist the clinician. It is by no means fool-proof and should not be analysed in isolation.

There will be a number of occasions when it will be difficult to achieve a tracing that is free from artefact. The coronary care nurse will need to be able first to identify artefact and second to remove this abnormality to obtain a more accurate account of cardiac rhythm. To do this the nurse will need to be able to troubleshoot (see Chapter 8).

Pain

Most patients with acute coronary syndromes will develop pain. This is typically central crushing chest pain radiating to the left arm and jaw. However, atypical presentations are not uncommon and some patients will not experience any type of pain. Patients with diabetes in particular are likely to present with atypical symptoms (Findlay 2003). This is thought to be related to the effects of diabetic neuropathy, which reduces the sensitivity of the cardiac nerve network.

The fact that most patients will develop pain at some point during their admission means that pain assessment and control are a major part of the CCU nurses' role. However, there is evidence to suggest that nurses do not always manage to assess or manage pain effectively (Thompson et al. 1994, Meurier et al. 1998). A pain thermometer is frequently used and is effective in establishing severity of pain by asking the patient to rate the pain on a 10-point Likert scale (Herlitz et al. 1986). This method is also helpful after administration of analgesia as a means of evaluating effectiveness of treatment. It is also reasonably easy to comprehend, although it does not consider a number of important additional variables such as the origin of the pain. Pain needs to be assessed thoroughly, establishing the type (stabbing, crushing, etc.), location, severity and any aggravating factors (exercise, food, etc.).

Only when a thorough assessment has been completed can the nurse consider management options. Patients in coronary care often complain of musculoskeletal pain resulting from the problems of bed rest. They may also have pain associated with pericarditis or even the aches and pains of a common cold. The nurse needs to ensure that the pain control is commensurate with the pain experienced. Using opiate analgesia for non-ischaemic pain may not be appropriate (Jowett and Thompson 2003).

Once pain is assessed adequately, if the origin of the pain is thought to be cardiac ischaemia then intravenous diamorphine should be administered as prescribed, usually 2.5–5 mg at a rate of 1 mg/min, followed by repeated doses until the patient is pain free. Diamorphine can now be administered (once only) by coronary care nurses using patient group directions. Caution is advised, however, because opiates can cause respiratory depression, although these effects can be reversed with the use of naloxone 400 µg.

Cardiac patients should never receive intramuscular medication. This method of administration can cause an increase in the levels of some cardiac enzymes, making the analysis of these enzymes futile, and also intramuscular puncture can result in marked haemorrhage into the tissue around the injection site. This risk is increased if the patient has received or is likely to receive thrombolysis or anti-platelet therapy.

Additional therapies that may be used in the acute phase include the use of nitrates. These drugs may be given sublingually, intravenously or via the buccal route. However, they frequently cause a sudden reduction in blood pressure. For this reason alone some doctors prefer to use intravenous or buccal nitrates, arguing that administration via either of these routes can be immediately terminated by removal of a tablet or discontinuation of intravenous therapy. Glyceryl trinitrate (GTN) spray has neither of these benefits. Oral mononitrates can also be used, although more as a means of pain prevention than treatment.

Although not regarded as analgesics pain control can often be achieved after the administration of β blockers and/or thrombolysis. The β blockers work by reducing heart rate and therefore myocardial demand and ischaemia. Thrombolysis works by degrading the fibrin clot and as a result improving coronary blood supply distal to the thrombus.

Another technique that can be used in the CCU is the use of relaxation therapy. During states of anxiety the body produces excess adrenaline (epinephrine). This free-flowing adrenaline stimulates the heart to beat at a faster rate and increases blood pressure, the net result being an increase in myocardial workload. The excess adrenaline can also stimulate arrhythmia. The use of relaxation therapy may reduce the state of anxiety and therefore the associated risks.

Communication

Although cardiac nurses are socialized into the technical environment, the CCU can be a daunting place to the uninitiated. It is important that the nurse is confident and able to communicate effectively to attempt to allay some of these fears. Time needs to be spent sitting and talking to the patient and the family. Only then are we able to understand their feelings. Although some studies have found that patients regard the most important element of the role as the nurse being competent in caring for the technical part of their care, others feel that the need for information was the most important feeling (Moser et al. 1993). The monitoring system that is frequently taken for granted by nurses may promote all sorts of anxieties for patients. It is important that the patient be aware that alarms may sound quite frequently and are not a cause for concern. Other patients may feel reassured if they are aware that the unit has a central monitoring system that allows the nurse to observe the patient's monitor while not at the bedside.

Anxiety is the most common emotional response to an acute MI (Jowett and Thompson 2003). However, nurses have a tendency to use blocking tactics to avoid discussing these anxieties. They are frequently guilty of making statement such as 'you're bound to be anxious, you've had a heart attack'. Although these statements are well meant and used in an attempt to alleviate suffering, they actually stop any discussion dead in its tracks. Cardiac nurses have to develop facilitation skills to allow patients to express their anxieties without assuming their origin. The use of open-ended questions that allow the patient to discuss their feelings in an appropriate environment may elicit improved communication. The use of the Hospital Anxiety and Depression Scales (HADS; Zigmond and Snaith 1983) in the acute phase may provide an insight into the patient's anxieties. It may also identify patients who are depressed and need referral to specialist services.

The nursing role does not end with the patient; it is generally acknowledged that chronic illnesses such as CHD affect the family members – particularly the spouse (Leske 1991, O'Farrell et al. 2000). This argument is supported in both qualitative (Thompson et al. 1995) and quantitative (Thompson and Cordle 1988) research studies. Frequently reported symptoms among family members of cardiac patients include anxiety, anguish depression, fatigue and insomnia (Hentinen 1983). In the acute phase there are feelings of shock, disbelief, anger and, understandably, the fear of losing a partner (Dhooper 1983). In the longer term, Thompson et al. (1995) noted that some partners remained emotional and tearful a month after the event, and Theobold (1997) noted that interviewees described a crushing uncertainty, turmoil and lack of information, which increased their anxiety. This increased anxiety level could have a detrimental effect on the patient's recovery (Waltz et al. 1988), rehabilitation (Moser et al. 1993) and ability to retain information, vital for that recovery (Cupples 1991).

Nurses are constantly told that communication is a two-way process, and yet asking patients and relatives for feedback is infrequently carried out. The assumption appears to be that, as long as the thank-you cards keep rolling in, we must be doing well. This view is far too simplistic. When being discharged patients are often just glad to be alive, yet on reflection they may feel that some elements of their care needed improving or that care was indeed faultless. This valuable feedback allows the service to develop in a way that meets the needs of the patient, not in a way that we think meets those needs.

Sleep

Coronary care units should be the ideal place for rest and recuperation. Unfortunately this is not always the case. During busy periods patients are often aware of the emergencies taking place around them and may find it difficult to rest while listening to the constant ringing of alarm bells. The coronary care nurse is able to reduce some of those environmental factors that inhibit sleep. Lighting within the unit should be at a minimum, alarm bells although audible should be turned down at night. The volume of telephone ring tones should be reduced and all staff should be aware of the need for patients to rest.

Patients may also be frightened to sleep for fear of not awakening or may be experiencing on-going pain. The nurse will need to discuss some of these issues while ensuring adequate pain relief. They should also minimize the need for routine observations. A number of patients will require regular half-hourly or hourly observation. Others will not need this level of input and observations could be taken during waking periods and allow the patient to rest in between. There is also no excuse for the lack of natural awakening in CCUs. Hygiene needs and bed making should be regarded as low priority when compared with the need for rest. Rest periods should be taken when the patient desires and not prescribed by nursing staff, although this may be more difficult in open plan units.

Dying

Although the in-hospital mortality rate has dramatically reduced over the last 40 years (Antman and Braunwald 1997), the fact remains that some patients will die while in the CCU. This death can be sudden in the event of a cardiac arrest or a slower process in such cases as cardiogenic shock. Although most CCU nurses spend time developing their skills in advanced life support and the technical elements of the role, the skills and knowledge in the area of breaking bad news are often lacking. This part of the role is often seen as the most difficult, and yet it receives the least amount of input. Although breaking bad news is more than bereavement care, it is one area in which nurses struggle.

In some of the earliest work in bereavement care, Parkes (1965) claimed that bereaved relatives progressed through stages of grieving that started with denial. This linear model of bereavement has been taught in schools of nursing for decades. However, it is now accepted that the grieving process is neither linear nor universal and relatives may experience a myriad of emotions. A number of articles have been written about the importance of breaking bad news in critical care and most highlight the impact that the sudden nature of the death can have on the grieving process (Worden 1991, Edwards and Shaw 1998). They also argue that the circumstances in which the news is broken are crucial, with some relatives experiencing traumatic memories (Wright 1996). The ability of the nurse to communicate effectively is crucial and, when this process has failed, it can have a detrimental effect on those concerned (Norbury 2003). Norbury (2003) suggests that, when being told of a death, relatives found that time stood still and they were unable to make sense of the information given. It could be argued that this is a form of denial. However, it is more likely to be an inability to comprehend the situation in which they find themselves.

The environment in which the news is broken also impacts on the experience. A number of authors (British Association for Accident and Emergency Medicine and Royal College of Nursing 1995) highlight the need for a designated area in which patients and relatives can be supported or counselled. This room should be close by and easily accessible at all times of day and night. The room itself should be private and reasonably well presented. There should also be access to a telephone where families can contact loved ones without being exposed to the busy hospital traffic and tissues should be made available to them. Once the setting has been prepared introductions should be made and the nurse should establish the identity of all parties, reducing the likelihood of informing the wrong relatives. Once introductions have been made the news may be broken. This part of the process is arguably the most difficult because of the sheer magnitude of the message. You will need to establish what the people already know and continue at their speed. Very often it is worth breaking the news in stages, e.g. 'As you know your father was admitted this morning with a heart attack and we started some treatment to help his heart through this critical stage. Unfortunately the treatment was unable to support his heart and despite all our efforts I'm sorry to have to tell you he died a few minutes ago'. Some people will want to be told outright and that is their right. However, others need time to come to terms with what is being said. You have to use the word 'died' because this is the only word that tells the story. Euphemisms, although helping us to deal with the situation, serve only to confuse the relative. There is also a great deal written about the use of touch in therapeutic relationships. Each case is, however, individual and while recognizing that some people prefer not to engage in a tactile relationship others benefit a great deal emotionally from the use of touch. After the breaking of bad news it is imperative to allow the family time to grieve.

There are a whole host of factors that influence the grieving process. Relatives who express a faith find that their spirituality gives them a sense of comfort (Norbury 2003) during this difficult time. The spiritual wishes of patients and relatives should therefore be considered when planning care. Other relatives comment on the need to 'be with their relative'. Until recently relatives have been excluded from CCUs during critical periods in an attempt to spare their feelings. However, the work of Hanson and Strawser (1992) found that over three-quarters of the relatives of people who had died, who had witnessed the resuscitation attempts, stated that the experience has helped them to adjust to the death. The Royal College of Nursing (2002) have now recognized the importance of this issue and published guidance to nursing staff in a document entitled *Witnessing Resuscitation*.

There are also a number of practical points that will need to be dealt with such as the issuing of a death certificate. Nurses need to ensure that they are aware of all these so that they can help the family during this difficult time. Most, if not all, hospitals now have a booklet to be given to relatives after a death. Nurses should familiarize themselves with this literature.

Some CCUs have adopted policies for contacting the relatives after the death to provide additional support and answer any questions that they have about the death. Small studies in this area have found these to be regarded as helpful to relatives (Wilson et al. 2000). However, we should err on the side of caution because these projects need to be handled with tact and time has to be devoted to them. It should also be noted that nurses are not counselling services; they are not trained counsellors and often lack the skills necessary for this relationship. A number of factors are thought to help the relative during this traumatic time. Norbury (2003) found that social support and bereavement support services from voluntary or hospital organizations were considered to be of great benefit to the bereaved, so it would seem logical that CCU nurses should familiarize themselves with the referral process for these organizations.

Breathing

A patient with an acute coronary syndrome may be breathless at rest as a result of pulmonary oedema. Conversely, in the absence of heart failure breathing may be within normal limits. There are a number of ways in which respiratory status can be assessed. The most common methods are respiratory rate and O_2 saturation monitoring. A rise in respiratory rate is often the first indication of the deterioration of a patient's condition. Yet frequently it is not recorded adequately. O_2 saturations are a more technical means of assessment through measurement of the levels of circulating O_2 in blood capillaries. An O_2 value of less than 90% is a cause for concern in the absence of respiratory disease (Braunwald et al. 2002). O_2 therapy is also administered to improve the circulating level of O_2 and increase myocardial oxygenation (Ryan et al. 1999).

When administering O_2 therapy the nurse needs to pay particular attention to oral care because piped O_2 lacks moisture and can cause ulceration of the mucosa in the mouth. Humidified O_2 is recommended for long-term O_2 therapy. Attention also needs to be paid to the delivery mode. In the critical phase O_2 may be delivered via an O_2 mask, which delivers high levels of O_2. However, if tied too tightly it can cause pressure ulcers around the ear. As soon as is practical, the patient may prefer to use nasal cannulae. This allows a greater freedom to drink, eat and speak. It may also make the patient feel more human.

Maintaining body temperature

The temperature may be raised as a result of the myocardial damage and inflammatory response. It may also be elevated if streptokinase has been the thrombolytic drug used. Use of this antigen-based drug produces an immune response, so a mild elevation of temperature should be expected. However, this should be monitored closely, because any further increase could indicate infection. In the presence of infection blood cultures should be taken and medical staff informed.

The patient may also feel cool to touch and look pale as a result of peripheral vasoconstriction. In this instance the first priority is to check the patient's blood pressure and, if reduced, strategies need to be developed to increase it to within normal limits.

Expressing sexuality

When patients are admitted to the CCU they frequently lack the tools of hospitalization, i.e. toiletries, pyjamas, night dresses, etc. They may therefore be dressed in gowns or hospital nightwear. In the past coronary care staff have encouraged such attire to ensure easy access during defibrillation. Although this may be acceptable in the first few hours, however, relatives should be encouraged to provide the patient's own nightwear and toiletries. This allows the patient to retrieve some of his or her identity that was lost on admission.

The diagnosis of acute coronary syndrome can have a dramatic effect on a person's life. Part of this effect may be on relationships. There is evidence to suggest that some patients struggle to maintain a sexual relationship with their partner after a cardiac event. This may be a psychological issue related to the loss of libido or in some cases this can be a physical problem. Erectile dysfunction caused by a lack of penile blood flow is more common than was first thought. It may also be compounded by the use of β blockers – these cardioprotective drugs can cause impotence. Yet, frequently patients are unaware of this side effect and assume that the problem has been caused by their heart attack. The nurse needs to broach this subject tactfully and allow the patient to discuss any problems. The use of written literature highlighting the problem may promote discussion.

Work and play

After a coronary event patients are likely to need time off work. In some occupations this need not be a problem. Other patients may be less fortunate. Self-employed people may find that they have very little income during their illness, which will obviously cause concern and anxiety for both the patient and the family. It is important that these issues are discussed tactfully and support offered. After discussion, it may be necessary to refer the patient to a medical social worker to discuss the entitlement of sickness benefit.

Most patients will return to a normal working life, although others may be anxious about returning to work and use this opportunity to retire or seek a career change. The coronary care nurse may not have the knowledge required to advise the patient at this point. It is therefore imperative that help be sought from a cardiac rehabilitation occupational therapist and physiotherapist. These specialist practitioners should be involved in the care of the patient at the earliest stage feasible.

Some patients rely heavily on the ability to drive for either occupational or leisure pursuits and, although there is often no reason why they will not be able to go back behind the wheel, they will need to refrain from driving for 4 weeks. When they return to driving they will need to inform their car insurance company of the heart attack. This should not increase their annual premium. However, if this is not the case the British Heart Foundation are able to provide a list of insurance companies with competitive rates for drivers after a heart attack. Other patients will rely on a higher class of driving licence, e.g. heavy goods vehicle (HGV) and, although having a MI does not automatically bar them from driving, the criteria are stricter for more advanced drivers. Up-to-date guidelines are produced by the DVLA in Swansea.

Although CCUs are likely to be quieter and calmer than most medical wards, this in itself can cause problems for the patient, because although these properties are desirable they can also lead to prolonged periods of boredom. A number of studies have investigated the effects of music and relaxation therapy in post-MI patients and found this approach to be favourable (White 1999, Biley 2000). Other units promote quiet periods that allow the patients to sleep during the day and, although these innovations may be suitable for some patients, there is a need to individualize care. At the very least nurses should use the time allocated to sit with the patient and offer support or facilitate discussion. On a number of occasions the author has found that some patients use the quiet time to worry about their condition or how they are going to manage when discharged. An individualized approach will allow the patients who want to sleep to do so while also allowing the patients who want to discuss their anxieties or worries with the nurse to do so.

Although most coronary care patients are not fixated on their leisure pursuits on admission, there are those who grieve for the life that they believe they have lost. Once again it is important that the nurse is able to discuss these matters. Patients may have a whole host of misconceptions that need to be dispelled before they are able to progress and during this process their mood starts to lighten. Exercise may be an important part of the patient's life and so he or she should be encouraged to continue with aerobic activity after a successful exercise tolerance test. The use of videos to show the patient a traditional cardiac rehabilitation programme may help to highlight the fact that a return to a healthy lifestyle is still possible in most cases.

Eating and drinking

When patients are admitted to the unit, they may experience nausea as a result of either the effects of opiate medication or diminished blood supply to the gut (which is often seen in hypotensive patients). The nurse should ensure that an appropriate antiemetic has been previously administered, e.g. metoclopramide 10 mg and that vomit bowls, tissues and mouthwashes are within reach of the patient. The nurse also needs to ensure that there are no environmental factors contributing to the patient's condition, e.g. offensive odours. If the patient continues to experience nausea and vomiting, the nurse should ask the medical staff to consider an alternative antiemetic.

When able to eat the patient may prefer to eat small, manageable portions. Conversely, some patients return to their normal diet very quickly. The nurse needs to discuss dietary requirements with the patient and assist when he or she orders meals. Patients should be encouraged to adopt a balanced, healthy diet, incorporating high fibre, low fat, high protein, low carbohydrate. The reason for specifying the word 'healthy' as opposed to 'specific requirements' is because the components of a healthy diet make up all the nutritional requirements for a cardiac patient. This philosophy also reduces the medical focus of patients' diets and allows them to think about diet as one measure in adopting a healthier lifestyle, as opposed to the medical model. The requirements of a healthy diet may need to be explained to the patient, and may also need to be explained to the partner, especially if the partner prepares and cooks the meals. It may also be easier for both parties to adopt a healthier diet.

Eating is often regarded as much more than merely stocking up on basic requirements, akin to putting petrol in a car. To many, eating is a pleasurable experience using all the bodily senses to see, smell and taste the food. In hospital there are a number of factors that influence this experience. The presentation of the food can have a dramatic affect on our perception of the taste and influence our enjoyment of the experience.

The timing of meals is equally important. Far too often meal times are squashed into a small part of the day, e.g. between 8am and 5pm. A heavy meal at lunchtime is hardly digested when the evening meal is served. Nurses should liaise with catering services and portering staff to ensure that meal times are patient centred and not led by the needs of ancillary staff.

A further disadvantage of bedrest is the need for patients to use commodes at the bedside. Ideally patients should be wheeled to the bathroom, but this is not always possible. We are then left with the situation where patients on CCUs frequently have to open their bowels at the side of their bed. Although this may be unavoidable there is a need to consider the effects that the aroma and noise generated during this act have on other patients, especially at meal times.

There is often no reason to restrict fluid in the patient with acute coronary syndrome, unless there is evidence of severe left ventricular dysfunction. However, the monitoring of fluid balance seems to be routinely practised in the first 24 h. The rationale for this practice is to ensure that the patient is not retaining fluid and therefore exerting undue pressure on the left ventricle at this critical period.

Elimination

A combination of diamorphine and immobility can reduce gastric motility, leading to constipation. If left untreated, this results in the patient straining to defecate. The effects of this exertion are to produce vagal stimulation and a dramatic lowering in heart rate, which could result in a cardiac arrest.

There may also be psychological reasons why the patient has not opened the bowels while in the CCU. The lack of privacy available to patients may mean that they are reluctant to do so. This issue is difficult to overcome in some units because the open expanse needed to see all patients does tend to mean that beds are separated only by curtains. Unfortunately these curtains are neither sound nor odour proof, resulting in other patients sharing the experience. Once again if a patient is stable he or she should be transferred to the toilet. When a patient does open the bowels, the nurse should visually check the stool for signs of fresh blood, which may signify the presence of a gastrointestinal haemorrhage secondary to administration of a thrombolytic.

The need to monitor strict fluid balance in the first 24 h will mean that patients have to use urinals or a commode at this stage. The urine volume is measured and documented accordingly, although the accuracy of fluid balance charts sometimes leaves a lot to be desired. In hypotensive patients there will be a need for catheterization. The hourly urine output is monitored and should be in excess of 30 ml/h. A reduction of urine output below this level can indicate renal impairment. The urine will also be required for a routine ward test. The presence of glucose and ketones is more significant in cardiac patients because this can highlight underlying diabetes (Malmberg et al. 1997).

Personal cleansing and dressing

On admission patients may not want to, or be able to, care for their own hygiene needs. However, they may wish the nurse to care for them in this way although, as their condition improves, they should be encouraged to become more independent. Conversely, other patients may just want to be left to rest and these wishes should also be respected.

Some older CCUs may not possess washing facilities because of the limited likelihood of patients needing them. However, some patients are now being cared for in the CCU several days after admission as a result of the shortage of beds on medical wards. Therefore, there is a need for CCU nurses to consider patients' needs and transfer them to the bathroom as soon as possible. There is no rationale for insisting that stable patients, several days after admission, continue to wash at their bedside.

The use of make-up is best avoided in the acute phase because of the ability of eye make-up, lipstick and nail varnish to mask the presence of cyanosis in peripheral and central tissues. However, once the patient is stable there is no reason why she should not be allowed to return to all the daily rituals. To the patient this may be regarded as being one step nearer to home.

Cardiac rehabilitation and secondary prevention

The CCU is very often the first phase of the cardiac rehabilitation process. During this phase it is important that patients be given time to discuss anxieties about the future and allowed to set their own agenda. Although it is important to ensure that patients understand the diagnosis, it is equally important to allow them to come to terms with this news in their own time. The use of written information is useful in facilitating this process. It cannot be stressed enough that the coronary care nurse has a major part in the rehabilitation process and that they should never abdicate responsibility by referring to the cardiac rehabilitation nurse. Cardiac rehabilitation is discussed in more detail in Chapter 12.

Transfer

There is evidence to suggest that length of stay for coronary care patients has increased over the last decade. This increase is more likely to be related to a lack of hospital beds than a result of the need for critical care. The effects of delayed transfer are unknown at this point. However, there is a need to ensure that nursing care reflects patient need and is individualized. Therefore, all stable patients who are more than 2 days after the event should be disconnected from a monitor and allowed to mobilize around the unit. Patients should be informed of their progress and explanations given about their transfer. Patients find it difficult to deal with the sudden change in environment from critical care to general care or even critical care to discharge. The nurse can play a pivotal role in preparing the patient and relatives for this transition.

Investigations

Full blood count: daily

Us&Es: at least daily, although should also be taken if patient develops arrhythmia or receives large doses of diuretics

Troponin: 12 h after admission

ECG: a post-thrombolysis ECG should be recorded 40 min after thrombolysis (Connaughton 2001); it would be hoped to see at least a 50% resolution of ST elevation in this ECG (Schroder et al. 1995); an ECG should then be recorded daily or if the patient develops pain or arrhythmia

Glucose: on admission and thereafter depending on the result

Lipid: within the first 24 h (preferably fasting)

Complications

Infarction, re-infarction or failed re-perfusion

The very nature of the CCU means that a large part of the nursing role is related to the early identification of complications of the underlying condition. The fact that most of the patients in CCUs have underlying CHD with acute plaque rupture means that they are at a 3–4% further risk of acute thrombosis (Ryan et al. 1996). This phenomenon can be identified in a large percentage of cases by recording an ECG. Any change in ST-segment shape or position can indicate a change in plaque dynamics. It is therefore imperative that the CCU nurse be able to identify these changes and inform the medical staff so that appropriate therapy can be commenced. The management of infarction after unstable angina would necessitate administration of thrombolytic therapy; however, the medical management of re-infarction is rather less straightforward and will often depend on local policy. The two options that are available are re-thrombolysis (although tissue plasminogen activator or tPA is the preferred option) or salvage angioplasty. Unfortunately the preferred choice is more likely to be affected by bed availability in specialist centres than by best evidence.

The administration of thrombolysis during an acute MI has quite rightly been afforded a great deal of discussion in documents such as the National Service Framework (NSF) for CHD (Department of Health or DoH 2000). However, it has been argued that thrombolysis will provide complete restoration of blood flow in only 50% of cases (Schroder et al. 1995). The coronary care nurse needs to be able to assess the efficacy of thrombolytic therapy through ECG analysis. Most CCUs routinely record post-thrombolysis ECGs. The optimum time period for these recordings is 40 min and 2 h after completion of therapy. Thrombolysis is deemed effective if ST-segment elevation has reduced by at least 50%. The management of failed re-perfusion is similar to that of re-infarction.

Post-MI angina

Post-MI angina is unfortunately quite common. Some authors have reported that up to 58% of patients (Schaer et al. 1987) experience this phenomenon. It should be suspected if the patient complains of a pain similar to the initial presentation. In the first instance an ECG should be recorded to assess ischaemic patterns and analgesia administered as appropriate. Anti-anginal therapy may be commenced or increased. However, if the patient remains unstable the subsequent medical management would be percutaneous coronary intervention (see Chapter 10).

Mitral valve involvement

After an acute anterior MI the papillary muscles of the left ventricle can become damaged. This typically occurs 3–5 days after an MI (Connaughton 2001). This injury can place undue strain on the mitral valve, which eventually starts to regurgitate. The regurgitation of blood into the left ventricle places excess pressure on the left ventricle and it starts to fail. The patient will become breathless and tachycardic as the heart and lungs attempt to compensate. An audible murmur is found in 50% of cases (Connaughton 2001); the other 50% will be diagnosed with the use of echocardiography. Treatment is decided based on the severity of the condition because all options carry a high risk, although patients often require urgent surgery.

Ventricular septal defect

If the septal area of the left ventricle is damaged during an acute MI, there is a danger that the ventricular septum can tear during systole. Necrotic tissue lacks mobility and therefore can tear away from more mobile surrounding tissue. The net result is a hole between the right and left ventricles. The danger of this scenario is that deoxygenated blood can pass across the septum into the left ventricle and is therefore transported into the peripheral circulation. The effects of this condition can once again differ. A patient with a ventricular septal defect (VSD) will become breathless and tachycardic as a result of the body's tissues being supplied with deoxygenated blood. A VSD can be diagnosed initially by the presence of a pansystolic murmur. To confirm diagnosis an echocardiogram should be requested and a cardiology opinion sought. The presence of VSD is associated with a high mortality rate (94%) if the condition is managed medically compared with 47% if treated surgically (Crenshaw et al. 2000).

Arrhythmia

Arrhythmia is probably the most common complication in an acute coronary syndrome. It ranges from benign ectopics to ventricular fibrillation and anything in between. The nurse needs to have developed a high level of skill in this area, not only being able to distinguish between the various arrhythmias but also having the knowledge needed to arrange immediate care. The role of the coronary care nurse has always focused on the prevention of complications rather than dealing with their effects. Arrhythmia management is a typical example of this principle. It is far more beneficial to administer atropine to the slowing heart than it is to manage an asystolic arrest. Although monitor alarms can alert the nurse to problems, there is no substitute for visual observation.

Left ventricular dysfunction or heart failure

A large proportion of patients experience some degree of left ventricular (LV) dysfunction after an acute MI. However, the extent to which their life is affected depends very much on the extent of myocardial damage. Patients can present with gross pulmonary oedema, which requires urgent oxygenation and may take the form of continuous positive airway pressure ventilation and diuretic therapy. Alternatively, the effects might be more subtle and present only as an increase in heart rate and a mild drop in blood pressure. Once again the effects are very individual. Every patient in a CCU should be assessed by a doctor at least twice daily. The doctor will need to listen to the patient's heart sounds and lung fields to detect the presence of oedema or valve incompetence. Any patient diagnosed as having heart failure should be prescribed an angiotensin-converting enzyme inhibitor.

Cardiogenic shock

Cardiogenic shock occurs in only a small number of patients with acute coronary syndromes. However, for those whom it does affect it has a mortality rate of up to 80% (Goldberg et al. 1999). Therefore, cardiogenic shock is a real issue for coronary care nurses and physicians. The key to reducing mortality from this condition is early identification and intervention. Cardiogenic shock can be defined as, and should be considered in all cases where the patient has, a blood pressure of < 90 mmHg systolic and a urine output of < 30 ml/h, and is pale, cold and clammy.

Post-MI cardiogenic shock is usually caused by the left ventricle being unable to eject enough blood to perfuse the body's tissues adequately. This process may be studied using echocardiography and is referred to in percentage terms as the ejection fraction. The normal ejection fraction is about 60%, but patients in cardiogenic shock have ejection fractions that are much less than this.

The medical management for this condition often involves the administration of cardiac inotropes such as dobutamine. Inotropes increase the contractility of the ventricle, thereby increasing stroke volume and cardiac output. However, inotropes will act only on viable myocardium and in a percentage of people will not be effective. The next step would be to introduce a pulmonary artery flotation catheter. This type of approach is not a treatment option but can provide an accurate account of fluid status and can be used as a guide when titrating therapy.

Some patients may benefit from coronary intervention and the use of an intra-aortic balloon pump should be considered as a means of stabilization. The augmentation of diastolic blood pressure and subsequent coronary filling and reduced LV workload can improve the short-term prognosis. However, an intra-aortic balloon pump is not a long-term option and is frequently used only to support the patient while awaiting surgery.

Pericarditis

Pericarditis can occur in isolation or in the post-MI period, although seldom within the first 24 h. The pain can be distinguished from ischaemic pain by the positional or respiratory effect. Pain may be eased by sitting forward or worsened on inspiration. An audible friction rub may be heard and ST-segment changes on the ECG are characteristically saddle shaped. This may be witnessed in a number of leads. Medical treatment consists predominantly of non-steroidal anti-inflammatory drugs. In the most severe cases a pericardial effusion may develop.

Haemodynamic monitoring

Generally haemodynamic status is monitored with the use of non-invasive blood pressure monitoring and pulse. Although this is acceptable with stable patients, the lack of continuous observation limits its use in critically ill individuals. Patients with single or multiorgan failure often require a more invasive approach, which allows haemodynamic changes to be immediately identified. Probably the most common invasive procedure witnessed by nurses in general settings is the use of central venous pressure (CVP) monitoring. This approach requires the patient to be placed in the supine position and the head of the bed to be lowered to allow easier venepuncture (Peters and Moore 1999). A central line is inserted by a doctor into either the jugular or the subclavian vein under aseptic conditions and then advanced into the vena cava. The jugular vein is probably easier to cannulate because of its proximity to the body surface. However, patients often feel restricted in their movement when they have a central line protruding from their neck and may prefer the subclavian approach (Waldman 2000), although the subclavian vein is deeper in the body and therefore more difficult to compress. When haemorrhaging it is also associated with a greater risk of pneumothorax so a jugular approach is often the preferred option. Central lines may also be inserted via the femoral vein, but the approach is rare because of the increased risk of infection and the inability to visualize the site easily

A CVP line can provide the nurse with details of pressures in the right atrium, which, in the normal adult, will be 3–10 mmHg. Care needs to be taken, when recording CVP pressures, that the transducer is level with the midaxillary line. Any deviation from this point can result in abnormal readings. A low reading is usually an indication of hypovolaemia caused by fluid loss or dehydration. A high CVP reading is more complex and may be associated with, among other things, LV or right ventricular failure, mitral valve failure, fluid overload and lumen obstruction.

A number of complications can occur during central line insertion. Although relatively rare compared with the number of central lines inserted, pneumothorax should always be considered if the patient becomes acutely short of breath during or immediately after insertion. Arrhythmia can occur if the cardiac wall is touched during insertion (Drewett 2000), so monitoring the patient's cardiac status during insertion should be regarded as best practice. Accidental arterial puncture can also occur during insertion, which may be identified by the production of bright red blood under a higher than anticipated pressure. This may, however, become difficult in the hypoxic and shocked patient whose arterial blood may be darker than anticipated as a result of poor oxygenation and under less pressure because of poor cardiac output. Blood gases may help to confirm the situation. If the position is uncertain, under no circumstances should any fluid be infused. The line should be removed and recannulation started.

The insertion of a central line increases the risk of infection at the entry site. The rates of infection have been estimated to be as high as 14% in some cases (Van Vilet et al. 2001). The insertion itself should be carried out under aseptic conditions, and the nurse should ensure that an occlusive but transparent dressing is used to cover the puncture site, allowing observation of the entry site. If infection is suspected at any time the line should be removed and repositioned. The central line should be removed as soon as it is no longer in use. When removing the line, the tip is often cut with sterile scissors and sent to microbiology for culture and sensitivity.

Pulmonary artery flotation catheters

Central venous pressure lines have a number of limitations in the care of the critically ill patient. The most widely accepted limitation of CVP lines is the poor correlation between CVP and left atrial pressure (Windsor 1998), resulting in poor correlation between CVP and LV function. This inability to measure the pressure on the left side of the heart has resulted in the development of the pulmonary artery flotation (PAF) catheter (frequently called a Swan–Ganz catheter). Such catheters are inserted in a similar way to CVP lines, but are advanced via the right atrium and ventricle into the pulmonary artery. PAF catheters have a balloon sited immediately before their tip. This allows the catheter initially to float into the artery during insertion and then into a pulmonary capillary. Once embedded in the capillary, the balloon obstructs any pressure influence proximal to this point, i.e. from the right ventricle, thus enabling the tip of the catheter to transduce the pressure from the left side of the heart. This reading is referred to as the pulmonary capillary wedge pressure or pulmonary artery wedge pressure, which correlates with left atrial pressure; this, in turn, reflects LV end-diastolic pressure, which is a far more accurate measurement of LV pressure. Another measurement that can be obtained using the PAF catheter is cardiac output from studies involving the injection of 10 ml iced water into the proximal port of the catheter. The monitoring system then measures the time taken for the fluid to reach the end of the catheter and, using a strict mathematical formula, it can estimate the patient's cardiac output.

There have been a number of studies that have questioned the use of this intervention in all groups of patients (Connors et al. 1996). However, a number of these studies lack randomization and incorporate a selection bias. In the author's experience PAF catheters can be used to guide medical treatment very effectively, but they are frequently inserted too late in the disease process and are managed by medical and nursing staff who lack fundamental skills. Although these catheters can be invaluable they are also dangerous in the wrong hands and should be inserted only by medical staff who have the skills and knowledge to care for the patient subsequently. The need for a PAF catheter has been greatly reduced with the advent of echocardiography.

Counterpulsation

Counterpulsation tends to be used for patients with a reduced cardiac output such as cardiogenic shock. Although it is not a treatment it can be used to stabilize the patient while awaiting treatment, e.g. transplantation, or while resting the heart. The most common method of counterpulsation is the use of an intra-aortic balloon pump. The principles of this approach are remarkably simple. A balloon catheter is inserted via the femoral artery and positioned in the descending aorta above the femoral bifurcation and below the subclavian arteries. Once in position, the patient has a radiograph taken to ensure accurate placement. The catheter is then connected to a machine that forces helium into the catheter which inflates the balloon during diastole. This inflation increases diastolic blood pressure (which is when the coronary arteries fill). The balloon then deflates just before systole, allowing the left ventricle to empty its contents into the aorta with reduced pressure, resulting in reduced workload for the left ventricle. The net results of the intra-aortic balloon pump are increased coronary perfusion and reduced LV workload and myocardial O_2 demand.

Conclusion

Patients with unstable coronary heart disease by definition are critically ill and require a commensurate level of care. The coronary care nurse has a vital role to play in minimizing the risk of further coronary events and assessing the efficacy of medical treatments. However, although the role has many technical components, it is vital that the coronary care nurse caters for all the patient's needs. To paraphrase Townsend and McCulloch, as far back as (1982), technical knowledge and expertise is useless unless delivered with compassion.

References

Antman EM, Braunwald E (1997) In: Braunwald E (ed.), Heart Disease: A textbook of cardiovascular medicine. London: WB Saunders Co., pp. 1184–288.

Bayes de luna A, Cornel P, Leclerq JF (1989) Ambulatory sudden cardiac death: mechanisms of production of fatal arrhythmias on the basis of data from 157 cases. Am Heart J 117: 151–9.

Biley FC (2000) The effects on patient well being of music listening as a nursing intervention: a review of the literature. J Clin Nursing 9: 668–77.

Bliss M (1990) Preventing pressure sores. Lancet 335: 1311–12.

Braunwald EB (1998) Evolution of the management of acute myocardial infarction: a 20th century saga. Lancet 352: 1771–4.

Braunwald E, Antman EM, Beasley JW et al. (2002) Guideline update for the management of patients with unstable angina and non-ST segment elevation myocardial infarction. A report of the American College of Cardiology/American Heart Association Task Force on Practice Guidelines (Committee on the management of patients with unstable angina). J Am Coll Cardiol 40: 1366–74.

British Association for Accident and Emergency Medicine and Royal College of Nursing (1995) Bereavement Care in A and E Departments. London: Royal College of Nursing.

Connaughton M (2001) Evidence-based Coronary Care. London: Churchill Livingstone.

Connors A, Speroff T, Dawson N, Thomas C, Harrell F (1996) The effectiveness of right heart catheterisation in the initial care of the critically ill patients. JAMA 276: 889–97.

Crenshaw BSGranger CB, Birnbaum Y et al. (2000) Risk factors, angiographic patterns and outcomes in patients with ventricular septal defect complicating acute myocardial infarction. Circulation 101: 27–32.

Cupples SA (1991) Effects of timing and reinforcement of preoperative education on knowledge and recovery of patients having coronary artery bypass graft surgery. Heart Lung 20: 654–60.

Day HW (1962) A cardiac resuscitation programme. Lancet 82: 153–6.

Department of Health (2000) The National Service Framework for Coronary Heart Disease. London: HMSO.

Edwards L, Shaw DG (1998) Care of the suddenly bereaved in cardiac care units: a review of the literature. Intens Crit Care Nursing 14: 144–52.

Dhooper SS (1983) Family coping with the crisis of heart attack. Social Work Health Care 9: 15–31.

Drewett SR (2000) Complications of central venous catheters. Nursing care. Br J Nursing 9: 466–78.

Findlay I (2003) Silent myocardial ischaemia in people with diabetes. In: Heart Disease and Diabetes. London: Martin Dunitz.

Goldberg RJ, Samad NA, Yarzebski J, Gurwitz J, Bigelow C, Gore JM (1999) Temporal trends in cardiogenic shock complicating acute myocardial infarction. N Engl J Med 340: 1162–8.

Hanson C, Strawser P (1992) Family presence during cardio-pulmonary resuscitation. Foote Hospital emergency department's nine year perspective. J Adv Nursing 18: 104–6.

Hentinen M (1983) Need for instruction and support of the wives of patients with myocardial infarction. J Adv Nursing 8: 519–24.

Herlitz J, Richter A, Hjalmarson A, Holmberg S (1986) Variability of chest pain in suspected acute myocardial infarction according to subjective assessment and requirements of narcotic analgesics. Int J Cardiol 13: 9–22.

Hill JD, Hampton JR, Mitchell JRA (1978) A randomised trial of home-versus-hospital management for patients with suspected myocardial infarction. Lancet i: 837–41.

Jowett NI, Thompson DR (2003) Comprehensive Coronary Care, 3rd edn. London: Baillière Tindall.

Jude JR, Kouwenhoven WB, Knickerbocker GG (1961) Cardiac arrest: report of application of external cardiac massage on 118 patients. JAMA 178: 1063–70.

Julian DG (1961) Treatment of cardiac arrest in acute myocardial ischaemia and infarction. Lancet ii: 840–4.

Julian DG (2001) The evolution of the coronary care unit. Cardiovasc Res 51: 621–4.

Killip T, Kimball JT (1967) Treatment of a myocardial infarction in a coronary care unit. A two-year experience with 250 patients. Am J Cardiol 20: 457–64.

Kouwenhoven WB, Jude JR, Knickerbocker GG (1960) Closed chest cardiac massage. JAMA 173: 1064–7.

Leske JS (1991) Overview of family needs after critical illness: from assessment to intervention. Clin Issues Crit Health Care Nursing 2: 185–226.

McGough AJ (1999) A systematic review of the effectiveness of risk assessment scales used in the prevention and management of pressure sores. MSc thesis, University of York.

Malmberg K, Norhammar A, Wedel H, Rydén L (1997) Glycometabolic state at admission: important risk marker of mortality in conventionally treated patients with diabetes mellitus and acute myocardial infarction. Long-term results from the Diabetes and Insulin-Glucose Infusion in Acute Myocardial Infarction (DIGAMI) Study. Circulation 99: 2626–32.

Marriott HJL (1988) Practical Electrocardiography, 8th edn. Baltimore, MA: Williams & Wilkins.

Mather HG, Morgan DC, Pearson NG (1976) Myocardial infarction: a comparison of home and hospital care for patients. BMJ i: 925–9.

Meltzer LE, Kitchell JB (1961) Intensive Coronary Care. New York: Robert J Brady.

Meurier CE, Vincent CA, Parmer DG (1998) Perceptions of causes of omissions in the assessments of patients with chest pain. J Adv Nursing 28: 1012–19.

Moser D, Dracup C, Marsden C (1993) Needs of recovering cardiac patients and their spouses; compared views. Int J Nursing Studies 30: 105–14.

Norbury E (2003) Sudden bereavement in a coronary care unit: a phenomenological study. MRes dissertation, Lancaster University.

O'Farrell P, Murray J, Hotz B (2000) Psychological distress among spouses of patients undergoing cardiac rehabilitation. Heart Lung 29: 97–104.

Parkes CM (1965) Bereavement and mental illness: part 1, a clinical study of the grief of bereaved psychiatric patients: part 2, a classification of bereavement reactions. Br J Med Psychol 38: 1–26.

Peters JL, Moore R (1999) Central Venous catheterisation. In: Webb AR, Shapiro M, Singer M, Suter P (eds), Oxford Textbook of Critical Care. Oxford: Oxford Medical Publications.

Proctor T, Yarcheski A, Orischello RG (1996) The relationship of hospital process variables to patient outcomes following myocardial infarction. Int J Nursing Studies 33: 121–30.

Royal College of Nursing (2001) Clinical Practice Guidelines: Pressure ulcer risk assessment and prevention. London: RCN.

Royal College of Nursing (2002) Witnessing Resuscitation: Guidance for nursing staff. London: RCN.

Ryan TJ, Anderson JL, Antman EM et al. (1996) ACC/AHA guidelines for the management of patients with acute myocardial infarction: a report of the American College of Cardiology and American Heart Association Taskforce on Practice Guidelines. J Am Coll Cardiol 28: 1328–428.

Ryan, Antman EM, Brooks NH TJ et al. (1999) The 1999 update: ACC/AHA guidelines for the management of patients with acute myocardial infarction. J Am Coll Cardiol 34: 890–911.

Schaer DH, Leiboff RH, Wasserman AG et al. (1987) Recurrent early ischemic events after thrombolysis for acute myocardial infarction. Am J Cardiol 59: 788–92.

Schroder R, Wegscheider K, Schroder K, Dissmann R, Meyer-Sabellek W (1995) Extent of early ST segment elevation resolution: a strong predictor of outcome in patients with acute myocardial infarction and a sensitive measure to compare thrombolytic regimens. A substudy of the International Joint Efficacy Comparison of Thrombolytics (INJECT) trial. J Am Coll Cardiol 26: 1657–64.

Theobald K (1997) The experiences of spouses whose partners have suffered a myocardial infarction; a phenomenological study. J Adv Nursing 26: 595–601.

Thompson DR, Cordle CJ (1988) Support of wives of myocardial infarction patients. J Adv Nursing 13: 223–8.

Thompson DR, Ersser SJ, Webster RA (1995) The experiences of patients and their partner one month after a heart attack. J Adv Nursing 14: 291–7.

Thompson DR, Webster RA, Sutton TW (1994) Coronary care unit patients' and nurses' ratings of intensity of ischaemic chest pain. Intens Crit Care Nursing 10(2): 83–8.

Townsend A, McCulloch J (1982) Affairs of the heart coronary care units and . . . the nurses' role. Nursing Mirror 155(15): 56–7.

Van Vilet J, Leusink JA, de Jongh BM, de Boer A (2001) A comparison between two types of central venous catheters in the prevention of catheter-related infections: the importance of performing all the relevant cultures. Clin Intens Care 3: 135–40.

Waldman C (2000) Cannulation of central veins for resuscitation and monitoring in the ICU. Anaesth Intens Care Med 1(3): 105–7.

Waltz M, Badura B, Pfaff H, Schott T (1988) Marriage and the psychological consequences of a heart attack, a longitudinal study of adaptation to chronic illness after 3 years. Soc Sci Med 27: 149–58.

White JM (1999) Effects of relaxing music on cardiac autonomic balance and anxiety after myocardial infarction. Am J Crit Care 8: 220–30.

Wilson A, Norbury E, Richardson K (2000) Caring for broken hearts — patients and relatives: three years of bereavement support in CCU. Nursing Crit Care 5: 288–93.

Windsor J (1998) Haemodynamic monitoring. Care Crit Ill 14(2): 44–9.

Worden JW (1991) Grief Counselling and Grief Therapy. London: Routledge.

Wright B (1996) Sudden Death: A research base for practice. London: Churchill Livingstone.

Zoll PM, Linenthal AJ, Gibson W, Paul MH, Norman LR (1956) Termination of ventricular fibrillation in man by externally applied electric countershock. N Engl J Med 254: 727–32.

Zigmond AS, Snaith RP (1983) The Hospital Anxiety and Depression Scale. Acta Psych Scand 67: 361–70.

CHAPTER EIGHT

Electrocardiography and cardiac rhythm recognition in practice – the basics

BRIAN PARR AND MIKE LAPPIN

The first section of the chapter discusses the basic principles of using electrocardiograph monitoring. This can be carried out in one of two ways: by 'real-time' 3- or 5-lead (sometimes 12-lead) cardiac monitoring and assessment of the heart's electrical events from a printed rhythm strip or a 12-lead electrocardiogram (ECG). The cardiac monitor is one of the most widely used devices in both the modern coronary care unit (CCU) and the general ward setting. It allows the nurse to observe the cardiac rhythm of the heart in a single lead. Alternatively a 12-lead ECG may be performed, which analyses the cardiac electrical activity from a number of electrodes positioned on the limbs and across the chest. This approach provides 12 different views of the electrical activity passing through the heart, allowing a wide range of abnormalities to be detected, including arrhythmias, myocardial ischaemia, left ventricular hypertrophy and pericarditis. A 12-lead ECG will provide much more information than is available on a cardiac monitor and should, where possible, be attached to any patient with suspected cardiac disease. However, this is not always possible and so health professionals regularly rely on the cardiac monitor.

The need for cardiac monitoring is great with cardiac arrhythmias and conduction defects occurring frequently after a myocardial infarction (MI) (Jacobson 1995). They also occur during anaesthesia and surgery in up to 86% of patients (Lee 2004). Many are of clinical significance and therefore their detection is of considerable importance. However it should be remembered that the ECG records only the electrical activity of the heart. It does not provide practitioners with information about mechanical function. The ECG monitor should always be connected to any patient with suspected heart disease, allowing the practitioner to detect any change in the appearance of the ECG complexes during the acute phase of admission.

Cardiac conduction system: an overview

The ECG displays the heart's electrical activity; it does not tell us whether the electrical activity is producing a mechanical (pulse) event.

For the heart to contract (pump) it needs to receive a signal. This signal is provided by the heart's 'specialized' cardiac conduction system. The cardiac conduction system is organized in such a way as to optimize the contraction and therefore the pumping efficiency of the four chambers of the heart.

The heart is electrically activated (depolarized) by an impulse generated high up in the right atrium. The generation of this impulse comes from a small group of cells that make up the sinoatrial (SA) node (Figure 8.1). The impulse then spreads across both right and left atria, much like the ripples seen when a pebble is dropped into a pool of water. When the impulse arrives at the bottom of the atrium, it cannot pass further because of the fibrous ring that separates the atrium from the ventricles. Low in the floor of the right atrium the impulse finds the next 'specialized' component of the conduction system: the atrioventricular (AV) node. The impulse is transmitted through this node down the bundle of His to the bundle branches of the right and left ventricles. Finally the impulse travels across the Purkinje fibres, which allow the spread of the impulse throughout the ventricular myocardium; this is activated from the bottom (apex) to the top (base) and from the inside (endocardium) to the outside (epicardium). The whole process of electrical activation and recovery of the heart is referred to as the cardiac cycle.

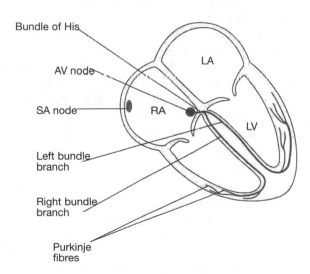

Figure 8.1 Cardiac conduction system. AV, atrioventricular; LA, left atrium; LV, left ventricle, RA, right atrium; RV, right venticle; SA, sinoatrial.

Connecting an ECG monitor (Figure 8.2)

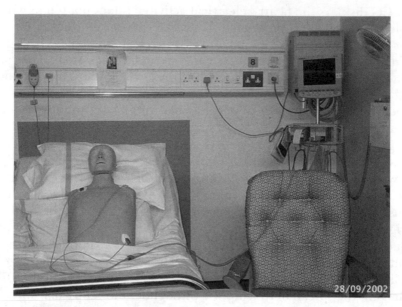

Figure 8.2 A manikin being monitored.

Hand (2002) describes the three electrodes that are used to monitor the
heart rate and rhythm: the negative (yellow) and the positive (red) electrodes detect the signal from the heart, whereas the black electrode is
neutral. The position of the black electrode has no influence on the configuration, but serves to reduce electrical noise or interference. The
position of the red and yellow electrodes significantly influences the
appearance of the signal on the ECG and it is, therefore, important to
ensure that the best position is used. Although an ECG trace may be
obtained with the electrodes attached in a variety of positions, conventionally for cardiac monitoring they are placed in standard positions each
time so that abnormalities are easier to detect. Thompson and Webster
(1992) state that ECG monitoring commonly requires three chest electrodes, usually two of which are placed in the right and left infraclavicular
spaces and the third may, for example, be placed at the right sternal edge.
In this position, a tracing with a configuration similar to lead I on the 12-
lead ECG is obtained (Figure 8.3). This configuration also allows a clear
area for application of chest electrodes for a 12-lead ECG, defibrillation
and external cardiac massage should these be necessary.

The cables from the electrodes usually terminate in a single cable,
which is plugged into the port on the ECG monitor. A good electrical connection between the patient and the electrodes is required to minimize the

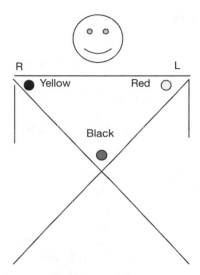

Figure 8.3 Although the positions refer to arms and legs, the electrodes are actually placed on the chest as described in the text. The reference to arm and legs is based on the historical positioning of electrodes, which is now rarely practised.

skin resistance. For this reason gel pads are used to connect the electrodes to the patient's skin. However, when the skin is sweaty the electrodes may not stick well, resulting in an unstable trace.

Leads versus cables

The term 'lead' when applied to the ECG does not describe the electrical cables connected to the electrodes on the patient. Instead it refers to the positioning of the two electrodes being used to detect the electrical activity of the heart. A third electrode acts as a neutral (Schamroth 1985). Goldberger and Goldberger (1981) liken the ECG to drawing a picture or taking a photograph of a person's head. If we want to explore the head we have to draw or photograph it from the front, sides, back: one view is not enough. Similarly, it is necessary to record many ECG leads to be able to demonstrate the electrical activity of the heart adequately. A 12-lead ECG therefore picks up the electrical stimulus from a number of angles. Notice that each lead records a different pattern; this arrangement reflects the different aspects of the overall recording. Continuous cardiac monitoring, on the other hand, uses one lead as opposed to the 12 leads of the electrocardiograph.

During the monitoring phase, one of three possible 'leads' is generally used; the leads are described by convention as follows (Goldberger and

Goldberger 1981, Lee 2004):

- Lead I: measures the potential difference between the right arm electrode and the left arm electrode. The third electrode (left leg) acts as
  neutral.
- Lead II: measures the potential difference between the right arm and
  left leg electrode.
- Lead III: measures the potential difference between the left arm and
  left leg electrode.

Electrical activity travelling towards an electrode is displayed as a positive
(upward) deflection on the screen and electrical activity travelling away as a
negative (downward) deflection (Marriott 1974, 1984, Schamroth 1985).

Most monitors in the general setting can show only one lead at a time
and therefore the lead that gives as much information as possible should
be chosen. The most commonly used lead is lead II (a bipolar lead with
electrodes on the right arm and left leg) (Figure 8.4). Lee (2004) com-
ments that this is the most useful lead for detecting cardiac arrhythmias
because it lies close to the cardiac axis (the overall direction of electrical
movement), allows the best view of P and R waves and is most commonly
used by nurses during cardiac monitoring (Sheppard and Wright 2000).

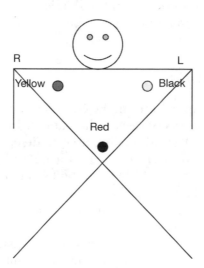

Figure 8.4 Lead II: the electrode position required to obtain a recording in lead II.

However, Marriott (1974) argued that, in order to get the most out of
monitoring, the precordial or chest leads are much more valuable than the
limb leads and it would be more appropriate to monitor on V1. Marriott
continues: 'for the last 20 years, people interested in arrhythmias have

always wanted to look at a V1 because it is an excellent lead for showing atrial activity and the QRS complex has a lot of information in it, much more than a lead II.' In his workshop text Marriott (1974) demonstrated a simple modification that had served him well when used with his patients (over 2000 individuals). The modified chest lead 1 (MCL1) hook-up consists of the positive electrode at the fourth right intercostal space and the negative electrode at the left shoulder, using the left arm as the indifferent electrode. As it is not on the arm, it is more convenient to put it out under the clavicle, modifying it to some extent (Figure 8.5 and Table 8.1).

Table 8.1 Marriott (1974) highlights the diagnostic advantages of modified chest lead 1 (MCL1)

1. Left ventricular (LV) versus right ventricular (RV) ectopy:

   – ectopic rhythms
   – pacemakers

2. Right bundle-branch block (RBBB) versus left bundle-branch block (LBBB)

3. LV ectopy versus RBBB-type aberration

4. Well-formed P waves

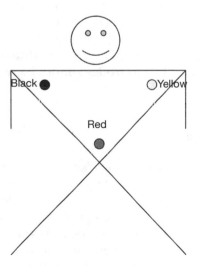

Figure 8.5 Modified chest lead 1 (MCL1): the electrode position required to obtain a recording in modified chest lead 1.

One further advantage of this lead is that it does not interfere with the position of defibrillation paddles if required in an emergency (Hand 2002).

Obtaining a quality recording

Tracing problems occur frequently and can usually be rectified easily. Poor electrode technique often appears as irregular fluctuations in the recording. Better contact is required here; examine the patient for excess body hair and remove if necessary. If the patient has an extreme diaphoresis it may be necessary to change the electrodes a number of times before appropriate contact is established.

Hand (2002) declares that where possible the electrodes should be placed over bone, e.g. the sternum, clavicles and lateral costals, to reduce electrical noise from skeletal muscle activity. If necessary the skin should be cleaned first to remove excessive body oil and perspiration. Body hair can prevent adequate contact between the electrodes and the skin, and so should be shaved where the electrodes are to be positioned. Sheppard and Wright (2000) also recommend preparing the skin by rubbing the area gently with dry gauze to remove loose dry skin and thus improve the conduction signal.

Defective cables may have been caused by 'overstretching' or damage from bedside equipment, e.g. cot sides or cabinets produce sharp waveform fluctuations or what appears to be an isoelectric waveform (Hand 2000). The cable may require replacement or, as in most cases, simple readjustment and further insertion into the monitor.

Muscular activity gives the appearance of fast fluctuations, with the amplitude exceeding that of the ECG tracing on the monitor. This is often rectified by ensuring that the patient is made more comfortable and by encouraging relaxation. A re-positioning of the electrodes over bone may also help. Skin integrity should be monitored throughout this period and any allergic reactions to the electrodes should be recorded and reported.

ECG waveforms

The cardiac cycle can be detected by special electrodes placed on the body of the patient, which are then displayed or recorded as a series of waveform shapes on the cardiac monitor, rhythm strip or 12-lead ECG (Figure 8.6).

As the first electrical event is the depolarization of the atria by the SA node, this is the first waveform to be seen. As the atria are small in comparison to the ventricles, the waveform is also small. This waveform is labelled the P wave. The next major electrical event is the depolarization of the ventricles. As these are bigger chambers (particularly the left ventricle), they produce the biggest waveform seen on the ECG. This waveform is labelled the QRS. The final waveform seen on the ECG is a smaller asymmetrical waveform labelled the T wave. This represents the

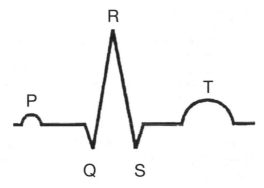

Figure 8.6 ECG waveforms of the cardiac cycle.

'electrical' recovery (repolarization) of the ventricles. Repolarization of the atrium is not seen on the ECG because it is effectively 'drowned' out by the electrical activity recorded by the depolarization of the ventricles. Occasionally a small wave is seen after the T wave – called a U wave. When seen it is thought to represent late repolarization of the ventricles.

From our knowledge and understanding of the cardiac cycle we can predict and measure how long each phase of the cycle should take, as the impulse journeys through the atria and ventricles along the cardiac conduction system. The waveforms are deliberately recorded on to 'graph' paper, which is made up of a number of large and small squares (Figure 8.7 and Table 8.2).

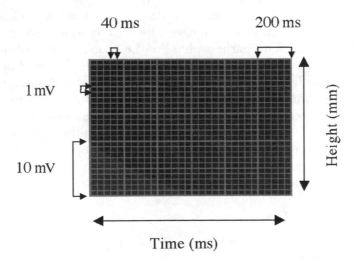

Figure 8.7 ECG paper showing timing and height markers and values.

Table 8.2 ECG complex measurements

Waveform	Height (mm)	Duration (ms)
P wave	≤ 2.5 (2.5 mV)	< 120 (< three small squares)
QRS complex	Variable	< 120 (< two small squares)
T wave	Variable	Variable

Each of the squares has been assigned a value according to whether it is measuring the height of an ECG waveform or a period of time the impulse of waveform takes:

- Time is measured in milliseconds (ms).
- Height is measured in millimetres (mm).

Segments and intervals

From the ECG complex a number of other important intervals and segment can be identified and measured (Figure 8.8):

- P–R interval: represents the time that the impulse generated within the atrium takes to penetrate the AV node and to be conducted to the ventricles via the bundle of His, bundle branches and Purkinje fibres. It is measured from the start of the P wave to the start of the QRS. The normal P–R interval is 120–200 ms (three to five small squares).
- QRS complex: represents 'electrical' activation of the ventricular myocardium. It is measured from the start of the QRS represented by a q, Q or r, R wave. The width of the QRS complex can vary in leads but must be < 120 ms (three small squares) for it to be considered normal.
- ST segment: represents earliest phase of the repolarization of the ventricles. It is measured from the end of the QRS to the start of the T wave. It is usually 'isoelectric' (at the same level as the baseline) and often merges imperceptibly into the T wave. The ST segment can sometimes be recorded 0.5 mm (half a small square) above the baseline in the limb leads or by 1 mm (one small square) in the V leads.
- Q–T interval: represents the total time taken to depolarize the ventricles. It is measured from the start of the QRS to the end of the T wave. Dependent on the heart rate, the Q–T interval varies between 0.25 and 0.50 ms.

Automaticity and intrinsic rates

The SA node, AV node, bundle of His and Purkinje fibres all possess the property of automaticity, which is the ability of a cell to produce its own

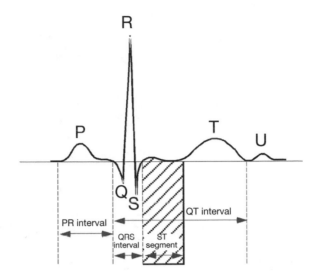

Figure 8.8 ECG complex showing intervals and ST segments.

electrical stimulus. This property acts as a fail-safe to protect the heart in case of failure of a higher pacemaker site.

The SA node, AV node and His–Purkinje system all possess differing intrinsic (natural) rates:

- SA node: 60–100 beats/min
- AV node: ≤ 50 beats/min
- His–Purkinje system: < 40 beats/min.

The SA node with its higher intrinsic firing rate is the natural pacemaker of the heart.

Cardiac axis

If you look at a 12-lead ECG (Figure 8.9) you will see that the P-QRST waveforms produced can look quite different in different leads. This is because each of the leads, while viewing the same electrical event, is doing so from a slightly different position. In general leads I and II normally show upright complexes, whereas lead aVR always shows negative (upside-down) complexes; likewise V1 normally shows mostly negative complexes whereas V6 shows positive complexes. This is because they are viewing the electrical activity from opposite sides of the heart. Developing the ability to calculate the cardiac axis in all the different leads precisely is quite an advanced skill and takes a fair amount of practice and experience, and therefore is not covered any further here.

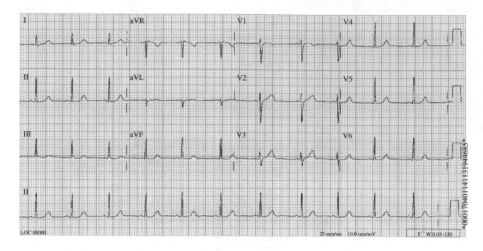

Figure 8.9 Normal ECG.

The ECG: what does it tell us?

Although the ECG reflects electrical and not mechanical events, changes in the anatomical structure or pathophysiological changes affecting the layers of the heart or conduction pathways can produce changes in the ECG complexes recorded.

Alterations in the size or thickness of either the atrium or ventricles as a result of enlargement or hypertrophy (Figure 8.10) can produce increases in the height and width of the corresponding P waves or QRS complexes.

Problems in conduction through either of the two main bundle branches as a result of ischaemic heart disease or chronic calcification will manifest as widened QRS complexes (Figure 8.11).

Acute coronary syndromes of acute ischaemia and infarction (Figure 8.12) as a result of coronary heart disease can produce very dramatic and noticeable changes to the ST segment and/or T wave. The ECG is crucial in diagnosis and treatment of these conditions.

Many other conditions such as pulmonary embolism, cerebrovascular events, and electrolyte or metabolic disturbances can alter and affect the complexes seen on the ECG.

One of the most common and important uses of cardiac monitoring and the 12-lead ECG is to provide us with important information about the patient's heart rhythm.

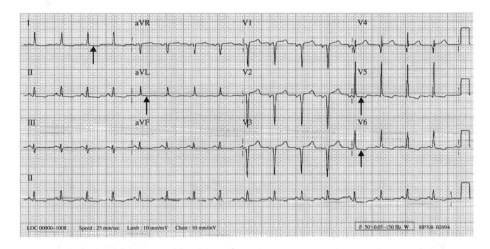

Figure 8.10 ECG showing increased amplitude of QRS complexes in leads V1–V3, and V5 and V6, indicative of left ventricular hypertrophy. Also note 'typical' ST strain pattern as indicated by the arrows.

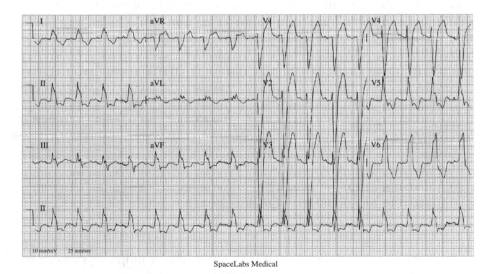

SpaceLabs Medical

Figure 8.11 Left bundle-branch block: note widespread QRS > 120 ms, and also 'typical' ST–T sloping off in opposite direction of main QRS deflection.

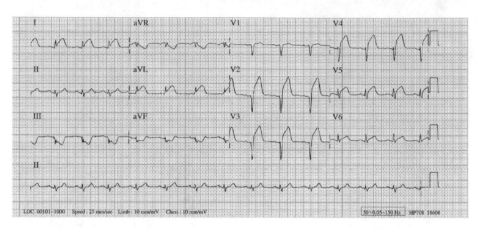

Figure 8.12 ECG showing ST-segment elevation of acute myocardial infarction in leads V2–V5, I and aVL. Note also ST-segment depression in leads III and aVF.

Assessing the cardiac rhythm

The ability to recognize and interpret both cardiac rhythms and analyse a 12-lead ECG takes time and practice. When developing this skill, the practitioner should always follow a systematic and structured approach; this will ensure the development of good habits from the outset and hopefully prevent too many wrong turns. The experienced practitioner can often interpret the rhythm by instant 'pattern' recognition; given time and practice the novice will also develop this skill. However, there will always be occasions when this is not sufficient, and a careful analysis of a printed rhythm strip or 12-lead ECG will be needed to avoid a misdiagnosis.

Disturbances in the cardiac rhythm can be the primary cause of the patient's deteriorating condition or may be a secondary problem as a result of another primary cause. Whenever assessing the cardiac rhythm it is important to remember the golden rule:

Always treat the patient not the monitor.

If a patient is not breathing and does not have a palpable pulse, cardiopulmonary resuscitation must be started without delay, even where the cardiac monitor is displaying a normal looking rhythm.

It is important to note that a patient's ability to 'tolerate' a cardiac rhythm disturbance is related to:

• acuteness of onset
• ventricular rate
• LV function.

A nine-step structured approach can be used in order to help diagnose cardiac rhythms (Table 8.3).

Table 8.3 Nine-step structured approach to diagnosing cardiac rhythm

Step	Rhythm characteristic assessed	Information obtained
1	Is there electrical activity?	There should recognizable P-QRST complexes. Absence of any electrical activity indicates that either patient is in asystole or equipment/interference problem exists (CHECK YOUR PATIENT)
2	Is the rhythm chaotic?	The electrical activity should be organized. Absence of recognizable 'organized' electrical activity indicates patient is in ventricular fibrillation or there is an equipment/interference problem
3	What is heart rate (QRS rate)?	The normal resting heart rate is between 60 and 100. Rates below or above this indicates the presence of bradycardia or tachycardia
4	Is the rhythm ('QRS') regular or irregular?	The 'rhythm' should be essentially regular (allowing for slight variation caused by inspiration and expiration) Possible causes of rhythm irregularity are: atrial ectopics ventricular ectopics AV node SA block atrial fibrillation atrial flutter
5	Are any P waves present?	There should be an upright P wave visible in lead II denoting normal atrial (SA node) pacemaker activation Absence of discernible P waves may indicate: junctional rhythm atrial fibrillation atrial flutter ventricular tachycardia
6	Is the 'P' wave upright (positive) in lead II?	Yes: indicates atrial depolarization from natural pacemaker (SA node) No: may indicate presence of: ectopic atrial rhythm junctional rhythm

Table 8.3 Nine-step structured approach to diagnosing cardiac rhythm (continued)

Step	Rhythm characteristic assessed	Information obtained
7	Is there a QRS for every P wave?	There should be a QRS complex after every P wave. Absence of a QRS following a P wave may indicate presence of: non-conducted atrial ectopics AV block
8	What is the P–R interval? Is it prolonged? Is it constant? Is it variable?	The normal P–R interval is between 120 and 200 ms This P–R interval should be analysed with the information gathered in question 7 Prolonged or highly variable P–R intervals may indicate presence and severity of AV block
9	What is the 'QRS' duration? Is it normal? Is it wide?	The normal QRS duration should be between 60 and 100 ms In the absence of bundle-branch block the width of the QRS complex indicates the origin of rhythm: < 120 ms: supraventricular (above the ventricles) > 120 ms: ventricular (tachycardia/bradycardia)

Calculating the heart rate

The heart rate corresponds with the electrical activation and contraction of the ventricles, which in turn corresponds to the QRS complexes seen on a cardiac rhythm strip or on the 12-lead ECG.

By counting the number of smaller or larger squares on the ECG paper, between the QRS complexes (R–R interval), and dividing this into 1500 or 300 we can calculate the heart rate per minute:

- One small square = 40 ms. Heart rate (HR) = 1500 divided by number of small squares between QRS complexes.
- One large square = 200 ms. HR = 300 divided by number of large squares between QRS complexes.
- Bradycardia means a slow heart rate of less than 60 beats/min.
- Tachycardia means a fast heart rate of more than 100 beats/min.
- The terms 'narrow complex tachycardia' and 'broad complex tachycardia' refer to the measured width of the QRS complex.
- QRS width < 120 ms = narrow complex tachycardia (Table 8.4).

- QRS width > 120 ms = broad complex tachycardia (Table 8.4).
- Remember the normal QRS duration = 60–100 ms.

Table 8.4 Examples of cardiac rhythms producing bradycardia, and narrow complex and broad complex tachycardia

Bradycardia	Narrow complex tachycardia	Broad complex tachycardia
Sinus Bradycardia	Sinus tachycardia	Ventricular tachycardia
Second- and third-degree atrioventricular block	Atrial tachycardia	Any tachycardia conducting with bundle-branch block
Ectopic atrial bradycardia	Atrial flutter	
Junctional bradycardia	Atrial fibrillation Re-entrant tachycardia	

In the addendum some algorithms of a systematic approach to cardiac rhythm interpretation are given, plus a series of figures of rhythm strips.

References

Goldberger AI, Goldberger E (1981) Clinical Electrocardiography: A simplified approach, 2nd edn. St Louis, MO: CV Mosby.

Hand H (2002) Common cardiac arrhythmias. Nursing Standard 16(28): 43–52.

Jacobson C (1995) Arrhythmias and conduction disturbances. In: Woods SL, Froelicher ESS, Halpenny CJ, Motzer SU (eds), Cardiac Nursing, 3rd edn. Philadelphia, PA: JB Lippincott, Chapter 20.

Lee J (2004) ECG monitoring in theatre: www.nda.ox.ac.uk/wfsa/html/u11/u1105_01.htm#card (accessed: 24/02/2004 and 30/06/2004).

Marriott HJL (1974) Workshop in Electrocardiography. Oldsmar, FL: Tampa Tracings.

Marriott HJL (1984) Practical Electrocardiography, 7th edn. Baltimore, MA: Williams & Wilkins.

Schamroth L (1985) An Introduction to Electrocardiography, 6th edn. Oxford: Blackwell Scientific.

Sheppard M, Wright M (2000) Principles and Practice of High Dependency Nursing. London: Baillière Tindall.

Thompson DR, Webster RA (1992) Caring for the Coronary Patient. Oxford: Butterworth Heinemann.

Addendum: Systematic approach to cardiac rhythm interpretation

Cardiac rhythm interpretation algorithm

In using these algorithms bear in mind that although they cover many of the more common arrhythmias, they are not intended to be exhaustive or claim to be completely 'foolproof'. They are intended to act as a guide for the student and practitioner developing interpretive skills.

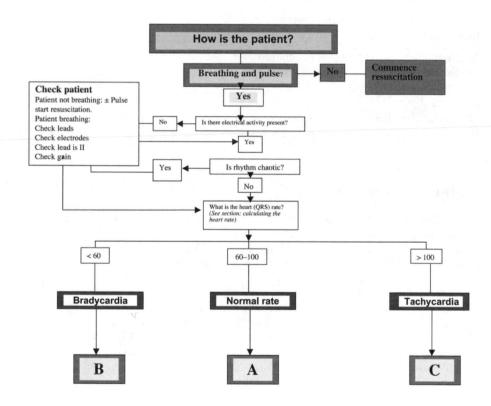

A   **Algorithm for heart rates > 60 – < 100**

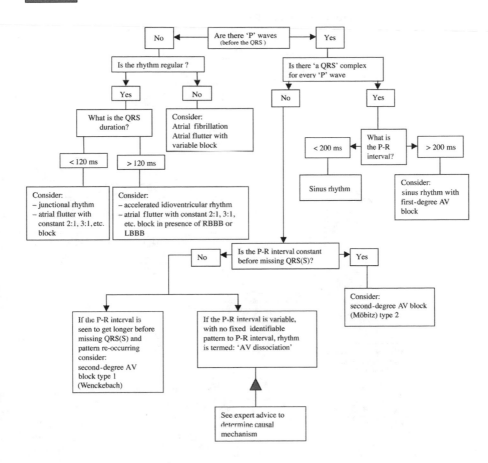

B   **Algorithm for heart rates < 60**

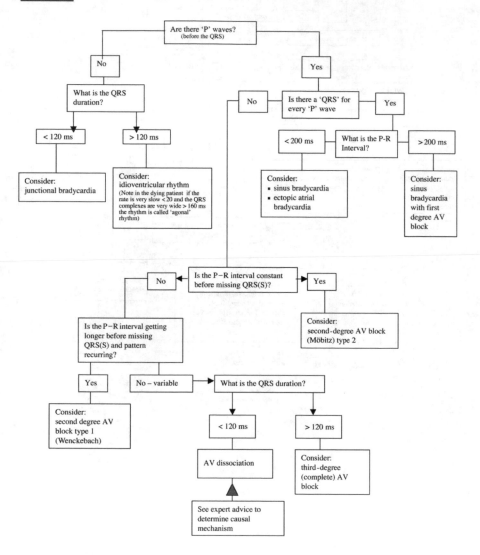

C   Algorithm for heart rates > 100

```
                    < 120 ms  ◄──  What is the QRS duration?  ──►  > 120 ms
```

Narrow complex tachycardia   **Broad complex tachycardia**

Is the rhythm regular?   Are there **clear** 'P' waves before **every** 'QRS'?

Yes   No   Yes   No

Are there 'P' waves present?   Is the baseline chaotic?

Yes   No   Yes   No

Are the 'P' waves upright in lead II?

Consider:
sinus tachycardia in presence of either right or left bundle-branch block
Seek expert advice

Is he rhythm regular?

Yes   No

Consider:
atrial fibrillation

Consider:
atrial flutter

SVT
Consider:
- **re-entrant tachycardia**
- **atrial flutter** (note 'saw-tooth' pattern of atrial flutter often mistaken for 'p' waves)

Treat as ventricular tachycardia (VT)
    Seek urgent medical review

If irregular consider:
AF with bundle branch block
  IF **ANY** DOUBT TREAT AS VT: SEEK EXPERT ADVICE

Consider:
- atrial tachycardia
- junctional tachycardia

Yes   No

What is the P R interval?

> 200 ms

Consider:
sinus tachycardia with first-degree AV block

< 200 ms

Consider:
sinus tachycardia

Sinus rhythm

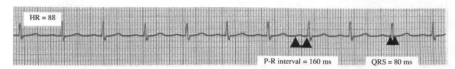

Key characteristics:

- ↪ HR: 60–100
- ↪ Rhythm: regular
- ↪ 'P' waves: visible
- ↪ 'P' wave for every 'QRS'
- ↪ P-R interval: constant
- ↪ P-R interval: 120–200 ms
- ↪ 'QRS': 60–100 ms (unless bundle-branch block present)

Sinus bradycardia

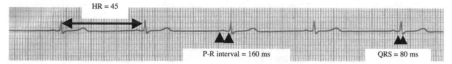

Key characteristics:

- ↪ HR: < 60
- ↪ Rhythm: regular
- ↪ 'P' waves: visible
- ↪ 'P' wave for every 'QRS'
- ↪ P-R interval: constant
- ↪ P-R interval: 120–200 ms
- ↪ 'QRS': 60–100 ms (unless bundle-branch block present)

Sinus tachycardia

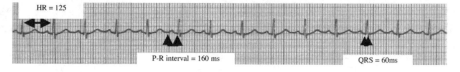

Key characteristics:

- ↪ HR: > 100
- ↪ Rhythm: regular
- ↪ 'P' waves: visible
- ↪ 'P' wave for every 'QRS'
- ↪ P-R interval: constant
- ↪ P-R interval: 120–200 ms
- ↪ 'QRS': 60–100 ms (unless bundle-branch block present)

First-degree AV block

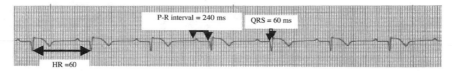

Key characteristics:

- ↳ H.R: as per underlying sinus rate
- ↳ Rhythm: regular
- ↳ 'P' waves: visible
- ↳ 'P' wave for every 'QRS'
- ↳ P-R interval: constant
- ↳ P-R interval: >200 ms
- ↳ 'QRS': 60–100 ms (unless bundle-branch block present)

Second-degree AV block (Möbitz type 1 – Wenckebach)

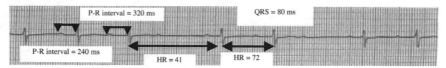

Key characteristics:

- ↳ HR: variable (caused by dropped beats)
- ↳ Rhythm: regularly irregular (caused by dropped beats)
- ↳ 'P' waves: visible
- ↳ Not a 'P' wave for every 'QRS
- ↳ P-R interval: not constant
- ↳ P-R interval: lengthing before dropped beat
- ↳ 'QRS': 60–100 ms (unless bundle-branch block present)

Second-degree AV block (Möbitz type 2)

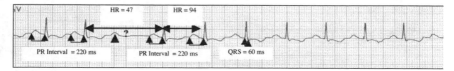

Key characteristics:

- ↳ HR: variable (caused by dropped beats)
- ↳ Rhythm: regularly or irregular (caused by dropped beats)
- ↳ 'P' waves: visible
- ↳ Not a 'P' wave for every 'QRS
- ↳ P-R interval: constant
- ↳ P-R interval: normal
- ↳ 'QRS': 60–100 ms (unless bundle-branch block present)

Third-degree AV block (complete heart block)

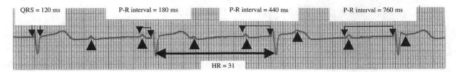

Key characteristics:

- ↦ HR: usually slow < 45
- ↦ Rhythm: regularly
- ↦ 'P' waves: visible
- ↦ 'P' waves 'QRS' complexes are not related to each other
- ↦ P-R interval: highly variable
- ↦ P-R interval: seen to be constantly changing
- ↦ 'QRS': > 120 ms as a result of ventricular origin of escape beat

Narrow complex tachycardia (SVT)

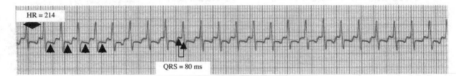

Key characteristics:

- ↦ HR: > 100 (often > 180)
- ↦ Rhythm: regularly
- ↦ 'P' waves: not readily visibly
- ↦ If 'P' waves not visible unable to determine 1:1 relationship
- ↦ P-R interval: indeterminable
- ↦ 'QRS': < 120 ms

Atrial flutter

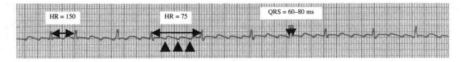

Key characteristics:

- ↦ HR: variable, sudden onset and uncontrolled atrial flutter often > 150
- ↦ Rhythm: can be regularly or irregular
- ↦ 'P' Waves: not readily visibly; 'saw-tooth' pattern – 'ff' waves
- ↦ P-R interval: indeterminable (no 'P' waves)
- ↦ 'QRS': < 120 ms (unless associated bundle-branch block present)

Atrial fibrillation

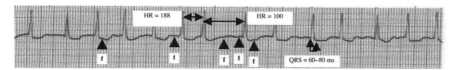

Key characteristics:

- ↪ HR: variable, sudden onset and uncontrolled atrial fibrillation often > 140
- ↪ Rhythm: irregularly irregular
- ↪ 'P' waves: not visible. Baseline 'chaotic' – 'FF' fibrillatory wave seen
- ↪ P-R interval: indeterminable (no 'P' waves)
- ↪ 'QRS': < 120 ms (unless associated bundle-branch block present)

Ventricular tachycardia

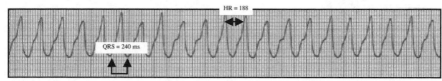

Key characteristics:

- ↪ HR: > 120
- ↪ Rhythm: regular
- ↪ 'P' waves: not readily visible. If seen they 'dissociate' from QRS
- ↪ P-R interval: indeterminable
- ↪ 'QRS': > 120ms

Idioventricular rhythm

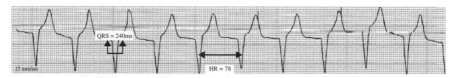

Key characteristics:

- ↪ HR: 50–110
- ↪ Rhythm: regular
- ↪ 'P' waves: not visible
- ↪ P-R interval: indeterminable (no 'P' waves)
- ↪ 'QRS': > 120 ms

Junctional rhythm

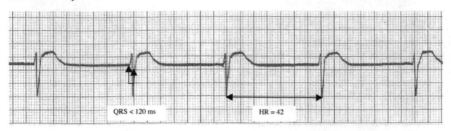

QRS < 120 ms

HR = 42

Key characteristics:

- ⮞ HR: 50-70
- ⮞ Rhythm: regular
- ⮞ 'P' waves: may not be not visible (if seen usually after or 'superimposed' on 'QRS')
- ⮞ P-R interval: indeterminable (no 'P' waves)
- ⮞ 'QRS': < 120 ms

CHAPTER NINE

Common investigations in the management of patients with coronary heart disease

GILL BLANCHARD AND IAN JONES

As part of the war against coronary heart disease (CHD), clinicians have a whole range of tests and investigations available to them to aid diagnosis and estimate prognosis. This chapter outlines the most common of these investigations and provides an introduction to their usage.

Biochemical markers for diagnosing CHD

For many years myocardial infarction (MI) has been diagnosed on the basis of clinical history, ECG changes, and elevation of cardiac enzymes or biochemical markers. The principle behind the monitoring of cardiac enzymes is a simple one. When there is myocardial damage, there is always a leakage of several particular intracellular enzymes through the damaged cell membrane, into the interstitial space. These are found in the circulating blood and are detectable by laboratory investigation (Hubbard 2002).

Creatine kinase

The primary function of this enzyme is energy production. Therefore, it is not surprising to find that there are higher concentrations of creatine kinase (CK) in the heart, skeletal muscle and brain (Hubbard 2002). As a result of this mass presentation, the detection of CK in circulating blood cannot always be attributed to myocardial damage, so CK is not regarded as cardiospecific. There are a number of isoenzymes that are more cardiac specific, including CK–myoglobin (CK-MB) (there are two types of assay: CK-MB protein is more specific and CK-MB activity is less specific but cheaper). CK-MB levels do not usually rise with angina, pulmonary embolism or heart failure. The advantages of using CK are that it can rule out an MI by producing a negative result and it is relatively inexpensive.

The rise in serum CK levels after MI peak between 12 and 24 h and remain elevated for 4–5 days. CK-MB levels are first detectable within 2–4 hours and peak at 6–12 h.

Lactate dehydrogenase

This enzyme is involved in the production of energy within a cell during periods of anaerobic metabolism. It is often used to support the diagnosis of acute MI made by CK-MB assay. It is quick and inexpensive to process. However, once again it is not cardiac specific and may be elevated in haemolysis, leukaemia, megaloblastic anaemia and renal disease (Woods et al. 1995). Lactate dehydrogenase (LDH) peaks in 24–48 h and remains elevated for 14 days. LDH is sometimes used in patients who present several days after experiencing pain.

Aspartate aminotransferase

This enzyme is found in the cytoplasm and mitochondria of all cells. There have been raised levels of aspartate aminotransferase (AST) found in 70% of patients who have had an MI (Hatchett and Thompson 2002). It is also inexpensive and quick. However, the enzyme is also elevated in liver disease, pulmonary embolism, skeletal muscle damage, shock and intramuscular injury. As a consequence it should not be relied on as a sole agent. AST levels peak between 24 and 36 h after infarction and remain elevated for 5 days.

Myoglobin

This is not strictly an enzyme and is not cardiospecific. The sensitivity of the test is poor and the process expensive, so it is not routinely used. However, elevation is noted between 1 and 2 h after infarction and some clinicians may request a myoglobin level if diagnosis is proving difficult in the early stages. Elevation peaks between 4 and 6 h and remains elevated for 1–2 days.

Troponin

The introduction of troponin testing was seen by many as a major breakthrough in the fight to become more cardiospecific. There are three types of cardiac troponins: troponins T, I and C, all of which are released into the bloodstream within 3 h, peaking at 12–24 h. Troponins I and T have similar efficacy (Maynard et al. 2000) and tend to be the most commonly used troponin test.

Troponin T

This is present in cardiac and skeletal muscle, but the cardiac type can be identified from those released by skeletal muscle. It is a highly sensitive marker, which has prognostic value in patients admitted with unstable angina as well as those with MI. It is cardiospecific and useful in ruling out an MI. It remains detectable for up to 14 days after the event. However, this could also be seen as a disadvantage, making it difficult to diagnose subsequent events. Troponin T is also of limited use in patients with renal impairment because it can often be elevated in the presence of uremia but as troponin is not found in healthy people a small increase indicates myocyte damage. However, it is expensive and difficult to perform.

Troponin I

This possesses many of the advantages of troponin T, but is very cardio-specific and not affected by non-cardiac factors. Similar to troponin T, it remains in the bloodstream up to 14 days after the event, but is expensive and therefore not always available in all hospitals.

Although troponin is of limited use in the first stages of assessment as a result of the time it takes to become elevated, it is of immense use when providing a diagnosis and stratifying the risk for the patient. An elevated troponin level is associated with a 30-day mortality rate almost three times the rate for patients with normal troponin levels. However, the use of troponin is not without problems. Troponin levels can be raised in patients with cardiac strain such as left ventricular dysfunction, pulmonary embolism and sepsis. The troponin value, based on which an MI is diagnosed, is also problematic, resulting in local variances.

Haematology

Full blood count

Haemoglobin
Coronary heart disease can be aggravated by the presence of anaemia. A low level of circulating haemoglobin leads to poor myocardial oxygenation and an increased heart rate, resulting in an imbalance between supply and demand causing chest pain. The presence of anaemia will need to be corrected.

White cell count

Although white cells may be raised 2–4 days after an acute MI the clinician needs to consider the possibility of infection. A white cell count (WCC) > 15 000/mm^3 is more likely to be a response to infection (Jowett and Thompson 2002) than infarction.

Platelets

These are usually normal in patients with CHD, but require close monitoring if the patient is to receive platelet inhibition after revasularization.

Biochemistry

Urea and electrolytes

Urea

Urea is a protein metabolite and is excreted from the body by the renal system. The presence of a high urea level can indicate dehydration. However, if the urea is elevated in the presence of an increased creatinine level, renal impairment should be suspected. The detection of renal impairment is crucial in patients undergoing angiography or intervention as a result of the nephrotoxicity of the contrast agent. In coronary care units this phenomenon is most often witnessed in hypotensive patients who have had cardiogenic shock as a result of hypoperfusion of the kidneys.

Potassium

Low levels of circulating potassium have been linked with a higher incidence of ventricular fibrillation in patients after an MI (Nordrehaug and Von der Lippe 1983). Despite 3.7 mmol being regarded as the lower level of the normal limit, a number of cardiologists advise that potassium levels be maintained above 4 mmol in the post-MI patient. Potassium levels can also be depleted quite quickly when receiving large doses of diuretics, so regular samples need to be taken to monitor potassium levels.

Magnesium

During the ISIS IV trial in 1995 the routine use of intravenous magnesium was not found to have any beneficial effect in patients after an MI. However, it is still believed that magnesium plays an important role in the prevention of arrhythmias. Although its routine use may not be particularly helpful, its use in patients with diuretic-induced hypomagnesaemia and hypokalaemia may still be worth considering (Connaughton 2001).

Sodium

Although sodium is vital for cardiac conduction it is frequently normal in cardiac patients.

Glucose

Patients with diabetes who present with acute coronary syndromes have a mortality rate almost twice as high as non-diabetic patients (McGuire et al. 2000). A high blood glucose on admission is also a prognostic indicator (Malmberg et al. 1997). The DIGAMI (Diabetes Mellitus, Insulin Glucose Infusion in Acute Myocardial Infarction) study (Malmberg 1997) showed that patients with a high blood glucose are best managed with intravenous insulin. The DIGAMI protocols have been adopted by most coronary care units and are used, with some local variations, for all patients with a blood sugar > 11 mmol. However, Jowett and Thompson (2003) argue that patients with a blood sugar > 9 mmol are more likely to experience complications than patients whose blood sugar is within normal limits.

Lipid profile

Cholesterol
There is little doubt that there is a correlation between high cholesterol levels (> 5 mmol) and the risk of CHD (Law et al. 1994). In high-risk groups such as patients with diabetes this level should be < 4.5 mmol. However, cholesterol levels are lowered 24 h after an acute MI, so a test should be obtained within those first 24 h of admission or left for at least 4 weeks (Carlson et al. 1995).

Although total cholesterol is a risk factor for CHD, the risk analysis becomes more accurate when considering the make-up of the total cholesterol. Cholesterol, similar to all lipids, is insoluble in water and so, to travel within the bloodstream, it is converted into water-soluble complexes called lipoproteins (Jowett and Thompson 2002). Explained in simple terms, there are two types of circulating cholesterol: high-density lipoproteins (HDLs) and low-density lipoproteins (LDLs). There is clear evidence to suggest that CHD risk increases with increased levels of circulating LDL-cholesterol. As a result, the European Society of Cardiology recommend that LDL-cholesterol should be < 3 mmol ((DeBacker et al. 2004). There is also a risk associated with low levels of HDL-cholesterol (< 1.05 mmol/l). Therefore the total cholesterol needs to be analysed to establish the ratio between HDL and LDL. The highest risk is associated with high levels of LDL and low levels of HDL.

Triglycerides
Triglycerides are another type of lipid which when elevated (> 1.7 mmol) are linked with an increased risk of CHD (DeBacker et al. 2004). However, treatment goals have not been defined for high triglyceride levels.

Echocardiography

Types of transthoracic echocardiography

This is a non-invasive tool that uses the velocity of sound, travelling through and then reflected from an acoustic interface, to provide an image of the heart and the surrounding structures. It is very useful for establishing a specific diagnosis and also in the estimation of severity, with no major risk to the patient. The usefulness of this tool relates to the quality of the images obtained from the individual. An air-free contact between the transducer and body wall is necessary. It is limited when used with patients who have chronic lung disease, chest deformities or morbid obesity.

M-mode echocardiography

This is a one-dimensional view (distance from the transducer versus time) of a cardiac structure, and was the original form of echocardiography. By using the changes of the cardiac structure over a cardiac cycle, i.e. mitral leaflet, it measures the distance between and the changes in distance to form a one-dimensional image. It is useful in depicting the size of the chambers, the thickness of the wall of the heart and the movement of the valves. There are some limitations because measurements are based on an assumption that the heart is positioned on the normal axis. Therefore, it should always be used together with the two-dimensional method.

Two-dimensional echocardiography

This uses a rapid movement of a one-dimensional ultrasonic beam across the heart to provide a real-time, cross-sectional image; therefore it has become the standard method.

Doppler echocardiography

This allows the measurement of intracardiac and intravascular flow, by detecting the changes in frequency of the ultrasound wave as it is emitted and received by the probe. As the ultrasound wave is emitted it hits moving red blood cells; the frequency of the ultrasound wave return is shifted in proportion to the velocity of the cells. The differences in the ultrasound waves are displayed as a function of time and direction of flow in relationship to the transducer. Flow mapping or colour Doppler is used to screen the heart flow in disturbances, such as those seen in valvular regurgitation and stenosis, or shunting as in atrial septal defects.

Transoesophageal echocardiography

Transoesophageal echocardiography (TOE) is a semi-invasive procedure that requires the placement of the ultrasound transducer into the oesophagus (similar to that of endoscopy), in close proximity to the heart. TOE can be done using a monoplane, biplane or multiplane. As a result of its invasive nature, it is a tool that should be used for specific indications rather than as a replacement for transthoracic echocardiography. It is mainly used for people with prosthetic valves because artefacts from the valve can create poor images in the standard method of M-mode or two-dimensional echocardiography, or if a specific structure, e.g. a left atrial appendage, needs reviewing and finally in patients who are not echogenic. The method is limited because patients need to swallow the probe and may therefore need sedation.

Stress echocardiography

This is a method of eliciting wall motion abnormalities as a result of inadequate myocardial perfusion. Although exercise was initially employed, currently pharmacological agents such as adenosine, dipyridamole and dobutamine are used to increase heart rate and blood pressure. It is mainly used where there is inclusive evidence of ischaemia. The test is not as expensive or as prolonged as a Myoview scan (see below), but it can promote allergic response to the pharmacological agents and is limited in the following:

• Patients with chronic lung disease, chest deformities or morbid obesity.
• Patients who have a history of an MI or acute coronary syndrome within 3 days of test should be avoided because of the risk of further events.

Although not contraindicated patients with known poor left ventricular function, broad complex tachycardia or ventricular tachycardia, it is not recommended.

Nuclear scans

MUGA (multi-gated acquisition)

This is a procedure that uses a radioactive substance, which tags itself to the red blood cells and then circulates through the body while a gamma camera records it. By taking pictures in both systole and diastole, they are able to compare and assess ventricular function. It is used in patients who are not echogenic, or who require assessment of ventricular function and transplantation assessment. However, it is more expensive than echocardiography, can promote allergic reaction, and is limited in people with chronic lung disease and not suitable for valvular information.

Myocardial perfusion imaging stress test (Myoview)

By injecting a radio-isotope (Cardiolite or Myoview), this investigation can demonstrate ischaemia by analysing the uptake of tracer by the heart muscle. Normal muscle will have a bigger uptake than that supplied by a narrowed artery. In other words, areas of the heart that have an adequate blood supply will quickly pick up the tracer whereas those vessels with reduced blood flow pick the tracer up slowly or not at all. By studying the images (taken by gamma camera) of the heart, it is possible to identify the location, severity and extent of the reduction in blood flow. This investigation requires the patient to be prepared adequately; they need to refrain from eating, smoking or drinking caffeine 4 h before the procedure. The test is usually performed for patients who are unable to undertake a cardiac exercise test or in whom the results are equivocal, for patients who have had a previous Myoview scan for comparison and to provide evidence of reversible ischaemia in patients. However, it is an expensive and prolonged (at least 3 h) procedure.

Cardiac exercise (stress) test

Exercise capacity is a strong predictor of outcome; in the last 50 years the cornerstone of diagnostic procedures for CHD has been the use of a graded exercise test. This is a non-invasive, relatively inexpensive tool, which can provide a wealth of clinically relevant diagnostic and prognostic information.

Indications

This test should be performed only when a specific question needs answering that has specific implications for the future clinical management. It is therefore a useful tool for confirmation of a diagnosis, establishing prognosis or finally as a baseline for rehabilitation or other physical activities:

- For the diagnosis of coronary artery disease in patients with suspected episodes of myocardial ischaemia
- For assessing functional capacity before cardiac rehabilitation.
- For evaluation of patients with variant angina pectoris.
- For evaluation of exercise tolerance and effects of medical therapy in patients with coronary artery disease or pump failure.
- For evaluation of patients with symptoms suggesting exercise-induced arrhythmias.
- For evaluation of asymptomatic people with specific professions (pilots, police, heavy goods vehicle/passenger-carrying vehicle [HGV/PCV] drivers).

Contraindications

The following conditions are absolutely contraindicated for exercise testing:

• unstable angina pectoris (chest pain at rest within 48 h)
• during the initial phase of an acute MI
• evident heart failure
• acute myocarditis
• recent pulmonary or systemic embolism or thrombosis
• severe aortic stenosis
• severe hypertrophic obstructive cardiomyopathy.

Preparation

Although there are no real preparations, it is ideal to stop β blockers for at least 48 h before procedure.

Interpretation

This traditionally is based on observation during excrise (Table 9.1).

Table 9.1 Diagnostic and prognostic variables during exercise or recovery

Observations during exercise

Maximal exercise capacity
ST-segment depression
ST-segment elevation
Angina pectoris
Inadequate blood pressure response
Inadequate heart rate response
Ventricular arrhythmia

Observations during recovery

ST-segment depression
Delayed slowing of heart rate
Ventricular arrhythmia

Angiography

For details of angiography, see page 233.

References

Carlson R, Lindberg G, Westin L et al. (1995) Serum lipids four weeks after acute myocardial infarction are a valid basis for lipid lowering intervention in patients receiving thrombolysis. Br Heart J 74: 18–20.

Connaughton M (2001) Evidence-based Coronary Care. London: Churchill Livingstone.

DeBacker G, Ambrosioni E, Borch-Johnsen K et al. (2004) European Guidelines on CVD Prevention in Clinical Practice. Third Joint Task Force of European and other Societies on Cardiovascular Disease Prevention in Clinical Practice. Atherosclerosis 173: 381–91.

Hatchett R, Thompson D (2002) Cardiac Nursing. A comprehensive guide. London: Churchill Livingstone.

Hubbard J (2002) The case of the man with myocardial infarction. In: Clancy, J Mc Vicar, A. (eds) Physiology and Anatomy. A homeostatic approach. London: Arnold.

ISIS 4 (1995) A randomized factorial trial assessing early oral captopril, oral mononitrate and intravenous magnesium sulphate in 58,050 patients with suspected acute myocardial infarction. Lancet 345: 669–85.

Jowett N, Thompson DR (2002) Comprehensive Coronary Care, 3rd edn. London: Baillière Tindall.

Law MR, Wald NJ, Wu T, Hackshaw A, Bailey A (1994) systematic under estimation of association between serum cholesterol and ischaemic heart disease in observational studies: data from the BUPA study. BMJ 308: 937–80.

McGuire DK, Emanuelsson H, Granger CB et al. (2000) Influence of diabetes mellitus on clinical outcomes across the spectrum of acute coronary syndromes. Findings from the GUSTO IIb study. Eur Heart J 21: 1750–8.

Malmberg K, Norhammar A, Wedel H, Rydén L (1997) Glycometabolic state at admission: important risk marker of mortality in conventionally treated patients with diabetes mellitus and acute myocardial infarction. Long-term results from the Diabetes and Insulin-Glucose Infusion in Acute Myocardial Infarction (DIGAMI) Study. Circulation 99: 2626–32.

Maynard SJ, Menown IBA, Adgey AAJ (2000) Troponin T or Troponin I as cardiac markers in ischaemic heart disease. Heart 83: 371–3.

Nordrehaug JE, Von der Lippe G (1983) Hypokalaemia and ventricular fibrillation in acute myocardial infarction. Br Heart J 50: 525–9.

Woods SL, Froelicher ESS, Adams Motzer SA (1995) Cardiac Nursing. Philadelphia, PA: Lippincott.

CHAPTER TEN

Cardiac intervention

GILL BLANCHARD, JAN KEENAN AND IAN JONES

Although coronary heart disease remains incurable, a number of therapies have been found to have a beneficial effect on quality of life and mortality. This chapter provides an overview of some of the interventions that are currently used in the battle against heart disease.

Cardiac catheterization and angiocardiography

In conjunction with other investigations cardiac catheterization is a gold standard invasive procedure which can establish a precise diagnosis. During the procedure the operator is able to:

- record pressure within the heart and the great vessels
- delineate the anatomy and functions so abnormalities can be seen.
- carry out the sampling of blood for gases so as to define the shunting of oxygenated blood
- allow for biopsy of the pericardium
- assess coronary flow.

The technique and procedures have remained similar to those of its forefathers (Sones 1959), but the recent refinements in technology have now meant that the procedure is normally performed as a day case, although there are some clinical reasons that may necessitate longer admission, e.g. severe disease, clinical instability or after intraoperative complications.

Venous and arterial sheaths have become standard kit (Figure 10.1), which has made access to the artery much easier, without sustaining massive blood loss. In addition the modern radiological equipment has allowed for smaller radiation doses and reduction in catheter diameter; this also means that they have been able to reduce the amount of contrast agent. All of these have helped in reducing recovery time. The procedure is usually done under local anaesthetic, although sedation can be given if necessary.

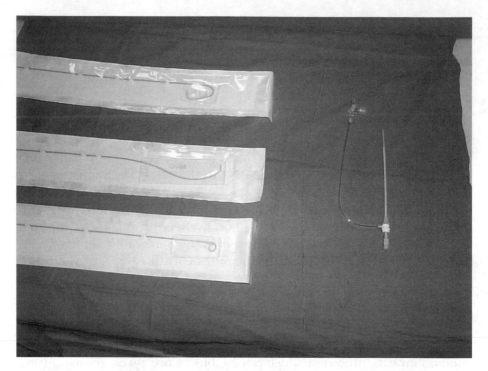

Figure 10.1 Cardiac catheter and introducer sheath: a femoral sheath, pigtail, and left and right Judkin's catheter.

Right heart catheterization

This uses the basilic, saphenous or femoral vein via a percutaneous stab or cut-down. The catheter is advanced up in to the right atrium, under fluoroscopic control (radiological guidance); this is then manipulated through the tricuspid valve into the right ventricle and out into the pulmonary artery, and from there it is wedged in the distal pulmonary artery. The pulmonary artery wedge (pulmonary capillary) pressure is an indirect measurement of the left atrial pressure and left ventricular end-diastolic pressure.

As the catheter is withdrawn from the pulmonary artery blood samples are obtained from each vessel and chamber. If there is a left-to-right shunt presence, the blood samples taken are found to be more oxygenated in the affected chamber and beyond than those from the great veins.

- Persistent ductus arteriosus (PDA): O_2 saturation in left pulmonary artery is higher than that in right ventricle.
- Ventricular septal defect (VSD): O_2 saturation in right ventricle and pulmonary artery is higher than in the right atrium.
- Atrial septal defect (ASD): O_2 saturation is higher than in the superior and inferior venae cavae.

As for all the blood samples, pressures are recorded as the catheter is withdrawn, and can demonstrate valve stenosis:

- Pulmonary stenosis is confirmed by demonstrating a systolic pressure difference between the pulmonary artery and right ventricle.
- Tricuspid stenosis is confirmed when the diastolic pressure is higher in the right atrium than in the right ventricle.

Left heart catheterization

This uses the femoral, radial or brachial artery. The catheter is advanced retrogradely up the aorta, until it reaches the aortic valve. It then can be manipulated across the valve into the left ventricle. Left heart catheterization is used for the following:

- Aortic stenosis: assessed by the pressure difference between the left ventricle and the aorta. In subaortic stenosis or hypertrophic obstructive cardiomyopathy (HOCM), the pressure drop lies within the cavity.
- Mitral stenosis: defined by the pressure difference between the pulmonary wedge and the left ventricle.

Angiocardiography

By injecting a non-ionic contrast medium it is possible to demonstrate the anatomy of the chambers of both the left and right heart, the coronaries and the great arteries, and also to observe the patterns of blood flow through the heart. This is achieved by revolving an image intensifier and camera which is positioned on a 'C' arm gantry around the patient's chest, as they lie on a radiolucent table. The injection of contrast medium is given either by a high-pressure infuser (ventricles, aorta or great vessels) or by hand injection (coronaries).

As the heart is a very mobile organ it requires a recording that is sufficient to produce a sequential image to rule out any motion artefact, so either a digitalized or a cine format is normally used. Figure 10.2 shows a cardiac catheter laboratory.

Appropriate injection site for definition of alleged abnormality

- VSD and mitral regurgitation: the site for injection is the left ventricle.
- Aortic valve disease: the site is the aorta.
- Coronary disease requires the operator to inject selectively into both left and right coronaries. To allow for the marked tortuosity of the coronary arteries and their multiple branch points, and the frequent eccentric nature of coronary stenoses, it requires multiple projections of each coronary.

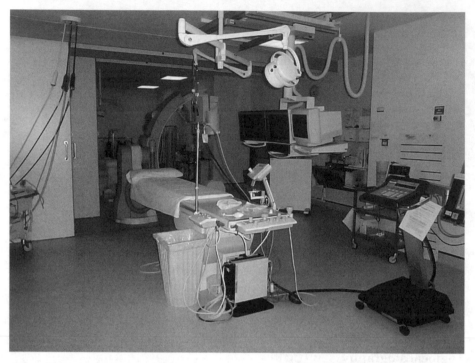

Figure 10.2 Cardiac catheter laboratory.

Clinical risks

This procedure is generally safe but as with all invasive procedures there are inherent risks (Gershlick 2002):

- Myocardial infarction (about 0.1%)
- Cerebrovascular accident (about 0.1–0.2% transient; 0.1% permanent)
- Arrhythmia (ventricular fibrillation in about 0.4% of all cases) or conduction disturbance (complete heart block in about 0.3% of cases)
- Vasovagal reactions
- Allergic reaction
- Peripheral complications including haematoma, pseudoaneurysm or fistula
- Nephrotoxicity
- Pulmonary embolism during right heart catheter
- Tamponade.

Of course these risks are more intrinsic in the sicker patient, e.g. the relative risk of a patient with left main stem disease is increased 20-fold more than for someone without.

Preparations

- Anxiety: this is natural but can be allayed by previous preparation and explanation, combined with a sedative if necessary.
- Blood tests:
  - urea and electrolytes: as a result of the nephrotoxicity of the contrast agent and the susceptibility of the myocardium to imbalances in potassium
  - full blood count: as a baseline for the operator.
- ECG: this provides the baseline for comparing against.
- Allergies: all allergies should be recorded but the most important to the operator is iodine because the contrast agent is an ionic preparation.
- Anticoagulation: should either be discontinued a few days before to allow for normal coagulation to occur or be changed to a heparin substitute, dependent on the need for anticoagulation. This needs to be discussed with the operator.
- Nil by mouth: although a general anaesthetic is not being used, it is preferable to refrain the patient from eating and drinking for a few hours before the procedure; because of the risk of inhalation an arrhythmia could occur.
- Pulses: evidence of peripheral vascular disease or absent pulses should be noted before the procedure.

Percutaneous coronary intervention

Balloon angioplasty (Gruntzig et al. 1979) has been around for the last 20 years and is the original non-surgical method of coronary revascularization in patients with angina that had been unresponsive to medical treatment, whether it be stable or unstable angina. Through the development of the balloon angioplasty other major developments have evolved from atherectomy, intravascular ultrasonography to intercoronary laser, and are now brought together under a heading of percutaneous coronary intervention (PCI). The major development to come out of the percutaneous transluminal coronary angioplasty (PTCA) is the stent, which has gone through numerous evolutionary changes until eventually in 2000 it became of age after the endorsement for use of stents in routine practice by the National Institute for Clinical Excellence (NICE 2000).

Coronary angioplasty

After angiography a PTCA requires a balloon catheter to be passed to the site of the coronary stenosis and inflated, under fluoroscopic control

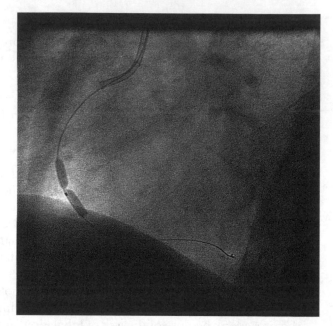

Figure 10.3 Coronary angioplasty: right coronary artery with the balloon inflated at the stenosis, This is demonstrated by the waisting in the middle of the balloon.

(Figure 10.3). This crude mechanism has five ways of improving the haemodynamics of the coronary:

1. plaque compression
2. plaque fracture
3. stretching of the plaque-free wall segment in eccentric lesions
4. stretching of the vessel wall without plaque compression
5. medial dissection.

Although the most important mechanism for improving the flow appears to be the rupture and dehiscence of the plaque, this results in numerous fissures forming and the emergence of blood-filled channels. The procedural success is a combination of the above mechanism, but is also related to the geometry of the vessel lumen which is determined by the resultant re-modelling of the vessel wall.

Limitations of procedure

- Abrupt vessel closure, occurring in the catheter or within the first 24 h. Path physiology behind this is (1) dissection (80%) of vessel wall, (2) thrombus formation (20%) and (3) coronary spasm. This has been associated with death in 0–8% and MI in 11–54% of cases. Previously > 20% of all patients with abrupt vessel closure were referred for emergency coronary artery bypass graft (CABG).

- Re-stenosis, which is defined as > 50% diameter stenosis at follow-up angiography, has been the single long-term limitation of this procedure, with an occurrence of 30–50% and a need for the target vessel to be revascularized in 20–30% of all patients. This does not occur until 4–6 months after the procedure and does not always cause further symptoms (Windecker and Meier 2002).

The RITA-1 (Henderson 1989) trial data compared single and multivessel disease that was considered suitable for PTCA or CABG. The results showed that the early mortality was similar but the 6-month data demonstrated that those randomized to PTCA had a greater need for re-intervention (38% versus 11% for surgery). This supported previous published observational data, which reported a re-stenosis rate in the PTCA patient of 40%. Although the 2-year follow-up data from the RITA trial demonstrated that the angina rate for PTCA had not changed dramatically (31% versus 32% at 6 months), it had risen in the surgical group from 11% to 22%.

Although over time there is a possible equalization of outcomes, PTCA alone remained an unsatisfactory treatment compared with surgery, as a result of the high incidence of further intervention in the first year (33.7 versus 3.3% requiring repeat surgery).

Coronary artery stents

As demonstrated in the RITA trial, there were two major limitations of PTCA in the short term. The high-pressure balloon inflations of PTCA induce a 'controlled plaque disruption' which at times can become uncontrolled, leading to abrupt closure, within the first 24 h.

Coronary artery stents have been developed as an important adjunct to balloon angioplasty and were endorsed in 2000 by the NICE. Their dual function of reducing acute complications and the long-term effect of re-stenosis has meant that the technique has now become an accepted treatment, challenging the surgical method of CABG.

The coronary angioplasty balloon catheter has evolved from a therapeutic tool to that of a complementary instrument that delivers the stent to the site. There are numerous varieties of stents on the market (Figure 10.4), although the basic principle underlying them remains the same. By scaffolding the vessel wall and tagging the intimal flaps between the stent and the vessel wall, sealing dissections, an effect of increasing the arterial lumen van be attained.

Re-stenosis after balloon angioplasty is centred on the neointimal (smooth muscle) response. Although at present there have not been any clinical drug trials that have shown any impact on smooth muscle hyperplasia, the impact of stents on the mechanical issues surrounding re-stenosis has been shown. This is a result of the luminal diameter gained when using a stent. The prevention of elastic recoil in conjunction with the

(a)

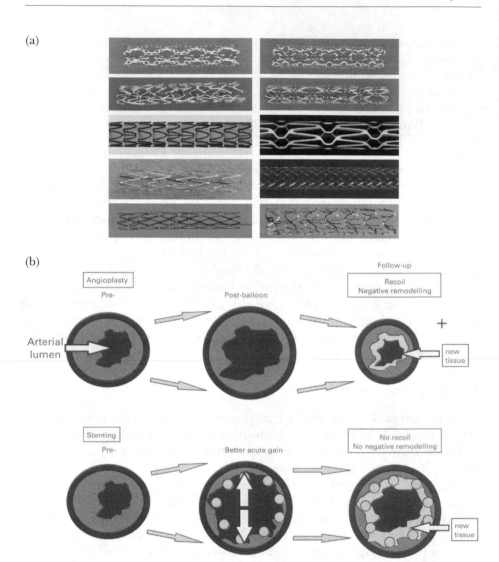

(b)

Figure 10.4 Role of stenting in coronary revascularization: (a) metal stents; (b) stents improve outcome by improving the acute gain and reducing recoil and negative re-modelling, although tissue growth is not affected and may even be greater with stents than with balloon angioplasty. Even so, the eventual lumen diameter is still larger after stenting. Reproduced with permission from Mills: Education in Heart Vol2:001, Blackwell Publishing.

negative re-modelling of the artery has been suggested by clinical data (Windecker and Meier 2002) to have reduced the risk of re-stenosis from 35% in PTCA to 15–20%.

Indications

The indication for PCI has grown over the last two decades and now no absolute contraindications remain, although single vessel coronary artery disease remains the main indicator (Table 10.1).

Table 10.1 Clinical and angiographic indications for percutaneous coronary intervention

Clinical indications	Angiographic indications
Angina pectoris • De novo angina pectoris • Stable angina pectoris • Unstable angina pectoris • Recurrent angina pectoris • After PCI (re-stenosis) • After CABG (graft attrition)	One to four lesions amenable to PCI • Not immediately life threatening • Vessel diameter > 2.5 mm • Lesion(s) subtending function, viable or collateral-dependent myocardium
Angina equivalent • Arrhythmias, sudden death survivors • Dyspnoea • Dizziness	Angiographic contraindications (relative) • Left main stenosis (except: protected by graft or collaterals, ideal lesions, inoperable patients)
Myocardial infarction • Acute myocardial infarction (primary PCI) • Post-infarct angina pectoris • Rescue PTCA (failed thrombolysis, cardiogenic shock)	Left main equivalent stenoses (exceptions: staged procedure, ideal lesions, inoperable patients) Lesion characteristics
Objective signs of reversible ischaemia • Resting ischaemia • Exercise-induced ischaemia	Chronic total occlusion • No collaterals to distal artery • Long and old • No stump
Clinical contraindications • Rapidly terminal cardiac or other systemic disease	• Extensive bridging collaterals • Thrombotic stenosis with non-significant underlying lesion • Diffusely diseased small-calibre native coronary artery

CABG, coronary artery bypass graft; PCI, percutaneous coronary intervention; PTCA, percutaneous transluminal coronary angioplasty.

There is no upper age limit to the applicability of PCI but there is a general shift in favour of PCI compared with CABG in elderly people, as a result of the higher perioperative morbidity and mortality in this group of patients with surgery.

Preparations

- As for angiocardiography with additional concentration on full blood count.
- Evidence of thrombocytopenia: operator should be aware of this because of the aggressive anti-platelet therapy.

Adjunctive pharmacological treatment

The therapeutic effect of PCI is accompanied by various degrees of arterial injury, with contact with all the thrombogenic agents causing platelet adhesion and aggregation, which may result in an intracoronary thrombus. The central treatment in all interventional investigations has been inhibition of platelets and the coagulation system. The following pharmacological therapies may be used to inhibit this effect.

Anticoagulation

Heparin
This is routinely used during the procedure although there is no general consensus around the issue of optimal dosage. Various studies have demonstrated the safety and efficacy of using low-dose heparin (5000 IU) through the procedure, although none has demonstrated any benefit of continuous heparin after the procedure.

Without increasing the risk of ischaemic complications, the low-dose heparin approach offers the advantage of lower incidence of bleeding complications, faster sheath removal and shorter hospitalization.

Direct thrombin inhibitors
These include hirulog, hirudin and argatroban. Although they have a lower incident of bleeding complications, the therapeutic effect is modest, so it is reserved for patients with adverse reactions to heparin.

Vitamin K antagonists
In the beginning coumarin derivatives were given alongside full-dose heparin, aspirin and dipyridamole as thromboprophylaxis. Various clinical trials established the superiority of an anti-platelet treatment over oral anticoagulation. The clinical benefit weighed against the reduction

in hospital stay has meant that this is not standard pharmacological treatment.

Antiplatelet

Aspirin
In the Montreal heart study it was demonstrated that aspirin and dipyridamole were beneficial in preventing peri-procedural ST-elevation MI, although in further studies the benefit of dipyridamole over aspirin has not been proved.

Low-dose aspirin (75–325 mg) is now recommended to all patients undergoing PCI, preferably started the day before procedure.

Thienopyridines
Ticlopidine and clopidogrel are the two thienopyridine derivatives used. They act by inhibiting platelet function independently of aspirin, through blockage of the ADP receptor. The understanding of the pathophysiological mechanism of stent thrombosis comes from the platelets rather than an abnormality in the coagulation activation. There have been numerous trials comparing the safety and efficacy of ticlopidine with clopidogrel, which demonstrated no difference in the rates of stent thrombosis or other major adverse cardiac events at 1 month, although the CLASSIC trial (Clopidogrel Aspirin Stent International Cooperative – Bertrand et al. 2000), which compared the two drugs, indicated a much superior safety profile with clopidogrel. There was a significantly reduced combined end point of major bleeding complications, neutropenia and thrombocytopenia, which has made clopidogrel the choice of thienopyridine.

A loading dose of 300 mg is preferably given 12 h before the procedure, and then a regimen of 75 mg is instigated for at least 28 days.

Glycoprotein IIb/IIIa inhibitors
These include abciximab (monoclonal antibody), eptifibatide (peptide molecule) and tirofibran (non-peptide molecule).

Platelet activation has numerous components, but the precondition for thrombus is the common pathway mediated by the platelet glycoprotein GPIIb/IIIa receptor. Therapeutic targets in the prevention of largely platelet-mediated ischaemic complications are to block these receptors. Although all the trials demonstrated, consistently across the board, the benefits in the reduction of early death, non-fatal MI and urgent revascularization, abciximab was the only preparation to show long-term protection. It is administered as a weight-adjusted bolus followed by an infusion over 12 h.

The contraindications are neutropenia and thrombocytopenia.

Pacemakers

Temporary pacemakers

The need for temporary pacing appears to have reduced since the advent of thrombolysis, but there are still times when patients present with conduction problems that require urgent pacemaker insertion.

What are pacemakers?

In essence a pacemaker is a device that produces electricity and transmits this energy into the heart to generate a heart beat. All pacemakers, regardless of their complexity are made up of a battery-powered generator that produces the electrical charge and a lead or leads that transmit this charge into a chamber or chambers of the heart to produce a heart beat.

Indications

There are a number of indications for temporary pacing (see box) but they all tend to centre on either the failure to generate an impulse or the inability to transmit the impulse to the ventricles. The insertion of a temporary pacemaker is not a simple procedure to the uninitiated and should be avoided unless it is absolutely necessary or specialist help is available. Connaughton et al. (1998) found that insertion of temporary pacemakers has a high complication rate if inserted by non-specialists or inexperienced staff.

Indications for temporary pacing

Anterior myocardial infarction (MI) with second or complete heart block or trifascicular block

Inferior MI with any of the above where the patient is compromised (BP < 90 mmHg)

Prophylaxis during surgery where the patient is at risk of conduction problems

Sick sinus syndrome

Treatment of tachycardia (the patient is paced in excess of the current tachycardia in order to establish control of the heart rate; once established the pacing rate is gradually reduced)

Patients with inferior MI often present with some degree of heart block caused by ischaemia of the atrioventricular (AV) node. However, this frequently resolves spontaneously when re-perfusion occurs. Unfortunately the presence of heart block in patients with anterior MI is often the result of necrosis of the bundle of His and the bundle branches; this effect also reduces the likelihood of an adequate ventricular escape rhythm. Therefore, asystole is far more likely and the need for pacing is increased.

Artificial cardiac pacing can be achieved by several methods including transcutaneous, transvenous and epicardial ones. The last is more likely to be reserved for patients undergoing some forms of cardiac surgery and therefore the average nurse is unlikely to care for patients following this approach. However, the former examples are reasonably common in most district general hospitals.

Transcutaneous pacing tends to be reserved for patients who undergo cardiac arrest or who are at risk of doing so. The approach is performed by attaching specially produced pacing/monitoring pads with connecting cable to the patient's chest and connecting the opposite end of the cable to a pacing machine. In modern units this machine is often part of the defibrillator, which allows the pads to be used for pacing and defibrillation if required. Once connected, the machine is able to transmit electricity down the cable into the pads across the patient's skin and into the heart. This will, it is hoped, produce enough electricity to produce a heart beat. Although these machines are invaluable, the small electric shocks that the patient experiences can be uncomfortable and distressing, so transcutaneous pacing should be time limited.

Transvenous pacing

Transvenous pacing tends to be the approach with which most health professionals will be familiar. This procedure involves a member of the medical staff accessing a patient's major vein and aseptically introducing a pacing wire. The choice of vein is dependent on a number of factors, which are highlighted in the box. The wire is then advanced ideally under radiological supervision, predominantly into the right ventricle, and anchored into its apex, although insertion into the right atrium would be more appropriate for patients with problems of the sinoatrial node. This procedure should be carried out in a room that caters for this type of procedure and performed by a suitably qualified health professional. The patient should be connected to a cardiac monitor for the whole of the procedure and should be cared for by a nurse who is able to identify the main cardiac arrhythmias.

Choice of vein

Brachial: appropriate for the inexperienced

Jugular: direct access into the right ventricle

Subclavian: more hazardous as a result of the risk of pneumothorax

Femoral: higher risk of infection, restricts the patient, but more appropriate for the inexperienced

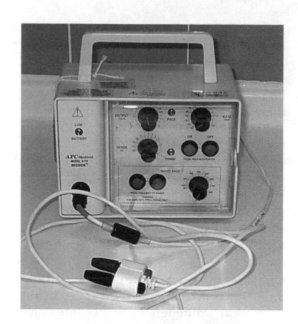

Figure 10.5 Temporary pacing box.

Once the wire is in place the proximal end is connected to a temporary pacing box (Figure 10.5), which is capable of transmitting a set amount of electricity along the pacing wire. The nurse will often carry out this procedure and set the box to transmit the desired output. Once enough electricity is produced, a paced heart beat will be seen on the cardiac monitor. The minimum amount of electricity required to produce the heart beat is termed the 'pacemaker threshold'. This threshold will often rise as the days go by and so the actual amount of electricity used for each beat is often double that of the threshold, allowing for some increase. As a result of this inevitable rise, the threshold should be checked daily. The box should also have the pacemaker setting adjusted according to the patient's condition. This pacemaker can be set to produce electrical charges and therefore beats at a desired fixed rate, e.g. 80/min, or can be adjusted to act only when the patient's own heart fails to beat. These two settings are termed 'fixed rate' or 'demand pacing'.

Following the procedure a chest radiograph should be obtained to serve as a record of the position of the pacing wire, to rule out pneumothorax and to provide a more accurate method of assessing the position of the wire.

Nursing care

Care plan for patient with temporary pacemaker *in situ*

Potential problem	The patient has a temporary pacemaker wire *in situ* and therefore at risk of developing complications

of arrhythmia, infection, displacement of pacing wire and equipment malfunction

Goal   To maintain and improve cardiac output and maintain patient safety

Nursing intervention

- Provide the patient with an explanation of the need for temporary pacing and provide reassurance
- Ensure all equipment used has been recently checked by medical electronics
- Record clinical observations (blood pressure, temperature (at least 4 hourly), pulse and respiration) as patient condition dictates
- Continue cardiac monitoring observing for signs of pacemaker malfunction (failing to sense or capture)
- Ensure pacemaker threshold is checked at least daily by a competent clinician
- Observe pacemaker site for signs of infection, bleeding or pain
- Dress site as required with a clear sterile dressing
- Assist the patient with any activities of daily living that may be compromised due to their condition
- Ensure safety of pacing box and accessibility of connections at all times

As well as the above the nurse should ensure that the pacing box itself remains safe and with the wires secure and visible, and accessible in case of disconnection.

Complications

There are a number of complications that can occur after insertion of a pacemaker (see box); probably the most common are those related to pacemaker activity. Failure of the pacemaker to sense occurs when it is unable to detect the patient's own heart beat and attempts to produce a beat of its own. This can be dangerous if the artificial beat occurs during the recovery phase of the patient's own heart beat. The pacemaker sensitivity settings may have to be adjusted.

Failure to pace is just that – the pacemaker is unable to produce a heart beat. This can be a result of the output being generated by the pacemaker being below threshold. In simple terms, if the pacemaker is set with an output of 2 V (2 V are discharged every time it wants the heart to beat), but the threshold is 2.1 V (the amount of electricity needed to produce a beat), then the heart will not beat. Additional problems can be related to the lead placement or more probably the movement of the wire in the ventricle. This may mean that the doctor has to reposition the wire in the right ventricle.

However, whenever a temporary pacemaker is not pacing as it should it is worth checking that the leads are connected to the pacing box and have not become dislodged. If a patient becomes dependent on the pacing box, disconnection can be fatal as a result of the lack of a heart beat. It is also good practice to ensure that a back-up pacing box is available in case the batteries in the first box fail or it malfunctions in some way.

Complications after insertion of a pacemaker

Failure to sense	Oversensitivity
Failure to pace	Proarrhythmic
Infection	Diaphragmatic twitch
Ruptured septum	Haemopericardium
Pneumothorax	

Permanent pacemakers

The principles of permanent pacing are similar to those of temporary pacing. However, instead of the wire exiting the body and connecting to a generator at the bedside, the permanent pacing wire connects to a generator implanted in the chest wall.

Indications for permanent pacing

Chronic complete heart block or after an anterior MI
Atrial fibrillation with slow ventricular response
Sick sinus syndrome
Vagovagal syncope
Carotid sinus syndrome
Tilt-positive patients
Heart failure

Different types

Permanent pacemakers are often described by their mode of action, which refers to the chamber of the heart in which the system is able to pace and sense. Some patients will have a pacing wire in their atria, which stimulates atrial contraction. This impulse is then transmitted to the ventricles in the normal way. However, the presence of AV node disease or necrosis will inhibit this effect. In these cases patients may require a lead in both the atrium and the ventricle, the first stimulating the atrium and the second stimulating the ventricle after a given time delay.

There are a whole host of combinations possible which makes it necessary to have a standard coding for all permanent pacemakers (Bernstein et al. 1987) (Table 10.2). The first two codes relate to the chamber paced and chamber sensed, and the third relates to the response of the pacemaker when a beat is sensed. Some texts will describe five functions of a pacemaker, including anti-tachycardia and programmable functions, but in

Table 10.2 Pacemaker codes

Chamber sensed	Chamber paced	Mode of response
Ventricle (V)	Ventricle (V)	Triggered (T)
Atria (A)	Atria (A)	Inhibited (I)
Dual (D)	Dual (D)	Dual (D)
None (0)	None (0)	None (0)

reality these functions are often omitted.

In the system in Table 10.1 atrial pacing would be classed as AAI, ventricular pacing would be referred to as VVI, and a system that is able to sense and pace both atria and ventricles would be referred to as DDD.

The procedure for implantation

Implantation of a permanent pacemaker is almost always carried out as a routine procedure, so it is much less fraught than temporary insertion. The patient is admitted for an overnight stay and, after receiving prophylactic antibiotics and the usual preoperative screening and care (fasting is required for only 2–4 h), is transferred to either a pacing room on the coronary care unit or theatre to undergo the procedure. The procedure itself is carried out under local anaesthetic and the patient is encouraged to inform the nurse if he or she develops light-headedness, breathlessness or chest pain. An electrode is introduced via either the subclavian or the cephalic vein, and the wire is progressed towards the chosen chamber under fluoroscopy. Once in position the generator box is attached and pacing is attempted. In addition, the threshold is checked. Ideally the lowest threshold possible is sought to preserve battery life. The battery will last about 8 years but may last longer if a smaller amount of electricity is required for each beat. The threshold will rise over the following days as a result of a number of factors, including tissue oedema surrounding the pacing wire tip (Kay 1996).

Once all tests have been completed satisfactorily, a pouch in the chest wall is made for the generator, and once appropriate positioning is achieved the site is sutured and the patient transferred back to the ward. On return to the ward, the patient should receive cardiac monitoring and the nurse should observe for signs of pacemaker use or malfunction. The wound should be observed for signs of haematoma, infection, etc. and routine observations performed dependent on local policy. A routine chest radiograph is also performed to ensure appropriate lead positioning and rule out pneumothorax. If uncomplicated the patient may be discharged the following day with a card specifying that he or she has a pacemaker and its mode of action. The patient should also receive some simple advice to dispel the myths surrounding pacemaker usage.

Electrophysiology studies in the management of cardiac arrhythmias

The development of cardiac electrophysiology was heralded by a series of breakthroughs in the understanding of the mechanisms of generation of cardiac arrhythmias. This understanding came from the recognition that intracardiac catheters could be used to record electrical activity inside the heart and to map cardiac activation (Wellens 2004). However, before the 1980s, cardiac electrophysiology was primarily used to confirm mechanisms of arrhythmia, with management primarily by pharmacological means (Kaye 2004). The efficacy of anti-arrhythmic drug therapy relies on several factors both intrinsic to the patient and imposed by the limitations of medication. Concordance with potentially complex and lifelong medical regimens is unpredictable, and is compounded by the effects of anti-arrhythmic agents that are notorious for their side effects, the most significant of which is their pro-arrhythmic activity, i.e. their ability to generate arrhythmias.

The shortcomings of anti-arrhythmic therapy have continued to spur the development of cardiac electrophysiology to its current status, in which it is possible to effect a cure for many patients with potentially life-threatening arrhythmias.

The generation of arrhythmias

Cardiac arrhythmias are generated by disturbances in automaticity and by re-entrant excitation. Automaticity refers to the unique ability of cardiac cells to initiate an electrical impulse. When this normal physiological function is disturbed, irregular cardiac activity may precipitate symptoms. Examples are the presence of ischaemic myocardial damage arising during acute coronary syndromes or MI, which most commonly gives rise to ventricular tachycardia (VT) or atrial tachycardia resulting from scarring of atrial myocardium after surgery. Re-entrant excitation is the more common source of arrhythmias, which arise as a result of the existence of two or more discrete pathways that are in electrical contact and capable of electrical conduction.

Supraventricular tachycardia (SVT) is a narrow-complex tachycardia, presenting with a narrow QRS complex (< 0.12 s) with rates between 150 and 250 beats/min. This arrhythmia is usually paroxysmal, or episodic, in nature and tends to present in young healthy patients who do not have heart disease (Bygrave 2002). The two common mechanisms involve re-entry as a result of either an accessory pathway, such as in Wolff–Parkinson–White syndrome, or junctional re-entry tachycardia (Kaye 2004) (Figure 10.6).

In normal physiology, the atria and ventricles are electrically separated by a fibrous ring, which allows transmission of the atrial impulse to the ventricles only via the AV node, the purpose of which is to delay conduction of the electrical impulse to the ventricles, in order to allow time for ventricular filling during diastole. In addition the AV node is capable only of unidirectional (one-way) conduction. An accessory pathway is the term

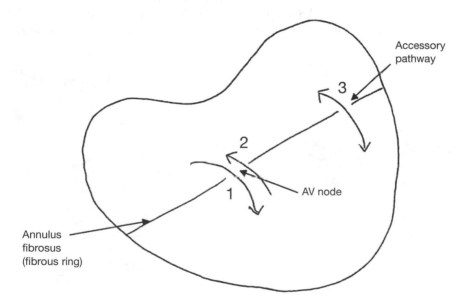

Figure 10.6 Wolff–Parkinson–White (WPW) syndrome: (1) normal conduction is from the atria to the ventricles via the atrioventricular (AV) node. (2) A junctional re-entrant pathway, located close to the AV node, allows fast or slow conduction in either one (unidirectional) or both (bidirectional) directions, setting up a fast or slow re-entry circuit. (3) In WPW syndrome, an accessory conduction pathway allows either uni- or bi-directional conduction between the atria and ventricles, in an area of the annular fibrosis separate from the AV node.

used to describe a discreet area of communication between the atria and ventricles, which is distinct from the AV node, and capable of electrical conduction, such as that which exists in Wolff–Parkinson–White (WPW) syndrome (Figure 10.6). This pathway will not have the same ability to delay conduction to the ventricles, may be capable of initiating ventricular contraction at rates up to 250 beats/min, and may allow electrical conduction from both atria to ventricles and ventricles to atria. Conduction from atria to ventricles via both the AV node and the accessory pathway gives rise to the characteristic 'slurring' of the upstroke of the R wave, known as the δ wave in the resting ECG (Figure 10.7).

In WPW syndrome, an atrial or ventricular extrasystole (ectopic) produces delay at the AV node and allows the electrical signal to pass back into the atria via the accessory pathway. This initiates a further atrial signal, which is transmitted via the AV node, and thus a re-entry 'circuit' is generated. This re-entry circuit accounts for 90% of SVT in WPW syndrome (Kaye 2004). Where the accessory pathway is capable of conducting impulses at a rate in excess of 250 beats/min, the risk to people with WPW syndrome is posed by atrial fibrillation (AF). Usually in AF, the AV node will control the ventricular response rate to a rapid atrial impulse. If the accessory pathway is able to conduct at a rapid rate, potentially lethal

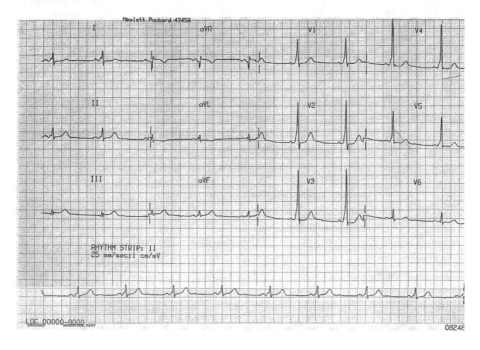

Figure 10.7 ECG in Wolff–Parkinson–White (WPW) syndrome, showing the slurred upstroke of the R wave, known as the delta (δ) wave.

haemodynamic instability or ventricular fibrillation (VF) can result. This arrhythmia is known as pre-excited AF and requires prompt correction (Bygrave 2002).

The most common cause of paroxysmal SVT is a junctional re-entry tachycardia. This occurs in individuals who have two, rather than one, conduction pathway in the region of the AV node. Although one pathway conducts rapidly and recovers slowly (the fast pathway), the other conducts slowly and recovers rapidly (the slow pathway). In most patients with junctional re-entry tachycardia, a circuit is formed by the conduction of the impulse from the atria to the ventricles (anterograde conduction) via the slow pathway, and from the ventricles to the atria (retrograde conduction) via the fast pathway (see Figure 10.6). The pathways are anatomically separate, with both inputting to an area known as the compact AV node. In junctional re-entry tachycardia, the ECG shows a narrow-complex tachycardia in which the P waves may be absent.

Atrial fibrillation and flutter

Atrial fibrillation is a common and recurrent arrhythmia associated with increased morbidity and mortality and is the most frequent sustained arrhythmia (Saad et al. 2002). In the 1980s and 1990s, it was commonplace to attempt electrical or pharmacological cardioversion in patients with AF, and to attempt to maintain sinus rhythm thereafter with anti-arrhythmic therapy (Wellens 2004). However, this is known for its limitations and is frequently unsuccessful. AF has been described by Peters et al. (2002) as one of the few challenges resistant to advances in clinical medicine. Recently, however, huge advances have been made in the understanding of the mechanism of AF. Two of these advances are the knowledge that AF is initiated and maintained in a large proportion of patients from an ectopic focus in the pulmonary vein, and that fibrillation of the atrial myocardium causes physiological changes in the myocardium, which make it progressively more unresponsive to treatment or electrical cardioversion (Peters et al. 2002). Atrial flutter arises from a re-entrant circuit, in particular from an area of slow conduction at the base of the right atrium in the area of the slow AV node (Kaye 2004).

The role of electrophysiological studies and catheter ablation

Actual or even perceived disturbance of the heart rhythm is a frightening experience, although, despite this, some patients may not seek help until such time as the symptoms are frequent or disabling. What drives the patient to seek medical help are symptoms such as palpitations, chest pain, breathlessness, fatigue, presyncope (dizziness) or syncope (loss of consciousness). It is important to gain a thorough understanding of the nature of the symptoms, including frequency, whether there is a sudden or gradual onset, their duration, at what time of day they tend to occur and whether at rest or during exercise. Bygrave (2002) also states that the physician should explore some strategies that the patient may use to control the symptoms, such as a Valsalva manoeuvre, position, rest or even exercise because this may offer a clue as to the origin of the arrhythmia. A 12-lead ECG is undertaken to rule out any abnormality that can be diagnosed from the surface ECG and, if the history or examination reveals any cause to believe that there may be underlying pathology (such as heart failure, cardiomyopathy, congenital heart disease), the patient may then go on to have further tests, e.g. exercise tolerance testing, in an attempt to find an ischaemic cause, and/or echocardiography in an attempt to identify a structural cause for the arrhythmia.

Angiography may be indicated if there are circumstances that lead the physician to suspect coronary artery disease either as a cause, or coexisting with, the arrhythmia. The assessment progresses to document evidence of the arrhythmia through Holter (24- or 48-h) ECG monitoring, or use of an R test or event recorder. If the symptoms are very infrequent, the patient may be encouraged to attend his or her GP surgery or an accident and emergency department to have an ECG recorded during the symptoms, or newer, implantable devices such as the 'reveal' may be used. When the arrhythmia has been documented, anti-arrhythmic therapy can be commenced.

It is at this point in the patient's journey that he or she may come into contact with an electrophysiologist. This will be because the symptoms are not well managed by anti-arrhythmic therapy or the patient's lifestyle makes long-term pharmacological management a poor treatment option, where there are persistent palpitations, or where recurrent syncope is the presenting symptom (Kaye 2004). The electrophysiologist will review the evidence of the arrhythmia and the patient's treatment, and proceed to electrophysiological study to guide a more interventional approach to treatment.

The electrophysiological study and ablation

The electrophysiological (EP) study allows identification and mapping of the location and cause of a re-entry circuit. Under local anaesthetic and light sedation, three to four quadripolar catheters are passed into the heart via the femoral and/or subclavian veins. These are positioned in the right atrial appendage, the apex of the right ventricle, close to the bundle of His and the coronary sinus. The catheters carry recording electrodes, which allow intracardiac electrical impulses to be mapped and accessory pathways to be identified and isolated, e.g. in WPW syndrome, the catheter will demonstrate separate atrial and ventricular activity close to the AV node, and proximity to the accessory pathway is indicated by the proximity of atrial and ventricular conduction waves (i.e. those not separated by conduction delay). Using quadripolar catheters and positioning these in the atria and ventricles allow the electrophysiologist not only to map the electrical pathways inside the heart, but also to pace the heart, locate a re-entry circuit and stimulate the arrhythmia. Ventricular pacing allows the electrophysiologist to assess for retrograde (ventricle to atria) conduction through a re-entry circuit. The conduction system is mapped without the presence of the arrhythmia, and the arrhythmia is stimulated by pacing to induce ectopic activity. The use of conscious sedation means that the patient can communicate with the electrophysiologist any similarity to previous symptoms that he or she experiences during the procedure.

In many cases it will be possible to proceed to ablation of the re-entry pathway. Using a catheter, radiofrequency energy is applied directly to the pathway. This creates heat of up to 50°C at the catheter tip, creating small areas of scarring and fibrosis in the myocardial tissue, through which electrical signals cannot pass. In the WPW syndrome, this will involve ablation of the accessory pathway, which effects a complete cure in 98% of cases (Kaye 2004). In junctional re-entrant tachycardia, this involves ablation of either the fast or slow pathway at the AV node. However, because of the proximity of the two, there is a 1–2% chance that both pathways will be disrupted, leaving the patient with no electrical communication between the atria and ventricles and totally reliant on a pacemaker.

It is precisely the complication of completely blocking conduction via the AV node that led to early electrophysiological attempts to control AF. In cases of refractory AF (unresponsive to cardioversion or anti-arrhythmic therapy) where the ventricular response rate is high, AF was in a few cases treated by creating a permanent conduction block at the AV node and using a pacemaker to manage the patient's heart rate. However, this is limited in that, although it can effectively control the ventricular rate in AF, it cannot restore atrial systole (Saad et al. 2002), meaning that the potential for thromboembolic complications of AF continues to exist. Latterly, through increasing understanding of the mechanisms of generation of AF and flutter, huge strides are being made in treatment by catheter ablation. Catheters are used to identify the arrhythmogenic focus (or foci) in the pulmonary veins, and these can be used to target radiofrequency energy at the arrhythmic foci. The disadvantage of this approach is that it requires the patient to be in sinus rhythm before the ectopic focus can be clearly mapped, a procedure that may require electrical cardioversion. More recently still, an alternative has been to ablate the tracts of myocardium, which extend from the pulmonary vein into the left atrium, thereby creating electrical isolation of the pulmonary vein from the myocardium (Peters et al. 2002).

In atrial flutter, a discrete line of ablation between the tricuspid annulus (valve ring) and the inferior vena cava gives a line of electrical block that is associated with a high degree of success sufficient to make it a standard treatment in terminating atrial flutter (Kaye 2004).

Limitations of radiofrequency catheter ablation

Although huge advances have come from development of the understanding of arrhythmia generation, radiofrequency (RF) energy has its limitations in the management of arrhythmias. To produce a continuous line of conduction block, it requires sustained contact with the myocardium. The depth to which RF energy can penetrate is also limited to the endocardium, which leaves arrhythmias deeper in the myocardium, such as ventricular arrhythmias, more difficult to treat (Keane 2002). Alternatives to RF energy are in the process of study, and include the development of laser, microwave, ultrasonic and cryothermy approaches to ablating the arrhythmia. One of the principal advantages of some of these alternatives is the ability to achieve deeper lesions without causing localized endothelial damage, which may improve the ability to control more refractory, or persistent, arrhythmias such as VT.

The internal cardioverter/defibrillator

DiMarco (2003) notes that despite advances in emergency medical systems and techniques in resuscitation, sudden death from cardiac arrest remains a significant problem. As adequate treatment is rarely readily available, the survival rate from a 'sudden death' event is dismal (Goldberger 1999). In the event that an individual does survive sudden cardiac death, this predicts a strong likelihood of a similar occurrence. One treatment option is the use of an implantable cardioverter–defibrillator (ICD), which is an implantable device that can automatically monitor and analyse rhythm and deliver shocks when it detects life-threatening arrhythmias such as VT or VF (Figure 10.8).

The ICD was first demonstrated to be clinically useful in the early 1980s (Cannom and Prystowsky 2004). Since that time studies have been ongoing to identify specific high-risk groups of patients who would be candidates for an ICD. Technological advances have enabled developments that allow it to have defibrillation, cardioversion, anti-tachycardia pacing, and single and biventricular pacing functions (Linde 2004).

An ICD system comprises a pulse generator and one or more leads for pacing and defibrillation. The pulse generator is made of titanium and encloses a lithium–silver vanadium oxide battery alongside the technology, which is able to sense, record, generate, cardiovert and defibrillate various

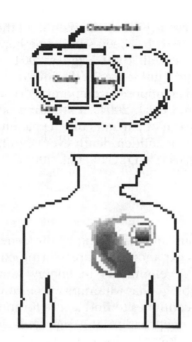

Figure 10.8 The internal cardioverter/defibrillator (ICD). (Reproduced with the permission of Medtronic.)

rhythms. The purpose of these functions is to maintain or restore rhythm-related cardiac function. The size of devices is now such that implantation in the chest wall, similar to that used for a pacemaker, is possible.

The evidence supporting the use of ICD devices in prevention of sudden cardiac death has been reviewed, in the UK, by the National Institute for Clinical Excellence (NICE 2000). This guidance suggests the use of ICDs for the purposes of primary prevention of sudden cardiac death in people who have sustained a previous heart attack, and one or all of: non-sustained VT on 24-h ECG monitoring; inducible VT on EP testing; or significant damage to the left ventricle. The NICE (2000) also advise on the use of ICDs for primary prevention in patients who have a familial tendency to sudden cardiac death, HCM (Hypertrophic Cardiomyopathy) and arrhythmogenic right ventricular dysplasia. Use of ICDs for secondary prevention is advocated in patients who present, in the absence of a treatable cause, with cardiac arrest caused by ventricular tachycardia or fibrillation, or sustained VT in people with a damaged left ventricle (NICE 2000).

The implanting of an ICD is a significant and frequently very frightening event for patients. Often they have survived cardiac arrest, and the suggestion of implanting a device is a stark reminder of the risk of recurrence. The psychological impact of implanting, and living with, an ICD has become the focus of descriptive research accounts of the patient experience, although the lifestyle impact has been studied perhaps to a greater degree (see, for example, James et al. 1999, Tagney 2004), with significant psychological and sociological influences of the imposed lifestyle change, e.g. changes in work life and an imposed (temporary) driving ban, which follows ICD implantation (James et al. 2001). Extending beyond the individual are the domains of concern of partners of ICD patients, which range from caring for the survivors of sudden death events, to uncertainty, financial and relationship concerns (Dougherty et al. 2001).

Conclusion

The development of our understanding of the generation and management of arrhythmias is expanding at a reassuring pace. The future looks set to see continued developments in energy sources for ablation of arrhythmias and technology that will improve our understanding further. Although the struggle continues to find a cure for more complex arrhythmias generated from deep within the myocardium, better control of arrhythmias, and better lifestyles for patients, as a result of the developments of electrophysiology, are within our grasp.

References

Ascoop CAPL, van Zeijl LGPM, Pool J, Simoons ML (1989) Cardiac exercise testing – I, indications, staff, equipment, conduct and procedures. Netherlands J Cardiol 2: 63–72.

Bernstein AD, Camm AJ, Fletcher RD et al. (1987) The NASPE/BPEG generic pacemaker code for anti-bradyarrhythmia and adaptive rate pacing and anti tachyarrhythmia devices. PACE 10: 794–9.

Bertrand ME, Rupprecht HJ, Urban P, Gershlick AH (2000) Double-blind study of the safety of clopidogrel with and without loading dose in combination with aspirin compared with ticlopidine in combination with aspirin after coronary stenting the Clopidogrel Aspirin Stent International Cooperative study (CLASSIC). Circulation 102: 624–9.

Bygrave A (2002) Electrophysiology studies. In: Hatchett R, Thompson D (eds), Cardiac Nursing. London: Churchill Livingstone, pp. 369–390.

Cannom D, Prystowsky E (2004) Evolution of the implantable cardioverter defibrillator. J Cardiovasc Electrophysiol 15: 375–85.

Connaughton M, Forsey P, Smith R, Gammage M (1998) The learning curve for temporary pacing: evidence from district general and teaching hospitals. Heart 79(suppl I): 51.

DiMarco J (2003) Medical progress: Implantable cardioverter-defibrillators. N Engl J Med 349: 1836–47.

Dougherty C (2001) The natural history of recovery following sudden cardiac arrest and internal cardioverter-defibrillator implantation. Progr Cardiovasc Nursing 16: 163–8.

Gershlick AH (2002) Role of coronary revascularisation. Intervention in coronary artery disease. In: Education in Heart, Vol. 1. London: BMJ Books.

Goldberger J (1999) Treatment and prevention of sudden cardiac death; effect of recent clinical trials. Arch Intern Med 159: 1281–7.

Gruntzig AR, Senning A, Siegenthaler WE (1979) Nonoperative dilatation of coronary-artery stenosis. Percutaneous transluminal coronary angioplasty. N Engl J Med 301: 61–8.

Henderson RA (1989) The Randomised Intervention Treatment of Angina (RITA) trial protocol: a long term study of coronary angioplasty and coronary artery bypass surgery in patients with angina. Br Heart J 62: 411–14.

James J, Albarran J, Tagney J (1999) Going home: the lived experiences of women following ICD implantation. Adv Clin Nursing 3: 168–79.

James J, Albarran J, Tagney J (2001) The experience of ICD patients and their partners with regards to adjusting to an imposed driving ban: a qualitative study. Coronary Health Care 5: 80–8.

Kay G (1996) Basic concepts of pacing. In: Ellenbogen K (ed.), Cardiac Pacing, 2nd edn. Cambridge, MA: Blackwell Science pp. 37–123.

Kaye G (2004) Percutaneous interventional electrophysiology. BMJ 327: 280–3.

Keane D (2002) New catheter ablation techniques for the treatment of cardiac arrhythmias. Cardiac Electrophysiol Rev 6: 341–8.

Kioka Y, Dallan L, Olivera S et al. (1991) Clinical experiences of emergency coronary bypass grafting following failed percutaneous transluminal coronary angioplasty. Jpn J Surg 21: 643–9.

Lincoff AM, Califf RM, Moliterno DJ et al. (1999) Complementary clinical benefits of coronary artery stenting and blockade of platelet glycoprotein IIb/IIIa receptors, Evaluation of platelet IIb/IIIa inhibition in stenting investigators. N Engl J Med 341: 319–27.

Linde C (2004) Implantable cardioverter-defibrillator treatment and resynchronisation in heart failure. Heart 90: 231–4.

Moses S (2003) Online resource:wwwfpnotebook.com/cv131.htm.

Nairs CR, Holmes DR Jr, Topol EJ. (1998) A call for provisional stenting: the balloon is back! Circulation 97: 1298–305.

National Institute for Clinical Excellence (2000) Guidance on the Use of Implantable Cardioverter Defibrillators for Arrhythmias. Technology Appraisal Guidance No. 11. London: NICE.

Peters N, Schilling R, Kanagaratnam P, Markides V (2002) Atrial fibrillation: strategies to control, combat and cure. Lancet 359: 593–603.

Saad E, Marrouche N, Natale A (2002) Ablation of focal atrial fibrillation. Cardiac Electrophysiol Rev 6: 389–96.

Sones FM Jr (1959) Acquired heart disease: symposium on present and future of cineangiocardiography. Am J Cardiol 3: 710.

Tagney J (2004) Can nurses in cardiology areas prepare patients for implantable cardioverter defibrillator implant and life at home? Nursing Crit Care 9: 104–14.

Wellens H (2004) Cardiac arrhythmias: the quest for a cure: A historical perspective. J Am Coll Cardiol 44: 1155–63.

Windecker S, Meier B (2002) Intervention in coronary artery disease. In: Education in Heart, Vol. 1. London: BMJ Books.

Chapter eleven

Cardiac surgery

Catherine Rimmer, Shonagh Senior and Ian Jones

This chapter discusses the main elements of cardiac surgery. It does not aim to discuss all variations of cardiac surgery, but predominantly focuses on coronary artery bypass graft (CABG) and valve replacement surgery as the most commonly performed major cardiac surgical procedures. There are, of course, many other surgical procedures involving the heart, including correction of congenital heart defects, intervention necessitated as a result of trauma, aortic aneurysm repair, surgery for tumours and growths, and pericardectomy. However, the cardiac surgery pathway discussed here, can be applied to most cardiac surgery patients regardless of surgical procedure.

There are many aspects to consider in the care of the patient undergoing cardiac surgery. Care must begin from when the patient is placed on a waiting list at the point of listing and continue well after discharge from hospital. This chapter aims to outline the priorities of this care and give an understanding of the needs, wants and expectations of the cardiac surgery patient and his or her carer.

In addition to practical aspects of surgical care, this chapter also discusses the current issues and recent changes affecting cardiac surgery service provision.

Indications for coronary artery bypass surgery

Coronary artery bypass surgery is indicated for symptom relief and/or to prolong life (Eagle et al. 1999). Coronary bypass surgery is designed to restore adequate blood supply to areas of myocardium affected by coronary artery stenosis (see Chapter 1), so reducing the risk of development of a myocardial infarction (MI) and relieving the patient of angina symptoms.

A patient is likely to have been treated medically for relief of symptoms and to help slow the progression of the disease process. The decision to proceed to surgery from medical management takes place after a consultation between the cardiologist and the cardiac surgeon. Patients who require urgent surgery may never have been treated medically and, by the time they present with symptoms of coronary heart disease (CHD), the condition is so far advanced that medical management is not an option.

There have been a number of studies to evaluate the effectiveness of surgery in symptom relief, prolongation of life and improvement of quality of life. The American College of Cardiology Foundation states: 'The evidence is complete that coronary artery bypass operation relieves angina in most patients' (Eagle et al. 1999, p. 1).

Indications for valve surgery

As with CABG, the patient with valvular disease is routinely referred to the cardiac surgeon by the cardiologist. The patient may have been under review or on medical treatment for valvular stenosis or regurgitation for some time by this point. However, if the valve has been damaged by infection, the disease process may have been more rapid and the patient may need to be referred to the surgeon as a matter of urgency. Often, patients who are listed for valve surgery, particularly elderly patients, will have preoperative angiograms to assess the condition of their coronary arteries. If the coronary arteries show signs of CHD the surgeon will discuss the benefit of undertaking a CABG with the patient. If the surgeon predicts the potential need for revascularization in the future, the decision may be made to perform a CABG while operating on the heart, thereby reducing the risk of damage or ischaemia to the myocardium, and hopefully preventing the need for repeated heart surgery in the future.

There are two types of valves that the surgeon may use for valve replacement operations: mechanical and tissue valves.

Mechanical valves

These valves are made of carbon fibre and are available in a variety of sizes, to fit into all valve positions. After the surgery the patient may become aware of a 'clicking' sound; this is the noise of the valve as it opens and closes. The patient should be reassured that it is quite normal to be able to hear the valve clicking.

Mechanical valve prostheses carry the risk of clot formation on their surfaces, because they are artificial material lying in the bloodstream. Patients who receive them are therefore required to take life-long anticoagulation. Anticoagulation can have complications of its own, however. Women who still wish to bear children risk fetal deformities. There are also some patients whose lifestyle is not compatible with anticoagulation. Mechanical valves are generally the valves that will predictably last the longest before the need for reoperation (Peterseim et al. 1999), but, because of the problems associated with anticoagulation, they are not suitable for all valve replacement candidates.

Tissue valves

Rather than being manufactured using a foreign substance (carbon fibre), these valves are made from animal tissue (xenografts), particularly from pigs (porcine) or cows (bovine), or from fresh or preserved human valves (homografts). This natural tissue is not associated with the problems of embolism as with the mechanical valves, so a recipient does not need to take life-long anticoagulation. Some surgeons, however, advise a short term of anticoagulation in the first few months postoperatively. Consequently, the lifestyle implications and potential complications of anticoagulation are avoided. However, these valves do not have the durability of the mechanical valves, so reoperation after around 10–15 years is possible (Peterseim et al. 1999). This is another consideration for younger patients when considering surgery.

Discussions between the patient and surgeon are crucial when choosing a valve prosthesis. There are recommendations available for choosing valves, according to age and risk factors (Peterseim et al. 1999), but the decision is ultimately with the surgeon and patient.

Assessing risk

Whatever the type of surgery, surgeons are required to follow guidelines when considering a patient for surgery.

In the UK, surgeons have adopted the guidelines of the American College of Cardiology Foundation (ACC) and the American Heart Association (AHA) (Eagle et al. 1999). In summary these organizations recommend that the benefits of surgery must be balanced against the risk of the operation. The guidelines include management of specific areas of acute coronary syndrome, as well as classifications of angina and left ventricular dysfunction. The ACC/AHA guidelines highlight the importance of the ability to 'predict the hospital mortality of the procedure and the risk of the complications of coronary bypass, including cerebrovascular accident, major wound infection and renal dysfunction' (Eagle et al. 1999, p. 1).

So that surgeons are able to calculate the risk associated with cardiac surgery, there have been a number of risk assessment tools developed by various bodies. Each has been studied for its accuracy and effectiveness in predicting mortality and morbidity (Geissler et al. 2000). It is widely recognized that geography has a role in risk prediction and that the scoring tool used should be one that represents the local population. The ACC advise: 'Although it may be possible to generalize the relative contribution of individual patient variables, rules must be calibrated to regional mortality rates and be updated periodically to maximize accuracy' (Eagle et al. 1999, p. 2).

Different scoring tools use a variety of guides and markers to calculate the risk of surgery. The ACC lists seven core variables, including urgency of operation, age, prior heart surgery, sex, left ventricular ejection fraction, extent of coronary stenosis and number of coronary arteries involved. Other factors often included in risk tools are diabetes, peripheral vascular disease, recent MI, cerebrovascular disease, chronic obstructive pulmonary disease and renal dysfunction.

The most widely, internationally accepted risk assessment tool is the Initial Parsonnet Score. However, this tool has been found to over-predict risk. At present, surgeons in the UK, use both the Initial Parsonnet Score and the Euroscore, which is a more realistic and accurate predictor for the British population and throughout Europe (Geissler et al. 2000). Whatever the risk assessment tool employed, however, it is essential that the surgeon evaluate the risk of surgery with the predicted outcome, symptom relief and quality of life (Eagle et al. 1999), and discuss the risks and benefits with the patient (with the involvement of any significant other, according to the patient's wishes). This will enable them to decide together whether the benefits outweigh the risks, and whether to proceed with surgery.

Consent

It is crucial that the risks of the surgery have been accurately assessed and explained to the patient in order that an informed consent is obtained to proceed with surgery. The Department of Health (DoH 2001a) published specific guidelines that clearly state the level of information a patient should receive when seeking consent for treatment. As the process of informing the patient of their surgery and care is ongoing after listing for surgery, it is essential that consent be an ongoing process that the patient is free to explore at any part of the surgical journey. The consent form should be completed by the surgeon and include the predicted risk for the patient. The DoH (2000b) stresses the importance of patient-focused consent procedures and outlines the action to be taken by clinicians in order to achieve this.

Waiting lists

The listing consultation appointment can be a time of great anxiety for patients and their families, no matter how well prepared they are for what the surgeon discusses with them (Gillis 1984, Artinian 1991, 1993, Moser et al. 1993). Many heart centres now provide a cardiac liaison or specialist nurse to support patients and relatives after this consultation. Cardiac liaison nurses are in a key position to support the patient and the family at his time (Foulger 1997) and their input can help prepare the patient both physically and psychologically. In addition, cardiac liaison input can also be very beneficial in reducing anxiety at this time (McHugh et al. 2001). In recognition of the value of continuation of care, cardiac liaison nurses are also often the providers of information, education and support throughout the cardiac surgery patient's journey.

Waiting times

Over the last 5 years cardiac surgery waiting times have fallen dramatically. In September 2001, 1804 patients waited longer than 9 months for their cardiac surgery, yet by March 2003 only one patient had been waiting longer than 9 months (CHD Collaborative and DoH 2004). Today, Trusts are achieving, the March 2005 National Service Framework (NSF) for Coronary Heart Disease target of waiting times of 3 months. Reduction in waiting times has been achieved through innovations in practice, both clinical and managerial, with developments in cardiology (NHS Modernisation Agency 2003a) and the Patient Choice scheme (DoH 2003) playing significant roles.

Booking

The aim of booked admission services is to let patients choose and pre-book the date of their admission or appointment (NHS Modernisation Agency 2003b). The National Booking Programme was launched in 1998 and asserts that trusts should be providing a booked admission service for all outpatient appointments, including pre-admission clinics, and all inpatient elective admissions, by December 2005 (NHS Modernisation Agency 2003b). Whether a trust is offering a full or partial booking system, however, it is imperative that some level of pre-admission preparation commences at the point of listing to ensure that patients are medically and psychologically fit for surgery, thus reducing cancellations for these reasons (Hind 1997, NHS Modernisation Agency 2003c).

Pre-admission preparation

The relevance and importance of pre-admission preparation are now widely accepted with pre-admission services forming an essential part of preparation for cardiac surgery, as well in other areas of surgery and medicine (NHS Modernisation Agency 2003c). There is no prescription for how pre-admission preparation should be provided and it is currently being delivered in a variety of ways, such as 'a face-to-face consultation in primary or secondary care, by postal questionnaire, by telephone, by using NHS direct or possibly by using a questionnaire on the internet' (NHS Modernisation Agency 2003c, p. 11). The development of national guidelines for preoperative assessment (NHS Modernisation Agency 2003c) may, however, help to establish standardization in this field if not in the form of its delivery, then perhaps in the quality of its provision.

Traditionally, much of the pre-admission preparation is carried out in the pre-admission clinic a few weeks before admission, but there is a strong argument for a degree of preoperative testing at the point of listing when waiting lists are so short (NHS Modernisation Agency 2003c). Clearly if the preoperative assessment is conducted on the day of listing, the obvious place for this to take place is at the secondary/tertiary centre (NHS Modernisation Agency 2003c). Whether this service is provided at the point of listing, in the weeks before admission, or as a service that is a mixture of them both, preadmission preparation serves several purposes: preoperative investigations, information provision, discharge planning and health education (Jones et al. 2002).

Preoperative investigations

As mentioned earlier, ideally many of the preoperative investigations required before surgery can be undertaken at the point of listing when the waiting lists are short. There are many factors that can lead to cancellations, such as hypertension, unstable blood sugars or abnormal blood results, which can be addressed in a waiting period of 2–3 months (NHS Modernisation Agency 2003c). However, if such factors are detected only at the preoperative clinic a few weeks before surgery, there is less time and opportunity to optimize that patient's health before admission, which can result in either postponement of surgery or the patient having surgery in a less than optimal condition (NHS Modernisation Agency 2003c). Conversely, it is just as important that irrelevant tests are avoided in order to avoid unnecessary inconvenience and discomfort to patients (National Institute for Clinical Excellence 2003). Standardization of preoperative guidelines should help to avoid this and would ensure patients receive the tests they require.

Preoperative investigations that the National Institute for Clinical Excellence (2003) recommends for patients awaiting cardiac surgery patients include those in Table 11.1.

Table 11.1 Preoperative recommendations recommended by the National Institute for Clinical Excellence (2003)

Patient	Recommended test
'Normal healthy patient (without any clinically important co-morbidity and without a clinically significant past/present medical history)' (National Institute for Clinical Governance 2003, p. 22)	Urea and electrolytes Full blood count Electrocardiogram (ECG) Chest radiograph Haemostasis, random glucose and urine analysis tests should be considered on an individual basis
Patients with other co-morbidities	HbA1c (glycated haemoglobin) for patients with diabetes Liver function tests

The National Institute for Clinical Excellence (2003) preoperative test guidelines are not exhaustive, however, and there are other investigations to consider. Cardiac operations obviously carry the risk of blood loss so blood tests for antibodies, group and save, and cross-match will also be required. From a health education angle, a lipid test can be very helpful, and can aid in tailoring dietary and secondary prevention advice. Informing patients of their cholesterol level can only help assist them to take ownership of this heart disease risk factor.

Although there is variation in the infection control practices and policies across British cardiac centres (Kendall et al. 2002), many follow guidelines that recommend the swabbing of nose, hairline, axilla, groin and perineum for methicillin-resistant *Staphylococcus aureus* (Report of a combined working party of the British Society for Antimicrobial Chemotherapy, the Hospital Infection Society and the Infection Control Nurses' Association 1998). If these tests can be conducted at the point of listing (which will give longer to treat the infection or colonization if identified), the likelihood of surgery being postponed because of positive swab results must be greatly reduced. Nevertheless, it may not always be appropriate for these tests to be carried out at the point of listing; a pre-admission clinic offers opportunities for these tests to be done (NHS Modernisation Agency 2003c). Early detection of abnormal results affords time to rectify them or order other appropriate investigations and treatments, or alternatively, if the patient is found to be unfit for surgery at this time, there is time and opportunity to prepare another patient and the valuable surgery slot is not lost (NHS Modernisation Agency 2003c). Field and Bjarnason (2000) claim that attendance at a pre-admission clinic also has a role in reducing the patient's risk of postoperative complications.

Preoperative information

Pre-admission clinics provide a forum and opportunity for the patient and family to find out information about the impending admission, in order to meet the physical, psychological and social needs (NHS Modernisation Agency 2003c). Artinian (1991, 1993) and Moser et al. (1993) studied the needs of patients and their carers and both concluded that, although both patients and carers expressed similar needs for information, the carers ranked this need higher than patients. If preoperative information can be delivered in a way that matches individual coping styles, it can reduce anxiety levels (Mitchell 1997, Lamarche et al. 1998, McDonald et al. 2003), which in some forms of surgery has been demonstrated to result in a less expensive recovery (Hough et al. 1991).

Preoperative discharge planning

Provision of information regarding surgery and the limitations that will be experienced afterwards are essential if patients and their carers are to make appropriate plans and provisions after discharge. Patients are not always able to make provisions independently for a safe post-discharge convalescence and so the pre-admission clinic provides an opportunity for staff to enquire into social circumstances. 'It also allows staff time to start making appropriate requests to social services or health authorities regarding funding for care packages' (Jones et al. 2002, p. 586). Not only will this type of proactive discharge planning reassure patients and their families about the post-discharge period, but it may also increase patient throughput and decrease length of stay (Sumer et al. 1997).

Preoperative health education

Cardiac surgery is not a cure for CHD and it is important to remember that it is a chronic condition. The NSF for CHD (DoH 2000a) stresses the importance of secondary prevention, and health education is now being provided earlier and earlier in the cardiac surgery patient's journey. The opportunity to address heart disease risk factors should never be over-looked and, although the pre-admission clinic may not necessarily be the most ideal occasion to commence health education, 'the situation may still lend itself to this' (Jones et al. 2002, p. 587). This early identification of predisposing risk factors will assist health-care professionals both in hospital and in the community in tailoring postoperative advice to the individual's needs (Jones et al. 2002).

Prehabilitation

Preoperative assessment should be considered as a process of preparation, however (NHS Modernisation Agency 2003c), and not just as a one-off task. This is being reflected in some areas with the establishment of 'prehabilitation' as a form of continuous pre-assessment from the point of listing through to admission for surgery.

Some cardiac centres have developed prehabilitation services where the initial testing is carried out by the tertiary centre at the point of listing and the primary care providers follow up abnormal results, health education, and social and psychological preparation. This system can be very successful if there is effective communication and partnership between the primary and secondary or tertiary care centres but has the potential for disaster without it. The advantage of this type of shared care is that the prehabilitation service is provided in the patient's own locality, therefore avoiding the need for repetitive travel to the tertiary centre (DoH 2000b). However, in other areas this type of service is not viable and some tertiary centres have established prehabilitation schemes where the cardiac liaison nurse or specialist nurse does the testing at the point of listing and then provides all the follow-up to the physical, social and psychological factors. Alternatively, some areas use primary care centres, which may not necessarily be the patient's own health-care centre but rather a specialist base for the provision of this type of treatment, with specialist health-care professionals (DoH 2000b).

Additional preoperative support

Many cardiac centres, recognizing the benefits of providing preoperative information (Hough et al. 1991, Mitchell 1997, Lamarche et al. 1998, McDonald et al. 2003), are continuing the information-giving process started in the listing consultation, and are providing preoperative 'information afternoons'. Although these information sessions can provide invaluable information about secondary prevention, heart disease, what to expect in hospital and discharge expectations, their location in tertiary care limits their accessibility. To provide equity of access to such information, patient videos have been developed and produced, which evidence has shown address patients' information needs as well as being a cost-effective method of preoperative teaching (Krouse et al. 2001).

Admission process

Admission to the ward

A warm welcome on to the ward by the admitting nurse and fellow members of staff is crucial in presenting a favourable first impression of the ward to the new patient and family members. The prospect of cardiac surgery can cause a great deal of anxiety and is a huge life event for many of the patients. A friendly nature and professional attitude may help to instil some confidence in the patient and loved ones. An introduction to neighbouring patients may be appropriate, ensuring patient confidentiality at all times.

Many patients admitted to hospital for cardiac surgery will be on a routine waiting list, hopefully having had the opportunity to attend a preoperative assessment service. However, many patients are admitted for surgery as urgent or an emergency, and so have not had the opportunity to have routine investigations performed. On admission to the ward, the nurse should ensure that investigation results are present in the notes or perform any outstanding investigations (Table 11.2).

Preparation for theatre

The patient is given a pre-medication on the ward and asked to remain in bed; the pre-med is designed to help the patient relax, induce sleep and reduce anxiety. The anaesthetist will often prescribe an antiemetic, analgesia, medication to reduce secretions and O_2 as well as a sedative. The combination of medication depends on anaesthetic preference.

Anaesthetic room

A nurse will accompany the patient to theatre from the ward to ensure safe handover of the patient to the theatre staff. In the anaesthetic room, heart rate, blood pressure and O_2 saturations are monitored by non-invasive techniques until an arterial line is inserted. A sample of arterial blood is analysed before a general anaesthetic is administered, to establish a baseline blood gas. Once Venflons have been inserted peripherally, the patient is anaesthetized and intubated. A central venous line is inserted, usually into the internal jugular vein or occasionally the subclavian vein, followed by a pulmonary artery catheter. Intravenous fluids will be commenced in the anaesthetic room. A urinary catheter is inserted before transfer into theatre. It may also be the preference of the anaesthetist to insert an

Table 11.2 Investigations on admission

Investigations	Rationale
Full blood count, urea and electrolytes, cholesterol, blood glucose, infection screen, chest radiograph	Those who have not been able to attend a preoperative preparation service will need to have these routine tests performed as soon as possible on admission, in order that any abnormal results may be addressed and resolved if possible. Those who have been preoperatively prepared will not need these investigations repeated (as long as they are current) but it will be necessary to check that all results are present in the notes
Urinalysis, blood pressure, temperature, O_2 saturations, pulse respirations	To ensure optimal preoperative health Early detection of preoperative problems or risks Establishment of baseline observations
Cross-match	Blood will need to be taken for cross-match. The amount required will depend on the surgery. Although practice varies, listed below are common requirements of units to be cross-matched in preparation for theatre: Single-valve surgery 2 units CABG 2 units Double-valve surgery 3 units Valve surgery and CABG 3 units Re-do CABG 3 units
Height and weight	Height and weight measurements are required to assist surgeons and anaesthetists to select appropriate lines, endotracheal tubes, nasogastric tubes and drug dosage Height and weight are crucial in the immediate postoperative period for calculations of cardiac studies using the pulmonary artery catheter (see Postoperative care)
Hair removal	The issue of hair removal has been controversial for some time. There is evidence to suggest that preoperative shaving can adversely affect surgical wounds (Sellick et al. 1991, Kjonniksen et al. 2002). However, dressing changes can be very uncomfortable on patients who have a lot of body hair. Hair removal should follow local guidelines in accordance with current research
Nil by mouth	Preoperative fasting should follow recent research. Local guidelines often have a fasting time of 2–6 h preoperatively (Brady et al. 2003, Mangiante et al. 2003)

Table 11.2 Investigations on admission (continued)

Investigations	Rationale
Consent	A current consent form should be filed in the patient's notes. It is good practice to check with the patient at each stage of the preoperative process that an informed consent has been obtained
Property	Patient's property should be listed and secured according to local policy for the period that the patient is out of the area, i.e. in theatre, ICU, etc.
Night sedation	The anaesthetist may well offer night sedation to the patient for the night before surgery
Communication with relatives	According to the wishes of the patient, family members or loved ones should be involved in the admission process. Trauma and stress for the relatives may be reduced by their inclusion and involvement
Medical clerking	The patient should be medically examined during the admission process, in order to establish that he or she is fit for surgery, and to identify any potential problems. This will also give the patient another opportunity to ask questions relating to surgery or hospital stay
Introduction to the physiotherapist, critical care nurse, liaison nurse	There may be an opportunity for the patient to meet with other members of the multidisciplinary team before surgery. This may help to reduce anxiety levels
Secondary prevention	The NSF for CHD (DoH 2000a) recommends that phase I of cardiac rehabilitation begins before discharge, and the benefit of early secondary prevention information has been discussed in pre-admission preparation. Risk factors including smoking, diet and lifestyle should be assessed and discussed on admission, although it may be prudent to make recommendations and discuss changes to lifestyle in the postoperative phase of admission, in order that the patient does not become overloaded with information at a potentially stressful time

CABG, coronary artery bypass graft; CHD, coronary heart disease; ICU, intensive care unit; NSF, National Service Framework.

epidural catheter to assist in postoperative pain relief; this is inserted in the anaesthetic room before surgery commences. The decision to use epidural analgesia is made by the anaesthetist in conjunction with the patient. It is important that the patient has an understanding of all infusions and invasive lines that are to be inserted.

Cardiac surgery

This section is designed to give a brief overview of the surgical procedures in this chapter. As discussed earlier, it is by no means meant as an exhaustive reference and further reading may be required for more detailed information.

Coronary artery bypass graft

So that surgery may be performed on the heart, the surgeon must have access to it. There are a number of surgical approaches that can be used to achieve this including sternotomy, mini-thoracotomy (MIDCAB) and bilateral anterior thoracotomy (Clamshell). The most common approach to date is the sternotomy, which involves using a sternal saw to cut the sternum, and then retracting both sides of the chest so that the surgeon has a clear operating field. The patient may or may not need to have cardiopulmonary bypass during the surgical procedure (see 'On pump' and 'Off pump'). An assistant will generally harvest the vessel to be grafted, either a saphenous vein from one or both legs, or a radial artery from the arm (see 'Donor vessels' below). Sections of the harvested vessel are anastomosed on to the aorta, and then on to the narrowed or blocked coronary artery, distal to the blockage. This provides an alternative route for blood to flow to the other side of the narrowing and supply the affected area of myocardium with oxygenated blood. However, if an internal mammary artery is used as a donor vessel (conduit), one end only is resected and attached to the diseased coronary artery. Blood flow then comes from the subclavian artery into the internal mammary artery and into the coronary artery, most commonly the left anterior descending (LAD) artery. The original coronary artery is not removed, merely bypassed in order to provide all the heart muscle with an effective blood supply.

Once the blood vessel has been resected, the anaesthetist will give a dose of intravenous heparin, 300 IU/kg for patients on pump, before they are put on to bypass, and 150 IU/kg for off-pump surgery (see below). The aim is for the activated clotting time (ACT) to be at least 350–400 s (Neema et al. 2004), sometimes lower (Cardoso et al. 1991), but often higher according to practitioner preference, throughout the rest of the procedure, by giving further doses of heparin as required. Once the surgery has been completed, a dose of protamine is given to counteract the heparin and bring the ACT to within normal limits. The risk of bleeding is greater while the patient is heparinized; this needs to be addressed before leaving the theatre.

The sternum is closed using steel sternal wires. This involves inserting a number of wires, often six or seven, through the sternal bone, effectively stitching the bone edges together. The muscle layers are then closed and finally the skin is closed, often using subcutaneous sutures.

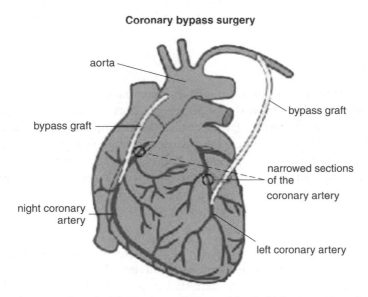

Figure 11.1 Reproduced with kind permission of the British Heart Foundation.

Donor vessels

Choice of vessel used as a conduit is dependent on many factors, including location of diseased artery, peripheral perfusion, previous bypass surgery, and patient medical and surgical history.

Internal mammary arteries

The left or right internal mammary artery (LIMA/RIMA) is widely used for coronary artery bypass surgery. Studies have found that the patency rates are generally higher than all other vessels of choice (Khot et al. 2004).

Using the LIMA or RIMA as a donor vessel, however, has its own complications. Pain can be increased down the affected side of the chest. Blood flow to the chest wall can be impeded and can have consequences for wound healing and muscle perfusion (Eagle et al. 1999).

Saphenous vein

Another common vessel used for coronary bypass is the saphenous vein from one or both legs. This can be harvested traditionally through open resection or endoscopically. Endoscopic harvest of the saphenous vein is reported to reduce the incidence of infective complications postoperatively compared with those harvested with the open technique (Perrault et al. 2004).

Radial artery

The radial artery is less commonly used for bypass surgery because of the complications associated with it. Studies report a reduced patency of grafts using the radial artery (Khot et al. 2004) compared with saphenous vein and IMA. There have also been postoperative complications associated with the harvesting of this vessel, as well as infection and pain; there are reports of donor arm weakness and persistent cutaneous paraesthesia (Budillon et al. 2003).

Other conduits

Alternative vessels that may be used include short saphenous vein, gastroepiploic artery and inferior epigastric artery. These vessels are often associated with complicated surgical techniques and less successful long-term outcomes.

Cardiopulmonary bypass

At present there are two techniques used by surgeons when undertaking cardiac surgery. To access the coronary arteries and effectively perform the surgery, the surgeon must decide whether or not the heart must be stopped.

On pump

If required, the heart can be stopped and the patient is put on to cardiopulmonary bypass. This involves cannulation of the aorta and the right atrium, thus enabling a bypass machine to maintain blood gases and general perfusion while the surgery is performed. Cardiopulmonary bypass has the potential for increased incidence of complications both peri- and postoperatively, including thromboembolism, atrial fibrillation (Athanasiou et al. 2004), and psychological and personality changes (Ganuschchak et al. 2004).

Off pump

The second option available to the cardiac surgeon is not to put the patient on to bypass at all, but to perform beating heart surgery. The surgeon will use a 'stabilizing devise' to keep sections of the heart still as they are operated on. The device is applied to the heart using suction and can be moved around to different sections of the heart as required. This equipment is designed to anchor an area of the heart that the surgeon is working on, keeping that area still while the heart continues to beat. The advantage of this technique is that the risks associated with the bypass machine are avoided; however, this technique is relatively new to the field and not all surgeons are proficient in its use. It is not suitable for all CABG surgery because often the heart needs to be stopped to access particular areas or if the patient's anatomy proves awkward. Surgeons using the 'off-pump' technique will always have a perfusionist and a bypass machine available for use in an emergency.

Minimal invasive direct coronary artery bypass

Coronary artery bypass surgery can be performed without a sternotomy, using a minimally invasive technique. An incision, approximately 7–9 cm long, is made on the left of the chest through the fourth intercostal space. The surgery is completed without the use of a bypass machine or a stabilizing device, with the heart beating throughout. The conduit most commonly used for a minimal invasive direct coronary artery bypass (MIDCAB) procedure is the LIMA.

The MIDCAB is perceived to have advantages over the traditional approach; it has been reported that intensive care time is reduced, hospital stay reduced and perceived health generally better (Al-Ruzzeh et al. 2004). Despite the potential advantages to the patient, it is widely acknowledged that the use of this procedure is limited. The approach may be performed only on patients whose disease affects vessels that can be accessed from this approach, particularly LAD artery. Although MIDCAB has been very successful in patients who are deemed high risk, i.e. cerebral vascular disease, renal disease and severely impaired left ventricular function, of reducing their postoperative complications (Diegeler et al. 1999a), MIDCAB is also reported to be more painful than the traditional sternotomy as a result of the intercostal muscle resection and often the breakage of ribs, particularly in the first 3 days postoperatively (Diegeler et al. 1999b).

Valve surgery

Access to the heart for valve repair or replacement is obtained by a sternotomy, as with CABG. There are a number of approaches used in order to
access the valves themselves.

Aortic valve replacement surgery

The aortic valve is accessed by cutting into the aorta and approaching it
from above. The valve is removed completely, including any fragments of
calcification to ensure that there is a clean area in which to attach the prosthetic valve. A number of sutures are sewn onto the inside wall of the aorta
and the other ends attached to the new valve. Once all the sutures are in
place, they are tightened and the valve is gently lowered into place. Each
suture is tightened and tied, and then cut. The valve is tested once in
place, then the wall of the aorta is carefully repaired. It is crucial that the
wall of the aorta is absolutely secure because the pressure exerted onto it
once the heart is beating again is immense.

Mitral valve replacement surgery

The mitral valve is either accessed through the left atrium wall directly, or
a cut is made into the wall of the right atrium and then through the septum. Each individual surgeon will decide on which approach to use, each
having his or her own preference, taking into account the condition of the
patient and the heart.

Valve repair surgery

Not all valves that require surgery need to be replaced, because it is possible to repair one or more leaflets of the valve to prevent the need for
total replacement. This procedure involves the same approach to access
the valve and the patient's recovery is much the same.

Ross procedure

The Ross procedure is a technically challenging surgical technique that
involves using the patient's own pulmonary valve (autograft) to replace
the aortic valve. The pulmonary valve position is then filled using a homograft. In normal situations, the pulmonary valve is likely to be almost
identical to the healthy aortic valve, even if the aortic valve is deformed.
The pulmonary valve position is better suited to contain a homograft,
because the pressure exerted on it is less than the aortic position. The
autograft is better suited to greater pressures and is therefore more
durable in the aortic position than that of a mechanical graft or xenograft.

The long-term outcome of patients receiving an autograft is favourable. This procedure is not suitable for all aortic valve replacement candidates; the surgeon will assess the suitability of each candidate on an individual basis. For the patient to be considered for a Ross procedure, the pulmonary valve should be trileaflet and identical in size to the aortic valve. Ideal candidates for the Ross procedure are those with a life expectancy of 20 years or more, women of child-bearing years and people for whom anticoagulation would be considered inappropriate or high risk.

Postoperative care

This section is a guide to the postoperative care of the uncomplicated cardiac surgical patient. We discuss the care that patients will require at each stage of their inpatient, postoperative journey, but there are certain complications of which the nurse should be aware when caring for the patient.

These complications of surgery are uncommon and an individual patient's risk will vary depending on underlying medical conditions and

Table 11.3 Postoperative complications

Potential complications	Details
Bleeding/haemorrhage	The patient is at risk of bleeding from the wound and from the operation site within the thoracic cavity immediately postoperatively. It may be necessary to re-open the sternum to investigate and treat the cause of bleeding. This complication can be very serious depending on the severity of the bleed
Cardiac tamponade	Cardiac tamponade is a collection of blood or fluid within the pericardium, which may restrict the movement of the heart muscle. This can be caused by an acute haemorrhage into the pericardium or a gradual collection of fluid that slowly constricts the heart. This complication can be very serious. Cardiac tamponade will necessitate surgical intervention, often re-opening of the sternum and evacuation, usually under urgent conditions
Cardiac arrhythmia	Arrhythmias can have a number of causes in the immediate postoperative phase, including medication, dehydration, cardiac stunning and electrolyte imbalance. Some arrhythmias are fairly common and can be dealt with easily, others are more serious needing urgent intervention

Table 11.3 Postoperative complications (continued)

Potential complications	Details
Hypovolaemia	Disproportionate fluid loss from haemorrhage or excessive urine output can cause dehydration. This will have an impact on blood pressure, cardiac rhythm, cardiac output and renal function, and should be corrected without delay
Chest infection	Mechanical ventilation and painful sternotomy wound can have a negative impact on respiratory status postoperatively. Inability to cough and expectorate sputum as a result of uncontrolled pain can increase the risk of chest infection (Tulla et al. 1991)
Wound infection	Sternal wound infection can occur in 0.4–8% of all cardiac surgery cases (Radford 1993). Leg wounds are also at risk of infection (Swenne et al. 2004). Cardiac surgery patients are often predisposed to wound healing complications, i.e. poor nutrition, diabetes, peripheral vascular disease and surgical wounds
Gastrointestinal disturbance/Injury	Risk of gastrointestinal injury is a well-documented complication following cardiac surgery (Simic et al. 1999, Byhahn et al. 2001, Jayaprakash et al. 2004). Gastro-intestinal haemorrhage, bowel ischaemia and gastric stress ulcers are among these complications. Extended bypass time has an increase in risk of such complications
Neurological event	Neurocognitive dysfunction is a complication associated with cardiopulmonary bypass (Knipp et al. 2004), in particular, with gaseous microemboli (Kurusz and Butler 2004). These complications cannot be avoided in the postoperative phase although monitoring of such complications is crucial for effective postoperative care
Thromboembolism	Pulmonary embolus and deep vein thrombosis are complications of cardiac surgery (Shammas 2000). They can result from cardiopulmonary bypass, reduced mobility or cardiac arrhythmias (Lahtinen et al. 2004). Prophylactic treatment is well documented (Kakkar and Stringer 1990, Agu et al. 1999, Prandoni et al. 2001)

previous medical and surgical history. Postoperative care of the patient is focused on prevention or early detection of these complications. It is anticipated that a patient will experience cardiac surgery without complication.

Awareness of the potential for complications will assist the nurse to care for her or his patient safely.

The following discussion provides a guideline to the care that a patient may require in the postoperative phase, starting from transfer from theatre through to discharge. The points are by no means an exhaustive list of the needs of the cardiac surgical patient and are designed for use as a guide to good quality postoperative nursing care.

Many areas use integrated care pathways to plan patient care, with a clear guide to what should be achieved at any point of the patient's surgical journey. It is intended that, if complications arise, this care pathway will be altered according to the individual needs of the patient. The patient's postoperative surgical care should always be individualized and holistic in nature.

Fast tracking

Historically, patients have been transferred to an intensive care environment from theatre for at least the first postoperative night. However, advancements in surgical technique and reduced need for cardiopulmonary bypass have presented the opportunity for patients to be 'fast tracked' to a high-dependency area for their first night, thus reducing invasive monitoring and length of time on a ventilator. The fast track will involve a short stay in an intensive care environment or a theatre recovery in order for the patient to be extubated. Accelerated recovery after cardiac surgery is reported to decrease duration of intubation and hospitalization for patients resulting in a more economical use of services (Flynn et al. 2004), although it is suitable for uncomplicated, elective patients (Kaplan et al. 2002). Fast tracking is not established at every cardiac centre and local areas will have policies and protocols regarding fast tracking with patient safety of the utmost importance.

Transfer from theatre

Immediately after surgery, the patient is transferred from theatre directly to an intensive care unit (ICU). Equipment is set up and monitoring established. A care plan for the patient needs to be activated. Care plans are often standardized; indeed, many may involve the use of integrated care pathways. The plan follows a nursing model favoured in that area, commonly that of Roper et al. (2003). It is vital that the nurse caring for the patient has performed equipment checks and reviewed alarm settings as soon as possible, to ensure patient safety. The anaesthetist generally accompanies the patient out of theatre and ensures that he or she is settled into the ICU.

Breathing

On arrival in the ICU, the patient is anaesthetized, and so requires artificial mechanical ventilation. It is usually the responsibility of the anaesthetist to ensure that the patient's airway is patent and establish him or her on the ventilator before leaving the bedside. Mechanical ventilation continues until the anaesthetic medication is discontinued and the patient is able to breathe effectively and independently. Arterial blood gas (ABG) analysis is often taken on arrival to the ICU to assess the effectiveness of ventilation after the transfer from theatre. ABG is then taken as required until effective ventilation is established by the patient, often with O_2 therapy. Continuous O_2 saturation monitoring is established via a finger probe. Respiratory rate, ventilator settings and peripheral O_2 saturation are monitored continuously and charted regularly. Regular auscultation of the chest assesses the need for suction via the endotracheal tube. Excessive secretions interfere with effective ventilation and should be removed as required.

Neurological status

Anaesthetic medication is administered intravenously until the patient is ready to be woken up. Pupil size and response to light are monitored in order that any neurological problems may be identified. Anaesthetic and pain medication alter neurological condition, but recovery from anaesthetic is closely monitored and intravenous analgesia adjusted according to its effects on neurological status. Once conscious the patient should be oriented to time and place, particularly to day and night, in order to reduce the potential for confusion and disorientation.

Temperature

A warming blanket is used in order that the patient's core temperature be normalized. This process is controlled and may take some time so that a sudden rise in temperature, which would result in vasodilatation, does not adversely affect blood pressure. Core temperature is likely to be low immediately after surgery as a result of cardiopulmonary bypass, including the method used to establish bypass. It is measured using the pulmonary artery catheter. Once warming has been successful and the core temperature normalized, the warming blanket is removed.

Heart rate and rhythm

Cardiac monitoring has been ongoing throughout the surgical procedure and continues in the ICU. Surgeons often routinely insert epicardial pacing wires so that some cardiac arrhythmias may be treated for the short term, while the heart settles after surgery. Patients often experience bradycardic arrhythmias or a degree of heart block immediately after surgery, which can be easily addressed by external cardiac pacing for a few days.

Arrhythmias are a common complication of cardiac surgery. External cardiac pacing may also be used to support blood pressure in the initial postoperative phase of recovery. A patient may also experience a tachycardic arrhythmia; this is treated with medication according to the rhythm and also the doctor's preference. Many local areas have protocols for the common arrhythmias after cardiac surgery, particularly for atrial fibrillation (AF). AF is a frequent complication for all cardiac surgery patients, particularly after valvular surgery – about 30–60% (Debrunner et al. 2004).

Blood pressure

Blood pressure is monitored continuously in the early stages of recovery via the arterial line. It should be recorded at least hourly and may well need to be supported with medication or pacing in the very early stages. Fluid balance influences blood pressure enormously and, as the patient begins to excrete any extra fluid from the bypass machine, the blood pressure may become affected. Intravenous fluids, crystalloid and colloid are administered accordingly. The anaesthetist may well have inserted a pulmonary artery catheter. The use of such monitoring must be limited to when necessary because of potential complications (McGee and Gould 2003). This catheter enables the nurse or doctor to measure and monitor cardiac output and cardiac studies. These readings may be useful when the blood pressure, urine output and heart rate are giving cause for concern or do not seem to be correlating with the overall clinical picture, although the reliability of such invasive monitoring has been widely questioned (Kumar et al. 2004).

Drains

All patients have cardiac drains that drain blood or air (dependent on site) directly into an underwater seal (similar to that used for a pneumothorax). Routinely the drains are mediastinal and pericardial. A pleural drain is used if the pleurae are breached during surgery. The output is measured initially every 15 min in order to establish any problems with postoperative bleeding as soon as possible. Local areas tolerate different amounts of drainage initially postoperatively. As a guide, about 100 ml/h is acceptable for the first few hours, dependent on blood pressure, urine output, heart rate and haemoglobin. Cardiac drains are generally used with low vacuum suction (−5 to −10 mmHg); this enables air in the thoracic cavity to be dispersed. The drains are removed when they have ceased to yield blood and air; often the drainage slows and a continuous haemoserous ooze presents. Again, local areas often have policies about their removal. Drainage of about 100 ml or less over 6 hours is generally acceptable. There must be no evidence of an air leak before the drains may be removed.

Urine output

Urine output must be monitored closely in the first few hours postoperatively. Initially it is prudent to monitor the output every 15 min, particularly if the patient has been on cardiopulmonary bypass. Patients experiencing 'on-pump' surgery are likely to have an excessive urine output in the first few hours, following the initial output; it should then settle down and the patient's fluid balance should be monitored closely. It is expected that the patient will retain some fluid in the early stage of recovery so a positive fluid balance of up to about 1 litre is acceptable. Intravenous fluid and diuretics are prescribed accordingly with this aim in mind. As well as the overall fluid balance (do not forget the drains!), hourly urine output must be considered. About 0.5 ml/kg per h is acceptable, so a 60-kg patient would expect 30 ml/h of urine. Urine output is affected not only by fluid balance. Blood pressure and kidney function should also be considered when setting targets.

Intravenous fluids

The anaesthetist or surgeon prescribes crystalloid fluid maintenance for adequate hydration of the patient. This is administered via the central line or peripheral cannulae. Any extra hydration fluid will be given according to the patient's condition. Blood transfusions are not always necessary. Again, blood is given according to the patient's condition, blood pressure, cardiac drainage and haemoglobin. Anaesthetic medication is given intravenously until no longer required, as well as some form of intravenous analgesia, often a morphine infusion. Any other medication needed, e.g. to support blood pressure, is also infused, usually through the central line. Other commonly used intravenous medications include an insulin sliding scale and prophylactic antibiotics (Kreter and Woods 1992).

Analgesia

Pain is controlled using a variety of methods; anaesthetists and surgeons have individual preferences. The following methods are often used at different points throughout the patient's hospital admission, continuing on to discharge.

Epidural

An epidural infusion may be established in the anaesthetic room before surgery and may continue according to local policy. The infusion contains local anaesthetic agents and can incorporate an opiate analgesia. Epidural analgesia is commonly used in the initial postoperative phase. The dose of analgesia is adjusted according to its effectiveness and the patient is usually weaned off it gradually as he or she is able to tolerate the pain level. The epidural catheter remains *in situ* until the patient is established on oral fluids and able to take oral analgesia.

Intravenous infusion

An intravenous infusion of an opiate analgesia is often initiated in the anaesthetic room preoperatively. Intravenous opiates are not used in combination with epidural opiate analgesia. Administration of intravenous opiates can have adverse affects on neurological status, so the infusion tends to be used in the initial postoperative phase only and the patient is weaned off as soon as possible.

Local anaesthetic

Some areas may advocate the use of a continuous local anaesthetic infusion at the sternotomy site (White et al. 2003). This is used in conjunction with oral or intravenous analgesia.

Oral

Once the patient has been extubated, he or she is encouraged to start drinking small amounts of water; any nausea needs to be settled and then they can be established on oral analgesics. A combination of oral analgesics may be used, including paracetamol, oral opiate, e.g. tramadol, codeine or anti-inflammatory analgesic. Choice of oral analgesic is by medical preference, patient tolerance and effectiveness. Whichever method of first-line analgesia is used, the patient should be well established on oral analgesia before discharge home is considered.

Analgesia should be regularly assessed for effectiveness and adjusted accordingly. It is vital that the patient is comfortable enough to move freely and breathe effectively. The sternotomy is likely to cause a great deal of discomfort and can impede breathing. The patient is encouraged to take regular deep breaths and expectorate any sputum that may be in the lungs or airways. If the patient has not received sufficient analgesia, the inability to cough may result in sputum retention or a chest infection.

Movement/Mobility

As with any patient who is unable to move independently, the sedated and ventilated patient requires regular pressure area care and possibly passive exercises. Antiembolic stockings are used according to local policy, usually started in the ICU. Once extubated and conscious, the patient is assisted out of bed and into a chair. The first time out of bed is usually hard work for the patient, so he or she is expected to sit out of bed for only a short period of time. Early mobilization is essential for an uncomplicated, speedy recovery after cardiac surgery, because it encourages deep breathing, gives pressure relief, encourages independence and can improve psychological well-being (Ng and Tam 2000).

Wounds

The sternal wound generally has a dry dressing to cover, which should remain *in situ* according to local policy, often 24 h in the initial postoperative stage (Wynne et al. 2004). Once that initial period is over, the wound should be assessed, kept clean and dry, and re-dressed as appropriate.

The leg wound has a similar dressing as well as a pressure dressing. This is applied to help prevent bleeding immediately postoperatively. The process of harvesting the saphenous leg vein is accomplished well before the bypass operation is completed but, as the patient is heparinized for the duration of the surgery, the closed and dressed leg wound is at high risk of bleeding until protamine is given and the risk of bleeding has been reduced. The pressure dressing is left on according to the preferences of the surgeon. In theory, the risk of bleeding is reduced once the effect of heparin is reversed; however, some practitioners request that the pressure dressing remain *in situ* for 24–48 h.

Blood tests

Baseline haemoglobin may be established soon after transfer from theatre, in order that fluids and blood products may be prescribed and administered accordingly. A baseline ABG will also help to assess ventilation and identify any problems early. It is advisable to monitor urea and electrolytes, immediately after surgery, particularly if blood loss or urine output is excessive. It is vital that potassium levels are kept within normal limits, usually 4–5 mmol/l. Serum K^+ levels can be affected by the cardioplegia used to put the patient on bypass, and then by the large diuresis immediately after coming off bypass. Problems with cardiac arrhythmias are more likely to occur in patients with lower serum K^+ (Johnson et al. 1999).

Hygiene

The patient is likely to require a level of hygiene care on return from theatre. Although this is low priority, mouth care, eye care, washing and hair care are all vital in providing holistic care. Privacy and dignity should be maintained at all times.

After the day of surgery, it may be appropriate to transfer the patient to a high-dependency area for the first postoperative day or to transfer directly to a ward environment from an ICU. The patient's clinical status is the most influential factor when allocating the area in which they will be nursed (Table 11.4).

Table 11.4 Day 1 after surgery – care

Potential problem	Action	Rationale
Ineffective breathing	Administer humidified O_2 via facemask as prescribed to maintain O_2 saturation within prescribed limits	Studies show humidification may not be necessary for low flow O_2 (Miyamoto 2004), but can increase comfort and prevent dehydration of airways (Pilkington 2004)
Chest infection	Chest physiotherapy and encouragement to expectorate sputum	Effective re-inflation of lungs To assist with deep breathing and sputum expectoration Expel air from thoracic cavity via cardiac drains
	Monitor arterial blood gases as required	Early identification of respiratory complications
	Remove arterial line according to local policy	To reduce risk of infection, haemorrhage or discomfort
	Monitor and record respiration rate	Early identification of respiratory complications
	Monitor temperature	To ensure that body temperature normalizes Early identification of infection
	Chest radiograph	To assess lung condition, particularly after cardiac drain removal
Haemodynamic instability	Monitor heart rate and rhythm Monitor blood pressure	To identify potential problems
	Secure epicardial pacing wires according to local policy	Reduce risk of infection and ensure easy access in emergency situation

Table 11.4 Day 1 after surgery – care (continued)

Potential problem	Action	Rationale
Haemodynamic instability (contd)	Administer intravenous fluids as prescribed	To maintain or correct haemodynamic status
	Remove pulmonary artery catheter, according to local policy	To prevent potential complications
Haemorrhage	Observe cardiac drainage	To detect bleeding and air leaks
	Remove cardiac drains according to local policy	To increase comfort and prevent potential problems
	Monitor haemoglobin as necessary	To detect and treat anaemia
Electrolyte imbalance	Monitor electrolyte balance	To identify, detect and correct electrolyte imbalance
	Monitor urine output according to patient need and local policy	To prevent, detect or correct ARF
Acute renal failure (ARF)	Monitor urea and creatinine levels	To detect early signs of ARF
	Monitor daily weight	To detect fluid retention
	Administer diuretic until weight is equal to preoperative weight	To ensure residual fluid from bypass has been excreted
Infection	Monitor regular temperature Monitor regular white cell count Monitor sputum and send for culture sensitivity as required	To detect early signs of infection
	Clean and dress wounds according to local policy	To prevent wound infection
	Administer prophylactic antibiotics as prescribed, according to local policy	To prevent infection

Table 11.4 Day 1 after surgery – care (continued)

Potential problem	Action	Rationale
Infection (contd)	Screen for infection when symptomatic	Identify and treat infection
Pain	Discontinue intravenous opiate analgesia as tolerated and prescribed	To prevent side effects of opiate medication, i.e. nausea, neurological impairment, constipation
	Establish regular oral analgesia as tolerated	To prevent discomfort and pain as far as possible
	Assess effectiveness of analgesia	To ensure adequate pain control
Reduced mobility	Assist and encourage mobility as tolerated	Reduce the risk of thromboembolism Encourage independence as soon as possible Improve psychological well-being (De Feo et al. 2002)
	Commence daily physiotherapy	To promote safe mobility
Poor nutritional intake	Encourage oral fluids as tolerated	To ensure adequate hydration
	Encourage diet as tolerated	To optimize nutritional status
	Treat nausea as necessary	To ensure patient comfort To promote oral intake of fluid and diet
	Administer intravenous fluids until oral fluid intake is adequate to maintain hydration	To avoid dehydration and associated complications
	Administer medication for stomach protection until oral intake sufficient	To prevent gastric ulceration while stomach is empty (Johnston et al. 1992)

Table 11.4 Day 1 after surgery – care (continued)

Potential problem	Action	Rationale
Thrombus formation	Fit antiembolic stockings	To prevent formation of deep vein thrombosis (Amarigiri and Lees 2000)
	Administer subcutaneous heparin	For thrombus prophylaxis (Kakkar and Stringer 1990)
	Encourage and assist early mobility	To prevent deep vein thrombosis
Inability to maintain hygiene needs	Assist with hygiene as necessary including mouth care, hair care and bathing	Maintain high standards of hygiene Ensure privacy and dignity
Instability of sternum	Prevent patient from excessive use of chest muscles that may loosen sternal wires and cause sternal instability Limit weight lifted according to local policy Assist support of sternum when coughing, sneezing and moving	Protection of sternum until healing provides some strength in the bone (about 6 weeks)

Postoperative care in the following days may well be delayed to resolve a complication or problem. Table 11.5 is a brief outline of routine care for a non-complicated cardiac surgery patient.

It is vital that the decision to discharge is not made on medical fitness alone, and a multidisciplinary ward round, comprising medics, nurses, cardiac liaison nurses, physiotherapists and pharmacists, can be very beneficial in a holistic assessment of the patient. There are so many factors to take into consideration at this time, not least the patient's social circumstances and the provision or availability of a safe discharge address. Ideally, the patient is discharged to the care of a friend or relative who is available to provide both the physical and the emotional support that the patient requires at this time. When this is not possible, plans should be made to discharge to convalescence, intermediate care teams or the local district general hospital. Choice of discharge location depends on the resources and policies of the patient's primary care trust. Social service input, if required, should also have been arranged by this point. These

Table 11.5 Routine care for a non-complicated surgery patient

Day 2

Reduce O_2 as tolerated
Remove intravenous infusions
Remove invasive lines including, central line, arterial line, urinary catheter and cardiac drains, according to patient condition and local policy
Remove cardiac monitoring
Reduce frequency of vital sign monitoring, i.e. heart rate, blood pressure, respiratory rate, O_2 saturation and temperature
Assist with shower
Assist to increase mobility
Encourage oral intake
Monitor fluid balance for 24 h after catheter removal, to detect urine retention
Monitor bowels
Monitor effectiveness of analgesia
Assess wounds and drain sites and dress appropriately
Assist with antiembolic stockings
Daily weight
Discontinue intravenous antibiotics
Daily physiotherapy
Encourage rest and sleep
Transfer to ward environment as appropriate

Day 3

Remove O_2
Remove epicardial pacing wires
Continue monitor of vital signs
Encourage increasing mobility
Encourage independent shower
Discontinue medication for stomach protection
Discontinue fluid balance monitoring
Assess wounds and drain sites and dress appropriately
Administer and assess analgesia
Encourage oral intake
Daily physiotherapy
Monitor bowel movement, treat as appropriate
Encourage rest and sleep

Day 4

Increase mobility
Climb stairs with supervision to ensure safety
Daily physiotherapy
Regular monitoring of vital signs
Encourage oral intake
Consider discharge

Table 11.5 Routine care for a non-complicated surgery patient (continued)

Day 4 or 5
Consider discharge: Are they medically fit? Is the analgesia effective? Has the patient had opened his or her bowels? Can the patient mobilize safely? If the patient could manage the stairs preoperatively, can he or she manage them now? Is there adequate support at home to facilitate a safe discharge?

arrangements can take time to finalize, which highlights the importance of discharge planning preoperatively. Whatever the discharge arrangement, however, the ability for patients to cope after discharge is greatly assisted if they are provided with realistic, practical information, presented in a form that matches their coping style.

Pre-discharge information

The provision of pre-discharge information is essential for the physical and psychological recovery, and well-being, of both the patient and the carer (Artinian 1991, 1993). Davies (2000, p. 319) studied 'patients' and carers' perceptions of factors influencing recovery after cardiac surgery' and found that there were significant differences between their perceptions throughout the recovery period, so ideally the carers should always be given the opportunity to be included in the pre-discharge information discussion.

The approach in delivering pre-discharge information depends very much on the resources and infrastructure that cardiac centres have in place, and ranges from individual patient and family discussions with specialist cardiac liaison nurses, to group sessions with physiotherapists, to more informal ad-hoc information provision by ward nurses. Whatever the form of its provision, however, it is essential that the verbal information is reinforced with written information (Johnson et al. 2003). There are significant numbers of qualitative and quantitative research studies that demonstrate that anxiety impedes learning and affects the ability to retain information (Cupples 1991).

As a result of the nature of cardiac surgery and the requirement for a sternotomy there are postoperative physical limitations. The sternum, as with any other bone, takes 6–12 weeks to heal and therefore patients are advised to avoid lifting, pushing or pulling anything heavy (with the definition of heavy generally being defined between 1 and 5 kg or 2 and 10 lb in weight) for at least 6 weeks. As a result of the physical limitations from the sternotomy, saphenous vein graft and/or radial artery graft wound, as well as the psychological impact that cardiac surgery has, it is essential that pre-discharge information equip the patient and carer with the information and resources to be able to cope after discharge. (Recovery from minimal invasive cardiac surgery, which has not required a sternotomy, is different from conventional cardiac surgery, as is the recovery from transplantation.) The following pre-discharge information guidelines focus on recovery from conventional cardiac surgery.

Initial discharge expectations

Patients and their carers need to be warned that it is normal to sometimes feel more tired for the few days after discharge than they perhaps felt in the days preceding discharge. This is partly the result of the journey home and the change in environment but it is perhaps also caused by the anxiety that many patients feel about returning home after such a big operation. The carers also often have feelings of anxiety at this time (Theobald 1997), although their fears and perceptions of problems frequently differ from those of the patient. Reassurance that these feelings of vulnerability are very normal for both patient and carer can assist them to accept this as a normal part of the recovery process. In addition, the provision of post-discharge support can be reassuring if they are not coping at home entirely on their own after an inpatient admission in a very acute environment.

Pain

Before discharge it is important that the prescribed analgesia is effectively controlling the pain in order to ensure adequate levels of pain relief after discharge. The importance of taking regular analgesia postoperatively should be explained and the value of reducing the level of analgesia slowly, according to the individual's pain threshold, emphasized. It is vital that pain be controlled in order for the patient to be able to breathe deeply, cough, expectorate, mobilize and rest, because an inability to perform these functions may lead to respiratory or circulatory problems (such as chest infection or deep vein thrombosis), poor posture or over-tiredness. Another factor to consider when discussing postoperative pain is whether the IMAs have been harvested. IMAs provide successful conduits for CABGs (Dietl et al. 1993), but can leave a short-term aching, burning or stabbing sensation in the harvested site (Holl 1995, Rowe and King 1998). Although this usually settles with time, it is important that the patient be informed of this potential occurrence so he or she is able to differentiate between these sensations and the preoperative angina.

Mobility, activity and exercise

The importance of regular mobilization postoperatively will have been stressed to the patient, ideally from pre-admission clinic and/or admission, but, if not, from operation day or day 1. Walking is the main form of exercise encouraged postoperatively because this does not interfere with the healing of the sternum. Patients should be encouraged to start off walking very short distances, e.g. around the house/flat and garden, but doing this several times a day, and then increasing the distances gradually as time goes on. Levels of activity to achieve obviously depend on the individual patient's preoperative level of activity and mobility, so an individual pre-discharge discussion can be beneficial in providing a tailored programme of activity. Written information that gives a guide to increasing activity week by week, and includes arm, leg and ankle exercise diagrams or pictures, can be particularly useful in providing a reminder of recommended activity. For the first 6 weeks the patient's activity is limited as a result of the healing of the sternotomy. After 6 weeks the patient is advised gradually to increase activity levels so that by 12 weeks postoperatively he or she has achieved the preoperative level of activity, if not more.

Antiembolic stockings

The use of antiembolic stockings in the area of cardiac surgery is fairly controversial and there is a lack of objective research about their efficacy in prophylaxis against pulmonary embolism (Ramos et al. 1996). However, support stockings are often used to ease symptoms of tenderness and oedema caused by removal of the saphenous vein (Jonker et al. 2001). Some centres advocate their use from the morning of surgery through to 6 weeks postoperatively, whereas others do not include antiembolic stockings in the pre- or postoperative treatment at all. Further research in this area is required to give a definitive answer to this question.

Hygiene

The pre-discharge discussion should include the importance of maintaining hygiene needs and appropriate care of the surgical wound. Continuing from discharge planning started in the pre-admission clinic and/or on admission, it is also important to establish that the discharge address has adequate and safe bathing facilities, and the patient is self-caring with these needs, so that if not occupational therapy referrals can be made.

Sense of taste

It is not unusual for the senses to be temporarily affected postoperatively, particularly the sense of taste (Beekmann-Ball and Grap 1992). This usually resolves with time (Beekmann-Ball and Grap 1992), although occasionally other factors such as neurological events may have caused some deficit or change in the senses, and so may take longer to resolve. Explanation about the normality of the change in senses can be very reassuring for carers as well as patients, particularly as it can often affect the appetite.

Appetite

As discussed above, it is not unusual for patients to experience a reduction or change in appetite (Tack and Gilliss 1990, Beekmann-Ball and Grap 1992), which often gives the carer more cause for concern than the patient. Patients and carers need to be educated about the different food groups and the amounts of food required in the immediate postoperative period for wound healing and energy. Information on this subject can help avoid conflict after discharge between patients and relatives if they have a shared understanding of dietary requirements. Gastrointestinal symptoms, such as nausea, poor appetite and lack of taste, decrease with time (Grap et al. 1996), and patients and carers should be reassured of this. Often, once patients return home, the appetite improves because they have access to their usual diet.

Elimination

Satisfactory urine output should have been established with 24 h of removal of the urinary catheter. However, it is often 3 days postoperatively before the bowels are opened, and with a reduction in length of inpatient stay it is important that this factor be checked before discharge. Appropriate advice should be given about the importance of avoiding constipation post-discharge, and when and how to seek assistance should this occur.

Emotional well-being

It is very common for patients to feel irritable or short-tempered, emotional and teary postoperatively (Goodman 1997), and patients seem to experience this at around 4 days postoperatively. The reduction in length of inpatient stay means that patients are less likely to witness other patients experiencing these emotional and psychological problems than they were several years ago. It is therefore very important that this potential component of the recovery is explained to patients and relatives so that they recognize it as a normal part of the recovery process. The patient should be encouraged to express feelings rather than to bottle them up and a supportive environment helps in this expression. Unfortunately many patients do not live in an environment conducive to expression of these feelings, or are not naturally emotionally expressive, and this highlights the relevance and benefits of specialist cardiac liaison and community cardiac rehabilitation nurses to support patients and carers after discharge.

Sleep

Many patients expect that when they return home they will be able to catch up on all the sleep that they did not have in hospital. This may be an unrealistic expectation, however, and it is common to experience a change in sleep pattern for several weeks after discharge (Tack and Gilliss 1990), perhaps waking as often as once an hour in the initial discharge period. It is important that this postoperative element is explained before discharge, as well as providing reassurance that this will settle with time. Encouragement to have a daytime rest is essential to avoid over-tiredness.

Returning to work

Advice about returning to work depends very much on the type of occupation and of course the specific type of cardiac surgery performed. Focusing on recovery from conventional cardiac surgery, the advice is to refrain from returning to work for 3 months. The rationale is that it takes 12 weeks for the patient to achieve a level of activity and fitness that matches or surmounts the preoperative level. At 12 weeks it should be possible for the patient to return to work but, if the job is very heavy or very stressful, he or she may benefit from returning on a part-time basis and then increasing the hours gradually.

Driving

The DVLA states that 'driving must cease for at least 4 weeks' after CABG surgery and 'may recommence thereafter provided there is no other disqualifying condition' (www.dvla.gov.uk/at_a_glance/ch2_cardiovascular. htm). Conversely, guidelines for postoperative valve patients say that this group of patients may continue to drive following their surgery provided that there are no other disqualifying conditions (DVLA 2004). Nevertheless, it is common practice for both postoperative CABG and valve patients to be advised to refrain from driving for at least 4 weeks. However, if at 4 weeks postoperatively the sternum is not stable or is continuing to click, the patient should avoid driving until so advised by the surgeon.

Sex

As a result of the physical limitations involved in the recovery from cardiac surgery, it is recommended that patients avoid sexual intercourse for the first 4 weeks after surgery (British Heart Foundation 2001), but if he or she can subsequently take the passive role then the patient should be able to engage in sexual relations without problems.

Secondary prevention

The NSF for CHD (DoH 2000a) recommends the delivery of phase I cardiac rehabilitation, and this includes the delivery of health education and a focus on secondary prevention before discharge.

In an ideal world the main focus for CHD risk factor education would be primary prevention, but in the real world and for patients requiring cardiac surgery this is too late, so the focus turns to secondary prevention.

The relevance and effectiveness of health education in the pre-admission setting have already been discussed, yet the timing of phase I postoperative health education is more controversial (Egan 1999). This controversy is perhaps reflected in the diversity of postoperative cardiac health education services received by patients before discharge, ranging from individual health education teaching, to group education sessions, to nothing at all – despite it being an NSF (DoH 2000a) recommendation that health promotion be delivered before discharge.

Salisbury (1994) claims that health education during hospitalization or in the 2 weeks after the cardiac event is too soon, and that patients are too anxious at this time (Gillis 1984, Artinian 1991, 1993, Moser et al. 1993) and more concerned with adjusting to their immediate future and limitations (Salisbury 1994), so health education may just be something else that they feel pressured to remember. This perception is, however, contradictory to other research which states that patients are actually keen to receive health promotion during a cardiac event admission, and that, despite their anxiety, lack of health education at this time heightens anxiety, rather than reducing it (Foulger 1997). The provision of information at this time can also assist patients and relatives to feel more in control of their recovery (Artinian 1991, 1993).

Research into health education provision does, however, provide consistent evidence that health education should be delivered in a form optimal to patient needs – and this differs from one patient, and the family, to another (Lane 1997, Theobald 1997). It must be recognized that cardiac surgery patients will have different needs and knowledge bases of heart disease risk factors and that their needs will alter throughout their CHD journey (Moynihan 1984, Nursing Times Professional Development

1995). The routine, elective post-cardiac surgery patient may have had cardiological treatment for many months if not years, and so his or her knowledge of cardiac risk factors may be significantly different to that of a patient who has had surgery carried out urgently, with no known previous cardiac history (Mullen et al. 1992). It is vital that patients and families understand that, although cardiac surgery provides relief from symptoms, it does not cure CHD (Kee et al. 1995). CABGs have a limited lifespan but can be protected in part by recipients managing their known risk factors (Pearson et al. 1994). It is widely documented that many of the CHD risk factors can be altered because they are often related to lifestyle, and Greenwood et al.'s (1996, p. 216) quantitative study is one of many to state that 'altering blood pressure, high cholesterol and smoking behaviour have been shown to have an effect on subsequent mortality from coronary heart disease'. If health education is to be successful, however, topics should also be based on an understanding of the individual patient's perception of risk factors in order to reduce his or her real fears and yet educate about the real risks.

Post-discharge support

As in most areas of cardiac surgery service, the range of post-discharge services provided is wide and varied. Some of the cardiac centres at the forefront of this field use the cardiac liaison nurse role to provide this support.

Telephone support

Many discharge problems relate to information needs, and telephone helpline services have proved an invaluable resource towards meeting them (Mistiaen and Poot 2003). The benefits of telephone support are numerous: it enables information to be reinforced, provision of health education and advice, and 'managing symptoms, recognizing complications early, giving reassurance and providing quality aftercare service' (Mistiaen and Poot 2003, p. 1). Mistiaen and Poot (2003, p. 1) continue, adding that this form of support 'is easy to organise and does not cost a lot of money or time'. Telephone support is probably the most common form of hospital-based post-discharge support and most centres, even if they cannot provide a nurse-initiated follow-up call service and a formal telephone helpline facility, encourage patients and relatives to call the ward if they have any queries or problems. However, this form of communication is difficult for the deaf or hard of hearing and those who do not speak English (Payne 1998). On balance, however, the advantages undoubtedly outweigh the disadvantages and patients certainly appreciate these calls (Moran et al. 1999).

Home visits

For some cardiac centres, home visits constitute the main form of post-discharge support. The advantage of a home visit is that it provides face-to-face contact and therefore enables the nurse to conduct a visual or physical examination of the patient, which is obviously not possible with telephone follow-up alone. Nevertheless, it does require a great deal of resources in terms of time and costs, and may mean that the service is provided at the expense of other cardiac services. However, phase II cardiac rehabilitation means that patients now receive more support from community nurses including community cardiac rehabilitation nurses than ever before, which helps the continual provision of this valuable home visiting service.

Whatever the form of post-discharge support, however, the factors in Table 11.6 are worth while considering when assessing the patient. (Note that patients who have undergone transplantation will have more complex factors to consider and Table 10.6 relates to postoperative CABG and valve patients.)

Table 11.6 Checklist of factors and problems to consider when discharging a patient

Checklist	Factors to consider	Problems to exclude
Pain	Is the pain controlled? Is the analgesia effective? Is the patient taking the analgesia appropriately?	Ineffective analgesia and/or inappropriate dosage
Breathing	Is the patient's breathing within safe, normal range for the patient? Is their breathing improving? Does their breathlessness resolve on resting?	Symptoms of heart failure, effusions or chest infection
Oedema	Is the patient experiencing oedema? Is it limited to the donor leg or both legs? Is the oedema within expected limits? How is the patient's breathing?	Symptoms of heart failure, fluid retention, deep vein thrombosis
Wounds	Are the wounds healing as expected? If required, is a district nurse visiting?	Wounds failing to heal, wound infection and/or inappropriate wound care
Mobility	Is the patient increasing his or her mobility levels gradually? Are the patient's mobility levels within expected limits?	Excessive/insufficient/ inappropriate levels of activity

Table 11.6 Checklist of factors and problems (continued)

Checklist	Factors to consider	Problems to exclude
Elimination	Is the patient's bowel pattern returning to normal?	Constipation, altered bowel pattern
Hygiene	Is the patient self-caring with his or her hygiene needs?	Inability to maintain own hygiene needs, lack of confidence maintaining own hygiene needs
Emotional/ Psychological Well-being	Does the patient/carer feel that he or she is coping with psychological impact of the surgery?	Depression, excessive irritability/tearfulness, inappropriate behaviour
Nutrition	Is the patient eating sufficient amounts to promote wound healing and sustain energy levels, and if not why not?	Insufficient dietary intake, nausea/vomiting
Sleeping and rest	Is the patient getting enough sleep (although disturbed sleep pattern is to be expected)? Is he or she having a daytime rest?	Insufficient levels of rest and sleep, inability to sleep, excessive lethargy

Outpatient review

Patients usually attend for a surgical follow-up assessment approximately 6–8 weeks after discharge (although occasionally this follow-up may be carried out by the cardiologist if the patient lives a long way from the tertiary centre). At the moment most of these clinics are medic led.

The NHS Plan (DoH 2000b) aims to break down the barriers and demarcations between staff. The reduction in junior doctors' hours and the introduction of the 10 key roles for nurses (DoH 2000b) have played a significant role in shaping the future of cardiac surgery follow-up clinics. As a result of these changes, it may soon become more commonplace for this service to be nurse led, running alongside consultant-led clinics (with the registrar or consultant seeing the patients with more complex conditions). Whoever assesses the patients, however, it is customary to review the items in Table 11.7.

After satisfactory assessment at the follow-up clinic patients can often be discharged back to the care of the GP, although those with ongoing

Table 11.7 Checklist for outpatient review

Checklist	Rationale
Blood pressure (BP)	Blood pressure is within safe and normal range. The 2004 British Hypertension Society recommends that drug treatment should be considered for individuals with BP ≥ 140/90 mmHg, and that optimal BP treatment targets are a systolic BP < 140 mmHg and a diastolic BP < 85mm Hg (130/85 mmHg, in people with diabetes); optimal BP level is now classified as < 120/< 80 mmHg (see British Heart Foundation 2004a and www.heartstats.org/topic.asp?id=881) Antihypertension medication is reviewed and appropriate for the patient
Wounds	The wounds have healed/are healing as expected If required, a district nurse is visiting/appropriate wound care is being provided Tissue viability advice is sought if required
Heart rate	Heart rate is within a safe range Heart rhythm is sinus rhythm/has returned to the preoperative rate and rhythm Anti-arrhythmic medication is reviewed/stopped/commenced
Sternum	The sternum is healing/has healed
Pain	The wound/bone healing/internal mammary artery/muscular pain is resolving Analgesia is effective/has been reduced/is being taken appropriately There has been no recurrence of angina
Breathing	The patient's breathing is within safe, normal range for the patient Breathlessness improving as expected for that individual patient Breathlessness resolves on resting
Oedema	Ankle/leg oedema is resolving Oedema is limited to the donor leg Oedema is within expected limits Breathing is within safe, normal range for the patient
Mobility	The patient is increasing mobility gradually within safe, appropriate levels for him or her Excessive/insufficient/inappropriate levels of activity are reviewed and discussed and advice given
Medication	Review of medications, to ensure that they are appropriately prescribed for the short term, particularly anti-arrhythmics and analgesia, and the long term, principally angiotensin-converting enzyme inhibitors, β blockers, statins and anti-platelets

Table 11.7 Checklist for outpatient review (continued)

Checklist	Rationale
Coronary heart disease (CHD) risk factors	The patient's individual CHD risk factors have been identified Appropriate CHD health education has been provided Appropriate referrals to other agencies such as dietitians, smoking cessation clinics, diabetes clinics, etc., have been made Appropriate secondary prevention medication has been prescribed
Cardiac rehabilitation	The patient has started his or her cardiac rehabilitation class or has heard from his or her cardiac rehabilitation provider about starting a class
Investigations	CABG patients: it is not customary to conduct chest radiographs or echocardiograms routinely at this point (unless clinically indicated) Valve replacement patients: again, routine chest radiographs or echocardiograms are not usually required at this point (unless clinically indicated) Valve repair patients: practice varies, with some consultants routinely ordering echocardiograms for all, whereas others are satisfied with the pre-discharge echocardiogram and do not order another at this point unless clinically indicated after examination
General progress	Reassurance for both patients and carers is vital at this point Advice about what to expect and how to progress in the next stage of the recovery process is also important

arrhythmia problems or who have had valve surgery may need to go back to the care of the cardiologist (care of the transplant recipient differs – needing closer follow-up treatment).

Cardiac transplantation

Cardiac transplantation has become a very effective treatment for severe cardiac failure with around two-thirds of patients living beyond 5 years after transplantation (Hosenpud et al. 2001). The availability of modern immunosuppressive drugs has dramatically reduced the risk of rejection and therefore increased the likelihood of patients returning to a fuller life.

Cardiac transplantation is indicated for all patients with end-stage heart disease without contraindications (Castle and Jones 2004). In reality this usually means patients in whom other medical and surgical options have failed. Prospective patients are referred to the transplant team for assessment before acceptance on the transplant register. The assessment process is extremely thorough and has to take into account co-morbidity and psychological state. The transplant team has to be sure that the patient will get the maximum benefit from the new heart. The assessment is carried out as an inpatient procedure over 3 days and has a variety of investigations including lung function, exercise tests, 24-h urine collection (Castle and Jones 2004), virology screen and angiogram. Once all the test results are available, the patient discusses the outcomes with the transplant team. This discussion includes timing of listing for transplantation. The cardiologist may decide that the patient is too well to be placed on a transplant list at this time and may prefer to observe the patient's condition. Conversely other patients may be too ill for transplantation or have additional underlying disease that limits their chances of survival.

Once listed the patient waits for a suitable donor heart to become available. This can be a testing time for the patient because in essence they are waiting for someone to die in order for them to live. When a donor heart becomes available, there are still some checks that need to be undertaken to establish whether it is suitable for the patient. The blood group and size of the donor and recipient need to be the same. Once a heart becomes available the patient is called to hospital but may find that the heart, after closer inspection by the transplant team, is unsuitable so he or she returns home to wait for another call. This may happen a few times before transplantation actually happens.

The procedure itself can be carried out in a number of ways, the more traditional method being referred to as orthotopic transplantation which is a straightforward removal of the patient's heart and insertion of the new heart by attaching it to the patient's own atrium. The domino procedure is sometimes a more attractive option for patients with high pulmonary resistance. This procedure involves the insertion of a heart from a patient who is undergoing a heart–lung transplantation for long-term pulmonary disease. This patient receives a new heart and lungs as one and the old heart is transplanted into the heart failure patient.

The patients are returned to a cardiac ICU where they receive high-level nursing care. A whole host of complications can occur in this stage, including arrhythmia, bleeding and renal failure. After the critical stage of this process, the main complications are rejection of the donor heart and cardiac allograft vasculopathy (Castle and Jones 2004). The risk of rejection can be reduced by the use of immunosuppressant drugs; however, this leads to a higher infection risk and so titration of medication is fundamental to outcome. Cardiac allograft vasculopathy manifests itself as a thickening of the lining of the artery, but this should not be confused with plaque formation such as in CHD.

Although these complications concerning modern-day drug regimens have become so effective that a large percentage of patients undergoing transplantation today will be alive after 5 years, the rates of cardiac transplantation have dramatically reduced over the last 10 years. The Department of Health (2001b) states that the 'fall in the number of transplants is a direct result of fewer organs being available for transplantation'. This reduction in availability of suitable donors is possibly related to the fall in number of fatal road accidents in the same period because most organ donors are cadaveric or patients who have been judged to be brainstem dead. Therefore although the possibility of cardiac transplantation provides hope for some people, there may never be enough suitable donor hearts for this type of surgery to become routine practice.

Rehabilitation

The NSF for CHD (DoH 2000a) emphasizes the importance of cardiac rehabilitation (see Chapter 12).

During the cardiac surgery admission, the relevance and benefits of cardiac rehabilitation should be discussed. This heightens patients' and carers' awareness of the support and education available to them, as well as helping them to understand its importance and significance in assisting both short-term recovery and its role in long-term secondary prevention.

Phase III of cardiac rehabilitation is probably the phase with which patients are most familiar because they may have been through a programme previously, perhaps after a MI or cardiological intervention. Depending on each hospital's system and patient caseload, cardiac rehabilitation classes for revascularized patients can start from as early as 6 weeks or as late as 4 months, postoperatively. Nevertheless, despite NSF targets aiming to get 85% of patients discharged after a heart attack or cardiac surgery into cardiac rehabilitation (DoH 2000a), only a third (33%) currently receive rehabilitation (British Heart Foundation 2004b).

It is hoped that areas leading the way in delivering successful cardiac rehabilitation will be able to share best practice with other areas, thus providing patients with the equitable access to quality rehabilitation for which the NSF is aiming.

Service user involvement

With so many changes taking place in the NHS and cardiac care, it is vital that the value of patient involvement be recognized when re-designing services (DoH 2000b). Many cardiac centres have acknowledged this and, although they may be at different points along the patient involvement journey, there have been some great results accomplished through collaborative working by cardiac surgery providers, patients and relatives. Patient and public involvement forums are having a great impact within the NHS as a whole, and patient forums have been established within cardiac services. However, in order for patient forums to be successful, staff must recognize patient input and involvement as more than just tokenism (Ward 2001), which only serves to alienate patients and carers who have taken the time and effort to be involved and take a role in improving patient services.

Although this concept of greater patient involvement may have seemed alien to many health-care providers a few years ago, many cardiac centres have now embraced this idea and both they and patients are reaping the benefits.

Conclusion

As discussed, this chapter aims to provide a guide to quality cardiac surgery nursing care. The needs of the cardiac surgical patient are varied and care planning should be initiated as soon as the need for surgery has been established in order to achieve excellence. A holistic approach is essential not only when planning individual care but also in the planning and development of service provision. This chapter has highlighted the many benefits of collaborative working of multidisciplinary team members, service users, and primary, secondary and tertiary care providers. To achieve and maintain best practice, regular auditing and measuring of standards are required in conjunction with collaborative working.

Practices in cardiac surgery and cardiology are constantly developing and evolving, which necessitates a flexible and adaptable approach from service providers when planning and delivering cardiac services. Such changes require the cardiac surgery nurse to be well informed and updated on developments and current best practice in order to provide the highest quality care.

Cardiac surgery centres have an obligation to maintain the highest standards of care for the cardiac surgery patient; however, this can be achieved only if the individual cardiac surgery nurse constantly strives to deliver holistic and evidence-based clinical practice.

References

Agu O, Hamilton G, Baker D (1999) Graduated compression stockings in the prevention of venous thromboembolism. Br J Surg 86: 992–1004.

Al-Ruzzeh S, Mazrani W, Wray J et al. (2004) The clinical outcome and quality of life following minimally invasive direct coronary artery bypass surgery. J Cardiac Surg 19: 12–16.

Amarigiri SV, Lees TA (2000) Elastic compression stockings for deep vein thrombosis. Cochrane Database of Systematic Reviews (3): Online CD001484.

Artinian NT (1991) Stress experience of spouses of patients having coronary artery bypass during hospitalization and 6 weeks after discharge. Heart Lung 20: 52–9.

Artinian NT (1993) Spouses' perceptions of readiness for discharge after cardiac surgery. Appl Nursing Res 6: 80–8.

Athanasiou T, Aziz O, Mangoush O et al. (2004) Do off pump techniques reduce the incidence of postoperative atrial fibrillation in elderly patients undergoing coronary artery bypass grafting? Ann Thorac Surg 77: 1567–74.

Beekmann-Ball G, Grap M (1992) Postoperative GI symptoms in cardiac surgery patients. Crit Care Nurse 12: 56–62.

Brady M, Kinn S, Stuart P (2003) Cochrane Database System Review (4). Online: CD004423.

British Heart Foundation (2001) Having Heart Surgery. Heart Information Series Number 12. London: British Heart Foundation.

British Heart Foundation (2004a) British Heart Foundation Statistics: Blood Pressure (www.heartstats.org/topic.asp?id=881 [17 June 2004]).

British Heart Foundation (2004b) British Heart Foundation Coronary Disease Statistics (www.bhf.org.uk/professionals/index.asp?secondlevel=519 [17 June 2004]).

Budillon A.M, Nicolini F, Agostinelli A et al. (2003) Complications after radial artery harvesting for coronary artery bypass grafting: our experience. Surgery 133: 283–7.

Byhahn C, Strouhal U, Martens S, Mierdl S, Kessler P, Westphal K (2001) Incidence of gastrointestinal complications in cardiopulmonary bypass patients. World J Surg 25: 1140–4.

Cardoso P, Yamazaki F, Keshavjee S et al. (1991) A re-evaluation of heparin requirements for cardiopulmonary bypass. J Thorac Cardiovasc Surg 101: 153–60.

Castle H, Jones I (2004) A long wait: How nurses can help patients through the transplantation pathway. Professional Nurse 19(12): 37–39.

Coronary Heart Disease Collaborative and the Department of Health (2004) Newsbeat. London: Department of Health Publications, p. 3.

Cupples SA (1991) Effects of timing and reinforcement of preoperative education on knowledge and recovery of patients having coronary artery bypass graft surgery. Heart Lung 20: 654–60.

Davies N (2000) Patients' and carers' perceptions of factors influencing recovery after cardiac surgery. J Adv Nursing 32: 318–326.

Debrunner M, Naegeli B, Genoni M, Turina M, Bertel O (2004) Prevention of atrial fibrillation after cardiac valvular surgery by epicardial, bilateral synchronous pacing. Eur J Cardiothorac Surg 25: 16–20.

De Feo S, Opasich C, Capietti M et al. (2002) Functional and psychological recovery during intensive hospital rehabilitation following cardiac surgery in the elderly. Monaldi Arch Chest Dis 58: 35–40.

Department of Health (2000a) National Service Framework for Coronary Heart Disease. London: Department of Health.

Department of Health (2000b) The NHS Plan. A plan for investment, A plan for reform. London: HMSO.

Department of Health (2001a) Reference guide to consent for examination or treatment (www.dh.gov.uk/PublicationsAndStatistics/Publications/Publications PolicyAndGuidlines.htm).

Department of Health (2001b) National Adult Heart and lung Transplant Service – Discussion Document. London: DoH.

Department of Health (2003) Waiting, booking and choice: Delivering more convenient care without delay website (www.doh.gov.uk/waitingbookingchoice/index.htm – 2 Feb 2004).

Diegeler A, Martin M, Falk V et al. (1999a) Indication and patient selection in minimally invasive and 'off-pump' coronary artery bypass grafting. Eur J Cardio-Thorac Surg 16: S79–82.

Diegeler A, Walther T, Metz S et al. (1999b) Comparison of MIDCAB versus conventional CABG surgery regarding pain and quality of life. Heart Surg Forum 2: 290–5.

Dietl CA, Madigan NP, Menapace FJ et al. (1993) Results of coronary artery bypass grafting using multiple arterial conduits. J Cardiovasc Surg 34: 513–16.

DVLA (2004) At a glance website (www.dvla.gov.uk/at_a_glancc/ch2_cardiovascular.htm – 17 June 2004).

Eagle KA, Guyton RA, Davidoff R et al. (1999) ACC/AHA Guidelines for CABG surgery: a report of the American College of Cardiology/American Heart Association Task Force on Practice Guidelines. J Am Coll Cardiol 34: 1262–347.

Egan F (1999) Cardiac rehabilitation into the new millennium. Intens Crit Care Nursing 15: 163–8.

Field J, Bjarnason K (2000) Dealing with the complications of upper-gastrointestinal surgery. Nursing Times 96(17): S11(suppl: NT Plus: Nutrition).

Flynn M, Reddy S, Shepherd W et al. (2004) Fast-tracking revisited: routine cardiac surgical patients need minimal intensive care. Eur J Cardio-Thorac Surg 25: 116–22.

Foulger V (1997) Patients' view of day-case cardiac catheterisation. Professional Nurse 12: 478–80.

Ganuschchak YM, Fransen EJ, Visser C, De Jong DS , Maessen JG (2004) Neurological complications after coronary artery bypass grafting related to the performance of cardiopulmonary bypass. Chest 125: 2196–205.

Geissler H, Holzl P, Marohl S et al. (2000) Risk stratification in heart surgery; comparison of six score systems. Eur J Cardio-Thorac Surg 17: 400–6.

Gillis CL (1984) Reducing family stress during and after coronary artery bypass surgery. Nursing Clin N Am 19: 103–11.

Goodman H (1997) Patients' perceptions of their education needs in the first six weeks following discharge after cardiac surgery. J Adv Nursing, 25: 1241–51.

Grap MJ, Savage L, Ball GB (1996) The incidence of gastrointestinal symptoms in cardiac surgery patients through six weeks after discharge. Heart Lung: J Crit Care 25: 444–50.

Greenwood DC, Packham CJ, Muir KR, Madeley RJ (1996) Knowledge of the causes of heart attack among survivors, and the implications for health promotion. Health Education J 55: 215–225, 216.

Hind M (1997) Advances in day surgery nursing. Br J Theatre Nursing 7: 17–18.

Holl R (1995) Surgical cardiac patient characteristics and the amount of analgesics administered in the intensive care unit after extubation. Intens Crit Care Nursing 11: 192–7.

Hosenpud JD et al. (2001) Eighteenth Annual Heart/Lung Transplant Registry data report. J Heart Lung Transplantation 20: 808–15.

Hough D, Crosat S, Nye P (1991) Patient education for total hip replacements. Nursing Management 22: 80I–80P.

Jayaprakash A, McGrath C, McCullagh E, Angelini G, Prober C (2004) Upper gastrointestinal haemorrhage following cardiac surgery: comparative study with vascular surgery patients from a single centre. Eur J Gastroenterol Hepatol 16: 191–4.

Johnson A, Sandford J, Tyndall J (2003) Written and verbal information versus verbal information only for patients being discharged from acute hospital settings to home (Cochrane Review). In: The Cochrane Library, Issue 2. Chichester: John Wiley & Sons Ltd.

Johnson RG, Shafique T, Sirois C, Weintraub RM, Comunale ME (1999) Potassium concentrations and ventricular ectopy: a prospective, observational study in post-cardiac surgery patients. Crit Care Med 27: 2581–2.

Johnston G, Vitikainen K, Knight R, Annest L, Garcia C (1992) Changing perspective on gastrointestinal complications in patients undergoing cardiac surgery. Am J Surg 163: 525–9.

Jones S, Rimmer C, Hatchett R (2002) The future of cardiac nursing. In: Hatchett R, Thompson D (eds), Cardiac Nursing: A comprehensive guide. Edinburgh: Churchill Livingstone, pp. 586, 587.

Jonker MJ, de Boer EM, Ader HJ, Bezemer PD (2001) The oedema-protective effect of Lycra support stockings. Dermatology 203: 294–8.

Kakkar VV, Stringer MD (1990) Prophylaxis of venous thromboembolism. World J Surg 5: 670–8.

Kaplan M, Kut MS, Yurtseven N, Cimen S, Demirtas MM (2002) Accelerated recovery after cardiac operations. Heart Surg Forum 5: 381–7.

Kee F, Gaffney B, Canavan C et al. (1995) Expanding access to coronary artery bypass surgery: who stands to gain? Br Heart J 73: 129–33.

Kendall JB, Hart CA, Pennefather SH, Russell GN (2002) Infection control measures for adult cardiac surgery in the UK – a survey of current practice. J Hosp Infect 54: 174–8.

Khot UN, Friedman DT, Pettersson G, Smedira NG, Li J, Ellis SG (2004) Radial artery bypass grafts have an increased occurrence of angiographically severe stenosis and occlusion compared with left internal mammary arteries and saphenous vein grafts (Report). Circulation 109: 2086–91.

Kjonniksen I, Andersen BM, Sondenaa VG, Segadal L (2002) Preoperative hair removal – a systematic literature review. AORN J 75: 928–38, 940.

Knipp SC, Matatko N, Wilhelm H et al. (2004) Evaluation of brain injury after coronary artery bypass grafting. A prospective study using neurophysiological assessment and diffusion-weighted magnetic resonance imaging. Eur J Cardio-Thorac Surg 25: 791–800.

Kreter B and Woods M (1992) Antibiotic prophylaxis for cardiothoracic operations. Meta-analysis of thirty years of clinical trials. J Cardiovasc Surg 104: 590–9.

Krouse HJ, Fisher JA, Yarandi HN (2001) Utility of video modeling as an adjunct to preoperative education. Southern Online J Nursing Res 2(8): 14.

Kurusz M, Butler BD (2004). Bubbles and bypass: an update. Perfusion 19(suppl 1): S49–55.

Kumar A, Anel R, Bunnell E et al. (2004) Pulmonary artery occlusion pressure and central venous pressure fail to predict ventricular filling volume, cardiac performance, or the response to volume infusion in normal subjects. Crit Care Med 32: 691–9.

Lahtinen J, Biancari F, Salmela E et al. (2004) Postoperative atrial fibrillation is a major cause of stroke after on-pump coronary artery bypass surgery. Ann Thorac Surg 77: 1241–4.

Lamarche D, Taddeo R, Pepler C (1998) The preparation of patients for cardiac surgery. Clin Nursing Res 7: 390–405.

Lane P (1997) Creating an education model for cardiac patients. Professional Nurse 13: 45–8.

McDonald S, Hetrick S, Green S (2003) Pre-operative education for hip or knee replacement (Cochrane Review). In: The Cochrane Library, Issue 2. Chichester: John Wiley & Sons, Ltd.

McGee DC, Gould MK (2003) Preventing complications of central venous catheterisation. N Engl J Med 348: 1123–33.

McHugh F, Lindsay GM, Hanlon P et al. (2001) Nurse led shared care for patients on the waiting list for coronary artery bypass surgery: A randomized trial. Heart 86: 317.

Mangiante G, Carluccio S, Nifosi F (2003) What is new in fasting guidelines of surgical patients? Review of the literature. Chirurgia Italiana 55: 849–55.

Mistiaen P, Poot E (2003) Telephone follow-up initiated by a hospital-based health professional, for post discharge problems in patients discharged from hospital to home (Protocol for a Cochrane Review). In: The Cochrane Library, Issue 2. Chichester: John Wiley & Sons Ltd.

Mitchell M (1997) Patients' perceptions of pre-operative preparation for day surgery. J Adv Nursing 26: 356–63.

Miyamoto K (2004) Is it necessary to humidify inhaled low-flow oxygen or low concentration oxygen? Nihon Kokyuki Gakkai Zasshi (abstract [electronic]) 42: 138–44. Available: Pubmed (16 June 2004).

Moran SJ, Jarvis, Ewings P, Parkin FA (1999) It's good to talk, but is it effective? A comparative study of telephone support following day surgery. Clin Effective Nursing 2: 175–47.

Moser DK, Dracup KA, Marsden C (1993) Needs of recovering cardiac patients and their spouses: Compared views. Int J Nursing Stud 30: 114–50.

Moynihan M (1984) Assessing the educational needs of post-myocardial infarction patients and their spouses. Nurse Education Today 14: 448–56.

Mullen PD, Maims DA, Velez RV (1992). A meta analysis of controlled trials of cardiac patient education. Patient Education Counseling 19: 143–62.

National Health Service (NHS) Modernisation Agency (2003a) Mapping the Future: Coronary Heart Disease Collaborative Summary Strategic Plan, pp. 7, 3, 8. London: HMSO.

NHS Modernisation Agency (2003b) Booking Homepage: Booking in the NHS Website (www.modern.nhs.uk/scripts/default.asp?site_id = 21 – 2 Feb (2004).

NHS Modernisation Agency (2003c) National good practice guidance on pre-operative assessment for inpatient surgery: Operating theatre and pre-operative assessment programme Website [(www.modern.nhs.uk/theatre/7511/11434/in%21pat%20 guidance%2014.3.03.doc, p11, – 19 June 2004).

National Institute for Clinical Excellence (2003) Preoperative Tests: The use of routine preoperative tests for elective surgery, Clinical Guideline 3. London: NICE, p. 22.

Neema PK, Sinha PK, Rathod RC (2004) Activated clotting time during cardiopulmonary bypass: is repetition necessary during open heart surgery? Asian Cardiovasc Thorac Ann 12: 47–52.

Ng JY, Tam SF (2000) Effect of exercise-based cardiac rehabilitation on mobility and self-esteem of persons after cardiac surgery. Perceptual Motor Skills 91: 107–14.

Nursing Times Professional Development (1995) Chronic cardiac disease: The role of the nurse. Nursing Times 24(suppl): 5–8.

Payne D (1998). Language barrier warning over NHS helpline. Nursing Times 94(5): 8.

Pearson T, Rapaport E, Criqui M et al. (1994) Optimal risk factor management in the patient after coronary revascularization: a statement for healthcare on professionals from an American Heart Association Writing Group. Circulation 90: 3125–33.

Perrault L.P, Jeanmart H, Bilodeau L et al. (2004) Early quantitative coronary angiography of saphenous vein grafts for coronary artery bypass grafting harvested by means of open versus endoscopic saphenectomy: a prospective randomise trial. J Thorac Cardiovasc Surg 127: 1402–7.

Peterseim DS, Cen YY, Cheruvu S et al. (1999) Long-term outcome after biologic versus mechanical aortic valve replacement in 841 patients. J Cardiovasc Surg 117: 890–7.

Pilkington F (2004) Humidification for oxygen therapy in non-ventilated patients. Br J Nursing 13: 111–15.

Prandoni P, Sabbion P, Tanduo C, Errigo G, Zanon E, Bernardi E (2001) Prevention of venous thromboembolism in high-risk surgical and medical patients. Semin Vasc Med 1(1): 61–70.

Radford KA (1993) Wound complications after cardiac surgery: a new approach to healing by secondary intention. J Cardiovasc Nursing 7(4): 82–7.

Ramos R, Salem BI, De Pawlikowski MP, Coordes C, Eisenberg S, Leidenfrost R (1996) The efficacy of pneumatic compression stockings in the prevention of pulmonary embolism after cardiac surgery. Chest 109: 82–5.

Report of a combined working party of the British Society for Antimicrobial Chemotherapy, the Hospital Infection Society and the Infection Control Nurses' Association (1998) Revised guidelines for the control of methicillin-resistant Staphylococcus aureus infection in hospitals. J Hospital Infect 39: 253.

Roper N, Logan W, Tierney AJ, Holland K (eds) (2003) Applying the Roper–Logan–Tierney Model in Practice: Elements of Nursing. London: Churchill Livingstone.

Rowe M, King K (1998) Long-term chest wall discomfort in women after coronary artery bypass grafting. Heart Lung 27: 184–8.

Salisbury H (1994) Health visitors' role in cardiac rehabilitation. Health Visitor 67: 262–4.

Sellick JA, Stelmach M, Mylotte JM (1991) Surveillance of surgical wound infections following open heart surgery. Infect Control Hosp Epidemiol 12: 591–6.

Shammas NW (2000) Pulmonary embolus after coronary artery bypass surgery: a review of the literature. Clin Cardiol 23: 637–44.

Simic O, Strathausen S, Hess W, Ostermeyer J (1999) Incidence and prognosis of abdominal complications after cardiopulmonary bypass. Cardiovasc Surg 7: 419–24.

Sumer T, Taylor DK, McDonald M et al. (1997) The effect of anticipatory discharge orders on length of hospital stay in staff pediatric patients. Am J Med Quality 12: 48–50.

Swenne CL, Lindholm C, Borowiec J, Carlsson M (2004) Surgical-site infections within 60 days of coronary artery by-pass graft surgery. J Hosp Infect 57(1): 14–24.

Tack B, Gilliss C (1990) Nurse-monitored cardiac recovery: a description of the first 8 weeks. Heart Lung 19(5 part 1): 491–9.

Theobald K (1997) The experience of spouses whose partners have suffered a myocardial infarction: A phenomenological study. J Adv Nursing 26: 595–601.

Tulla H, Takala J, Alhava E, Huttunen H, Kari A, Manninen H (1991) Respiratory change after open-heart surgery. Intens Care Med 17: 365–9.

Ward M (2001) Patient involvement is more than tokenism: Report from the Canadian federation of psychiatric nursing. Mental Health Practice 5: 18–21.

White PF, Rawal S, Latham P et al. (2003) Use of a continuous local anaesthetic infusion for pain management after median sternotomy. Anesthesiology 99: 918–23.

Wynne R, Botti M, Stedman H, Holsworth L, Flavell O, Manterfield C (2004) Effect of three wound dressings on infection, healing comfort, and cost in patients with sternotomy wounds: a randomised trial. Chest 125: 43–9.

CHAPTER TWELVE

Cardiac rehabilitation

PAULA BITHELL AND MIRIAM GASTON

The principles of the cardiac rehabilitation framework have mostly been applied to the care of patients with acute myocardial infarction (AMI) or to those who have been referred for or undergone cardiac surgery. However, it should be acknowledged that these principles can be applied to meet the needs of patients with other cardiology conditions, including cardiac transplantation, stable angina, heart failure and with automated implantable cardioverting defibrillators (AICDs). Therefore, it is important that health-care professionals understand these principles and the underpinnings of the cardiac rehabilitation process.

This chapter aims to explore these principles further, outlining the definition, history and individual components of cardiac rehabilitation, and finally examining the benefits, thus enabling health-care professionals to develop and deliver an evidence-based cardiac rehabilitation programme.

History and definition of cardiac rehabilitation

The vast majority of health-care professionals view cardiac rehabilitation as a purely exercise-based process. It should be acknowledged that, although exercise does play a large part in the process, it is not the only facet; this belief reflects back to cardiac rehabilitation's historical roots.

Cardiac rehabilitation began as a formalization of the concept of early ambulation post-AMI. Early in the twentieth century, post-MI patients were generally confined to bed rest for up to 2 months, in fear that physical activity would lead to the formation of ventricular aneurysm, heart failure, cardiac rupture and sudden death (Froelicher 1988). The modern correlate of this concern is the concept of myocardial re-modelling after an infarct. There is a concern that expansion of the infarcted and non-infarcted tissue with inappropriate physical activity may lead to aneurysm formation. Jugdutt et al. (1988) observed this phenomenon in patients with large anterior wall infarcts. (This is discussed further under 'Exercising special groups'.) It was not until the 1940s that researchers began to question the efficacy of prolonged bed rest (Levine 1944, Taylor et al. 1949). This research continued throughout the twentieth century and now early ambulation is an accepted form of management. During this time the concept of the cardiac rehabilitation process has also shifted to incorporate these changes, which has enabled other areas of care to be addressed, such as the patient's psychosocial needs, and identifying patient's risk factors for developing underlying coronary artery disease and incorporating secondary prevention measures, such as the management of the lipid profile, weight and blood pressure reduction, smoking cessation and diabetic control. Ensuring that the proven secondary prevention therapies are applied and that the appropriate lifestyle advice is provided is an integral part of the cardiac rehabilitation process.

The cardiac rehabilitation process consists of activities that include exercise prescription, education, risk stratification and a reduction of modifiable risk factors, which will lead to a more normal state of cardiovascular health. The most common and widely used definition of cardiac rehabilitation is from the World Health Organization (WHO 1993, p. • •), which reads as follows:

> The rehabilitation of cardiac patients is the sum of activities required to influence favourably the underlying cause of the disease as well as the best possible physical, mental and social conditions so that they may by their own efforts preserve or resume when lost as normal a place as possible in the community. Rehabilitation cannot be regarded as an isolated form of therapy but must be integrated with the whole treatment of which it forms only one facet.

It should be acknowledged that, in order to achieve a service that incorporates many factors, a multidisciplinary team of health-care professionals must be prepared to examine a varied and flexible approach. This may include close collaboration of many disciplines and the exploration of cross-boundary working. The way to achieve the successful delivery of cardiac rehabilitation is via a clear process of coordination and facilitation between the various disciplines, and primary and secondary care teams.

Professionals who may be involved in cardiac rehabilitation include nurses, physiotherapists, dietitians, pharmacists, occupational therapists, psychologists and physiologists.

Although cardiac rehabilitation was slow to develop in the UK, in the 1970s and early 1980s, it has gradually received investment and is now an integral part of the cardiac patient's care. The first large-scale controlled trial of cardiac rehabilitation in the UK was published by Carson (1982, cited in Coats et al. 1995) and since then there has been a gradual growth in exercise-based cardiac rehabilitation programmes. In 1988 the Coronary Prevention Group commissioned a secondary prevention and rehabilitation advisory committee. In 1989 the British Heart Foundation (BHF) began to fund the development of new cardiac rehabilitation programmes. This led to an expansion of cardiac rehabilitation services in the UK. Although this funding led to some further development and expansion of existing programmes and contributed to better provision, it did not provide comprehensive cover across the UK.

The British Cardiac Society (Davidson et al. 1995, Horgan et al. 1995) published a survey that found that, although there had been some expansion in services, this was only small in comparison to the percentage of patients who might be eligible to attend such a service and that the provision of service varied considerably. Following this the British Cardiac Society set recommendations for service provision and access to cardiac rehabilitation programmes in the UK. To address some of the points raised in the report and to provide clear guidelines, the British Association for Cardiac Rehabilitation (BACR) (Coats et al. 1992) was born.

Since the publication of the BACR guidelines, there have also been a number of additional guidelines published, which include guidelines from the Scottish Intercollegiate Guidelines Network (SIGN 2002), the National Institute for Clinical Excellence (NICE) and the Association of Chartered Physiotherapists Interested in Cardiac Rehabilitation (ACPICR 2002). These helped to form the basis of a high standard of service provision and provide a useful evidence base into the effectiveness of cardiac rehabilitation programmes. Following the publication of the National Service Framework for Coronary Heart Disease (NSF for CHD – Department of Health or DoH 2000), interest in the field of cardiac rehabilitation has increased significantly. Chapter 7 of the NSF for CHD is specific to cardiac rehabilitation and states that patients with the following conditions/circumstances will benefit from accessing it:

- After an AMI
- Before and after revascularization procedures (coronary artery bypass graft or CABG and angioplasty)
- With stable angina
- With heart failure
- For other specialized interventions such as cardiac transplantation.

Evidence to support the benefits of cardiac rehabilitation

There have been a number of papers written to support the benefits of cardiac rehabilitation (Oldridge et al. 1988, O'Connor et al. 1989, Wannamethee et al. 1998); these include an improvement in risk factor status, better compliance with medication, return to a normal lifestyle, return to previous occupation and psychosocial improvements. Some studies (Oldridge et al. 1988, O'Connor et al. 1989) have also shown a reduction in mortality and morbidity after attendance of cardiac rehabilitation programmes. These improvements and the reduction in mortality and morbidity may be attributed to better surveillance. However, there is some evidence to suggest that there is still a lack of scientific evidence in favour of the long-term benefits of cardiac rehabilitation programmes. There is no controversy about the benefits of risk factor intervention after an MI. Indeed treatment of arterial hypertension and hypercholesterolaemia, as well as the motivation to stop smoking, may be the most effective measures in the prevention of re-infarction.

Individual components of cardiac rehabilitation

Traditionally cardiac rehabilitation programmes have been divided into four phases:

1. The inpatient phase: involves information and education, psychological assessment, risk factor assessment, early risk stratification and suitability to attend the exercise component of cardiac rehabilitation, in-hospital mobilization, discharge planning and the implementation of evidence-based secondary prevention measures.
2. Immediate post-discharge phase: may be undertaken in many ways. This phase allows for the continued follow-up of a patient, providing an opportunity to raise any concerns or anxieties that have occurred since discharge. The coordinator assesses the patient's symptoms and applies symptom management often within the patient's own home environment, and reinforces any discharge advice and lifestyle management.
3. Intermediate post-discharge phase: this phase is usually when the patient attends a formal education and exercise programme in an outpatient setting.
4. Long-term maintenance phase: this phase usually comprises the long-term maintenance of lifestyle changes.

Although these phases provide a defined structure, their boundaries are becoming blurred as a result of the individual needs of each patient and new ways of working. Therefore, the duration of each phase may vary, as may the content. It is important that there is close collaboration between secondary and primary care clinicians throughout the four phases. Furthermore, when setting up a cardiac rehabilitation programme it is important to consider the personnel who will be involved in the delivery of the service. It is also important that the service meets the individual needs of the patient at the different phases of the disease and recovery process. These two important factors can help to address the following questions:

- What is it that should be done?
- How should this be applied and by whom?
- How will it be achieved?
- How will those achievements be monitored?

Phase I: inpatient phase

Traditionally phase I is carried out during the patient's hospitalization; however, as a result of shorter hospital stays and the volume of information given during this phase, some information may be given to the patient during phase II. It is important that certain areas are covered while the patient is still in hospital and that an individual plan of care be established. The topics that should be covered while the patient is hospitalized include: understanding the disease process and the diagnosis: discharge preparation including advice on symptom management; and activity, driving, vacation and lifestyle changes. It is important that the family are included in this planning and that the patient understands and feels involved in any future care and management. Initially the needs of the patient may be focused on reassurance and information. It is understandable that early into this process the patient will feel anxious; these anxieties should be heard and dealt with sensitively.

Once the initial anxiety has lessened or subsided, the patient may be more receptive to information and education. It is important that the specialist involved in the delivery of this information is able to assess a patient's readiness and receptiveness to information, so any verbal information given should be supported with written information and when at all possible family members should be involved. The specialist should allow the patient and the family to guide the information-giving process by asking questions that are pertinent to their lifestyle. Often this information will be retained more clearly. The patient and the family should feel involved in any lifestyle changes recommended by the specialist. These lifestyle changes can be supported with evidence-based medication. It is important that patients acknowledge that, although the prescription of these medications will help reduce further events in the future, it is still important that they modify their lifestyle to complement these therapies (risk factor advice and treatment are discussed in more detail later in the chapter).

Early risk stratification after an MI is extremely important and some patients may receive an exercise test pre-discharge or a coronary angiogram. There are a number of guidelines available outlining the management of

ST-elevation MI (STEMI) and non-ST-elevation MI (NSTEMI; British Cardiac Society 2001, 2004, European Society of Cardiology 2003). During the discharge planning phase, it is important that the specialist involved in the patient's care ensures that there is a smooth transition from phase I to II. Often patients and their families become anxious at the prospect of caring for themselves at home after they have been in the reassuring hospital environment. These fears can be alleviated by offering the patient a contact number, ensuring that the patient has clear advice on symptom management and when to return to the hospital should symptoms persist, and that the patient may receive a home visit from a secondary or primary care professional involved in cardiac rehabilitation. If the patient's care is being transferred to a primary care professional this should be done promptly to enable an early post-discharge visit and to provide the primary care team with the appropriate advice about the patient's condition and further management.

Phase II: immediate post-discharge phase

The phase II stage of cardiac rehabilitation may be carried out in a number of ways. First, the patient can be contacted by telephone; second, the patient may be visited by a primary or secondary care professional involved in cardiac rehabilitation; or, third, the patient may be invited to attend a hospital clinic run by a cardiac rehabilitation professional. Whichever method is being used the patient should be clearly informed about this before discharge. Although home visits can be time-consuming and not as cost-effective they do provide the clinician with an insight into the patient's well-being within his or her own home environment. Often the patient feels more relaxed in this setting and is able to express concerns or anxiety. However, there is little research examining the benefits of home visits post-MI.

Telephone contact can be more cost-effective and timely; however, it may be less personal and the patient may not be willing to express any concerns or anxieties during a telephone conversation. If a primary care clinician visits the patient at home, it is important that that clinician receives all the information relating to the patient, including any assessments carried out in hospital and the advice given. Phase II offers the clinician the opportunity to reinforce any information that the patient may have misunderstood or was not receptive to at the time it was given. This phase also provides the clinician with the opportunity to assess the patient's physical progress and adjust any management plans as appropriate.

Phase III: intermediate outpatient phase.

The content and duration of the phase III outpatient programme will vary depending on local resources and patient needs. Usually the exercise programmes are conducted in an outpatient setting and this may be a physiotherapy gym or a community-based setting. Recently, there has been a trend to move low-risk patients out into community programmes and to reserve hospital programmes for higher-risk patients. The length of the programme may also depend on the patient's needs and local resources. Usually programmes can last anything from 6 to 12 weeks and patients may exercise once or twice a week. Current guidelines recommended twice weekly (Coats et al. 1995, ACPICR 2002). These programmes should be multidisciplinary and involve physiotherapists, nurses, dietitians, physiologists, psychologists, pharmacists, occupational therapists and patient representatives.

There are two facets to a phase III programme: the first, which is purely exercise based, and the second, which is health education and secondary prevention. Some programmes may hold these components together and some are separate. If possible it is recommended that a multidisciplinary team should deliver the health education component including input from dietitians, pharmacists, physiologists, occupational therapists, patients, nurses and physiotherapists in relation to education on dietary advice, medications, stress management including anatomy and physiology, exercise, education and vocational assessment. Most patients will be able to attend the education-only sessions; however, not all patients may suit the exercise component.

Screening for exercise programmes is an integral part of the specialist's role in phases I and II. The patient should undergo careful medical examination before being referred to the exercise programme. A medical history should be taken from the patient, including any past history of cardiovascular disease or pulmonary disease, any neuromuscular problems or orthopaedic problems, current symptoms and medication, family history, lifestyle information including smoking history, nutrition and weight history, exercise habits and psychosocial information. All hospitals should have a local protocol clearly defining the entry criteria into the exercise component of the cardiac rehabilitation programme. Usually patients with uncomplicated AMI are suitable for attending the programme at 3–4 weeks after the event and patients who have under gone re-vascularization or other cardiac surgery would be suitable to attend at 6–8 weeks, as long as the sternum bone is stable and there are no other postoperative complications.

Exclusion criteria usually include uncontrolled hypertension, uncontrolled cardiac arrhythmias, significant valve disease such as aortic stenosis and mitral stenosis, uncontrolled medical conditions such as uncontrolled asthma or diabetes, severe musculoskeletal problems and severe neurological problems. There is usually no age restriction to the programmes; however, patients must be able to complete an exercise programme using a variety of equipment. They should undergo further assessment on their first visit, which may be carried out on an individual basis or as a group. There should be some kind of audible exercise measurement such as a 6-minute walk test or shuttle walk that can be performed before and after the exercise programme to measure the patient's outcomes. Most of these tests have demonstrated a correlation between exercise duration and ventilation (Vo_2) (Cahalin et al. 1995, Raul et al. 1998, Zugck et al. 2000). A number of research trials (Lanenfold et al. 1990, Rejski et al. 2000, Zugck et al. 2000) have shown these tests to be a reliable and valid tool as an outcome measure. Some exercise programmes may require a full Bruce protocol exercise test before starting the exercise component. The exercise tolerance test (ETT) has become an important assessment tool in the evaluation of individuals participating in adult fitness and cardiac rehabilitation programmes. It is a useful diagnostic and exercise capacity tool. The diagnostic exercise test is performed to resolve questions about the presence or absence of myocardial ischaemia, which can be useful post-MI. Functional testing is used to evaluate physical working capacity. Both the diagnostic and the functional tests are useful and may guide the clinician to referral for more invasive investigations, such as coronary angiography. It is a useful risk stratification tool for both the clinician and the cardiac rehabilitation specialist.

Functional capacity is usually measured in metabolic equivalents (METs) (e.g. 1 MET is about 3.5 ml/kg per min of O_2 intake). METs can be useful for prescribing certain recreational and everyday activities (Table 12.1), e.g. if a patient attending a cardiac rehabilitation programme achieves 10 METs on a maximal exercise test then the prescription of activities < 10 METs would be suitable. However, the cardiac rehabilitation specialist should remember that METs are only an estimate of energy expenditure, calculated automatically by an ETT machine and, unless Vo_{2max} is actually measured, METs should be used cautiously. Furthermore, activities that require skill may use more METs than have actually been allowed; environmental factors, such as wind and temperature, may also alter METs.

Another way to determine functional capability and then prescribe training intensity is by calculating the target heart rate. There are a number of recognized ways to achieve this, e.g. the Karvonen formula or heart rate reserved (maximal heart rate or MHR) method. However, the simplest way to do this is to use the target heart rate range of 70–90% of MHR attained on the most recent exercise test. Most exercise programmes prescribe exercise related to submaximal heart rate (SMHR), e.g. a 50-year-old woman would have an MHR of 200 – age = 150. A prescribed 70% intensity would equal an SMHR of 105 beats/min. Whichever method

Table 12.1 MET values for recreational and everyday activities

Activities	METs
Badminton	4–9
Bed exercise (arm movement, supine or sitting)	1–2
Bicycling	3–8
Bowling	2–4
Dancing	3–7
Fishing	
bank, boat or ice	2–4
stream (wading)	5–6
Football	6–10
Golf	
using power cart	2–3
walking (carrying bag or pushing cart)	4–7
Swimming	4–8
Gardening	
hoeing	4–8
digging, shovelling and pushing	4–8
wheelbarrow	4–10
weeding	3–5
raking	3–8
mowing the lawn	4–6
snow shovelling	8–15
Home improvements (painting, plumbing, etc.)	3–8
Heavy house work (scrubbing floors, making beds)	3–6
Light housework (sweeping, polishing, ironing)	2–4
Walking	
horizontal or slight grade	3–5
steep grade	6–8
up stairs	6–8
down stairs	4–5

MET, metabolic equivalent. Adapted from Fox et al. (1972).

is being used, this should be clearly documented on the patient's first appointment to a phase III programme.

On attending the programme the patient undergoes an assessment, which includes the results of the risk stratification process, ETT results, BP, heart rate, symptoms since discharge and exercise since discharge. Once these factors have been considered, the patient may have his or her risk further stratified into a low-, intermediate- or high-risk group.

Depending on the exercise performance on an ETT, 6-minute walk test or shuttle walk test, a prescribed exercise schedule is given that is suitable for the patient's level. Further guidelines for risk stratification are outlined in Table 12.2.

Table 12.2 Guidelines for risk stratification

Low	Uncomplicated clinical course in hospital, no evidence of myocardial ischaemia, functional capacity > 7 METs, normal LV function, ejection factor > 50% and an absence of significant ventricular ectopics
Intermediate	ST- segment depression > 2 mm flat or down sloping, reversible thallium defects, moderate-to-good LV function, ejection fraction 35–49%, changing pattern or new development of angina
High	Patients with prior myocardial infarction or infarct involving > 35% of the left ventricle with an ejection faction of < 35% at rest, a fall in exercise systolic blood pressure or failure of systolic blood pressure to rise more than 10 mmHg on ETT, persistent or recurrent ischaemic pain ≥ 4 h after admission, functional capacity < 5 METs with hypertensive blood pressure response or > 1-mm ST-segment depression, congestion heart failure syndrome in hospital > 2 mm ST depression at peak heart rate < 35 beats/min and high-grade ventricular etopics

ETT, exercise tolerance test; LV, left ventricular; MET, metabolic equivalent.
From American Association of Cardiovascular and Pulmonary Rehabilitation (1995).

The last two groups in Table 12.2 may not be suitable to attend the conventional exercise programme because these patients may require further investigations such as coronary angiography, and high-risk patients who have developed symptoms of heart failure should not be referred until their heart failure is settled and controlled on medication. (Exercise of high-risk groups is discussed later in the chapter.)

Exit criteria from the phase III programme will depend on the individual patient objectives and if these have been achieved. At the end of the programme patients should have an understanding of the benefits of exercise, be able to carry out exercise safely and effectively, recognize limitations and exercise free of any anginal symptoms. They should have an understanding of lifestyle modifications and have achieved a change in their lifestyle during the programme; their final assessment should be a clear and accurate account of their progress, which is then communicated to their local GP and practice nurse. Regardless of the setting, cardiac rehabilitation programmes should adhere to current safety standards of care. The current guidelines recommend that there is a one to five staff:patient ratio and that there is emergency resuscitation equipment within the exercise setting. Cardiac rehabilitation specialists should also hold a current Advanced Life Support Certificate.

Phase IV or long-term maintenance phase

This is an extremely important part of the cardiac rehabilitation process; it should be made clear to patients that, although their formalized programme of rehabilitation has now ended, the continuation of their lifestyle modifications and exercise schedules should continue in the community setting. Many areas now offer exercise on prescription courses for suitable patients, which are normally held in local sports facilities. This prescription would be available for those patients who have undergone all invasive tests, do not require any further intervention and have achieved all of their objectives during the phase III exercise programme. It is extremely important that patients understand that the maintenance of exercise and other lifestyle changes and the monitoring of these risk factors should continue in the primary care setting. This is a lifelong commitment from the patient. Communication between primary and secondary care is crucial during this phase and the patients' GPs and practice nurses should have a clear understanding of their progress and the objectives that they have achieved, so that they are able to plan their long-term follow-up in the community.

The acute and chronic responses of cardiovascular endurance exercise

During exercise, the following responses occur in healthy individuals: the release of neurotransmitters and adrenaline (epinephrine) and noradrenaline (norepinephrine) causes an increase in sympathetic activity, which in turn causes an increase in the heart rate; at the same time parasympathetic activity decreases caused by reduced levels of the neurotransmitter acetylcholine (Figure 12.1). Their combined effects cause an overall rise in the heart rate and an increase in stroke volume and cardiac output. The rise in sympathetic activity causes venous constriction and thus increases venous return (preload), giving a stronger contraction (Figure 12.2). There is then redistribution of the blood to the skeletal muscle and other tissues. At rest 15–20% of the cardiac output goes to skeletal muscle and the remainder to the visceral organs, heart and brain. During exercise this progress is reversed: 85–90% of cardiac output goes to the working skeletal muscle and is shunted away from the other organs such as the spleen, renal vascular beds and skin, with the exception of the brain and heart; 5% of the cardiac output goes to the coronary system. There is an overall increase of blood flow to the coronary system during exercise, caused by two main factors: the increase in sympathetic activity causing vasodilatation along with the build-up of waste products and laxative acids, which also contributes to coronary dilatation. Exercise capacity can be measured in metabolic values, which are a good way to prescribe exercise to healthy uncompromised individuals.

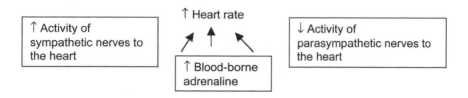

Figure 12.1 Response to exercise: heart rate.

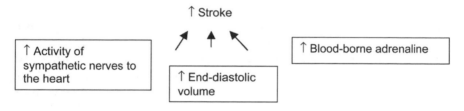

Figure 12.2 Response to exercise: stroke volume.

Exercising special groups

Although the prescription of exercise is well established in uncomplicated AMI, after revascularization there has been a reluctance to prescribe exercise for special groups of patients, particularly those with heart failure. Over the last 15 years published reports have shown that training not only improves exercise capacity but can also reverse skeletal muscle metabolic derangements, increase maximal cardiac outputs and improve quality of life (e.g. Coats et al. 1992, Keteyian et al. 1996, Myers et al. 2000).

The benefits include improved exercise tolerance, an increase in peak oxygen uptake (VO_{2max}) and in some cases partial relief of breathlessness, undue fatigue, sleep disturbances and muscle weakness. However, despite these findings physicians are often reluctant to refer patients for exercise rehabilitation. There may be a number of explanations: a cautious approach is often adopted as a result of the ominous nature of the condition. The Framingham Study suggests that 50% of patients die within 5 years of diagnosis (Wong et al. 1989). A study by Jugdutt et al. (1988) suggests that exercise training in patients with large anterior MIs and those with low ejection fractions and ST depression on exercise testing may not benefit from exercise training and might be adversely affected by further dilatation of the myocardium. However, research by Ginannuszzi et al. (1993) acknowledges that patients with low ejection fractions after MI are prone to further global and regional dilatation. Long-term exercise showed a significant improvement in physical work capabilities and did not have any additional negative effect. Furthermore, the NSF for CHD (DoH 2000) suggests that the benefits gained from a cardiac rehabilitation programme should be considered for patients with stable heart failure including the prescription for exercise.

Developing a programme for special groups including heart failure

Although there has been increased attention given to the prescription of exercise and the management of patients with heart failure, there are few published guidelines. Guidance on exercise prescription for individuals with heart failure focuses around recommendations from papers outlining exercise regimens in a general cardiac population and modified to meet the needs of the patient with heart failure. General cardiac rehabilitation guidelines tend to focus on relatively low-risk groups of patients after uncomplicated MI and coronary surgery, which bears little resemblance to the population with chronic heart failure.

Based on the complicated nature of the disease, the type of exercise should be given careful consideration, particularly in relation to central, peripheral and skeletal changes in heart failure. An exercise programme should be sensitive to the nature of the disease, allowing a combination of both aerobic and strength training, focusing on large muscle groups to offer enough stimulants to the skeletal muscle but not overloading the cardiovascular system. Other considerations include medical and non-medical factors, such as blood pressure, heart rate, symptoms of perceived exertion, medication and current New York Heart Association (NYHA) classification.

Non-medical factors include personal goals and preferences and behavioural characteristics. An exercise programme should not be generally prescriptive but tailored to meet the individual needs of the patient.

Risk factor modification and secondary prevention

Evidence-based strategies for the secondary prevention of coronary artery disease were originally introduced after the publication of the British

Cardiac Society's ASPIRE survey (ASPIRE Steering Group 1996). The results of the survey clearly demonstrated that, despite a wealth of guidelines and compelling clinical evidence, risk factor management and secondary prevention interventions that are of proven benefit have not been widely adopted into general hospital and general clinical practice. However, since then the NSF for CHD (DoH 2000) has helped focus the clinician's attention on the modification of patient's risk factors. Patients' risk factors can be classed as modifiable, such as smoking, hyperlipidaemia, hypertension, diabetes, and lifestyle factors, e.g. obesity and physical inactivity, or non-modifiable, such as family history of CHD, personal history of CHD, age, sex and ethnic origin (Sivers 1999). The main target of secondary prevention is to retard the progression of arteriosclerosis, the underlying cause of coronary artery disease, and to preserve left ventricular (LV) function after an MI. By implementing secondary prevention strategies far fewer patients need to be treated to save a life or a clinical event than with primary prevention strategies and there has long been evidence (Shaper et al. 1985, Norris et al. 1998) to indicate that risk factor modification is effective in reducing the risk of recurrent CHD events in patients who clinically manifest with the disease. More recently, evidence has demonstrated that this can lead to a retardation or even cessation of the progression of coronary arteriosclerosis and subsequent hospitalization for cardiac events (Wood et al. 1998). A number of studies have demonstrated that secondary prevention may have a major role in further reducing mortality rate (e.g. Norris et al. 1998).

Secondary prevention strategies can be divided into non-pharmacological interventions and pharmacological interventions. These are discussed in relation to individual risk factors.

Smoking

Smoking is a significant contributory factor for developing coronary artery disease, leading to acute MI (Shaper et al. 1985). A study by Wilhelmssion et al. (1975) suggested that giving up smoking will reduce the risk of further MI and reduce cardiovascular mortality by up to 50% over a 2-year follow-up. Another study by Daly (1983) also suggested that giving up smoking after an MI reduces the incidence of post-infarct angina. Although smoking cessation strategies have been shown to reduce the risk of recurrent events, these strategies are often difficult to achieve. Identifying the patient's readiness to change is the key to the implementation and success of these strategies. The effective delivery of advice and support is paramount in helping patients achieve their goal. The use of nicotine patches to aid smoking cessation has been proved effective without increasing the risk of cardiovascular events (Silagy et al. 1994).

The management of hyperlipidaemia

There are two methods available to the clinician to assist with the management of hyperlipidaemia: the first, which is non-pharmacological, is based on dietary modifications and the second is pharmacological intervention using statin therapy. Hyperlipidaemia has been shown to be a significant risk factor for the development of underlying ischaemic heart disease (Shepherd 1995) and the treatment of hyperlipidaemia using statins has shown a significant reduction in CHD, morbidity and mortality (Scandinavian Simvastatin Survival Study Group [4S Study] 1994). Before the publication of this landmark study, there had been some controversy over the reduction of lipids in the population with CHD. This was mostly as a result of earlier studies (Rossouw et al. 1990, Smith et al. 1993), which were either conducted on too small a population or lacked insufficient duration and statistical power. Since the publication of the 4S Study the pharmacological reduction of lipids by statins has become commonplace. The 4S Study was the first randomized, placebo-controlled, secondary prevention trial to have sufficient power to demonstrate that cholesterol lowering with simvastatin significantly reduced cardiovascular mortality after an MI and in patients with angina. Since then this study has been supported with two further studies: Sack et al. (1996) and the Lipid Study Group (1998). Current guidelines (British Cardiac Society 1998) recommend total cholesterol < 5 mmol or low-density lipoprotein (LDL)-cholesterol < 3 mmol for patients with established CHD. However, other studies (Pekkanen et al. 1990) suggest that patients with established CHD are at a high absolute risk whatever their level of serum cholesterol.

Dietary recommendations are still useful in the management of hyperlipidaemia and there have been a number of studies in this area (Oliver 1996, Tang et al. 1998). Tang et al.'s (1998) study demonstrated that, the more intense the diet, the greater the reduction in cholesterol achieved. This study demonstrated up to a 6% reduction in total cholesterol with an intensive diet. However, Oliver (1996) suggests that, although a 6% reduction in cholesterol may be beneficial to reduce CHD, it is too small to have an impact on the reduction of CHD mortality and morbidity in higher-risk individuals. Therefore, joint management should be applied with the use of statins and dietary advice to complement this. The most effective diet for secondary prevention appears to be one that is low in saturated fats but higher in polyunsaturated fats particularly omega-3 (ω-3) and -6 (ω-6) fatty acids, which are found in oily fish, vegetables and nuts. The Dart study (Burr et al. 1989) supports this by showing that a daily intake of oily fish resulted in a 29% reduction in total mortality rate during the first 2 years after an MI. A number of other studies, which have investigated diet alone, have also shown reductions in cardiac events and coronary deaths (Singh et al. 1992, De Lorgeril 1994). It should be noted that, although these studies have shown significant reductions in CHD mortality, they have not shown any significant change in total plasma cholesterol levels.

Obesity

Obesity is a contributory factor for CHD for a number of reasons. Being overweight is associated with raised blood pressure, raised blood cholesterol, glucose intolerance, type 2 diabetes and low levels of physical activity. Research has shown (Shaper et al. 1997) that there is an increase in mortality with a rise in body mass index and evidence suggests that central obesity is more significantly related to cardiovascular disease (Lawrence et al. 1996). Although there have not been any randomized, controlled trials investigating the effect of weight reduction on prognosis in patients with AMI, there has been evidence to suggest that the link between obesity and other risk factors is of significant concern to patients with CHD (Wood et al. 1998).

The management of hypertension

A number of studies have suggested that patients with hypertension have a worse prognosis after an MI than normotensive patients and that the treatment of hypertension can reduce morbidity and mortality from cardiovascular disease (Framingham Study – Wong et al. 1989, Collins et al. 1990). The Joint British Recommendations on the Prevention of Coronary Heart Disease in Clinical Practice (British Cardiac Society et al. 1998) recommend that hypertensive patients with CHD should have a sustained systolic BP < 140 mmHg and sustained diastolic BP of 85 mmHg. Patients with established heart disease and diabetes should have a sustained systolic BP < 135 mmHg and a diastolic BP < 80 mmHg. After an MI, β blockers have been shown both to reduce mortality, sudden death and re-infarction, and to be effective in the reduction of hypertension (Yusuf et al. 1985); in patients with impaired left ventricular function, angiotensin-converting enzyme (ACE) inhibitors should be used.

Diabetes mellitus

Diabetes is a significant risk factor for CHD, and CHD has been shown to be the major cause of mortality among patients with diabetes. The Framingham Study (Wong et al. 1989) showed that the risk of re-infarction was increased by 50% in post-MI patients who had diabetes. Furthermore, the Minnesota Heart Survey (Sprafka et al. 1991) showed that patients discharged after an MI with diabetes mellitus had a risk of death that was 40% higher than that of non-diabetic patients after 6 years of follow up. The DIGAMI (Diabetes Mellitus, Insulin Glucose Infusion in Acute Myocardial Infarction) study (Malmberg 1997) demonstrated that the long-term survival of post-MI patients with diabetes was increased by almost a third if they received insulin and glucose infusion followed by long-term insulin treatment. This showed an overall reduction in mortality rate of 11%. The management of patients with diabetes and CHD is paramount. There should be good control of blood glucose and rigorous CHD risk factor management, in particular smoking, hyperlipidaemia and hypertension. The improved management of these other risk factors can produce an overall reduction in morbidity and mortality (Webster 1997).

It is important that patients with CHD understand the importance of reducing modifiable risk factors. The patient should be given clear advice relating to smoking cessation, weight management, BP reduction, reduction of alcohol intake, reduction of hyperlipidaemia and control of diabetes mellitus. Patients should understand that dietary advice complements drug therapy and should be implemented into their lifestyle.

Pharmacological interventions in the secondary prevention of CHD

There is overwhelming evidence to demonstrate that pharmacological interventions have produced a significant reduction in mortality and morbidity in patients with established CHD. The NSF for CHD (DoH 2000) states that patients with CHD should, unless otherwise contraindicated, be discharged from hospital on anti-platelet, β-blocker, ACE inhibitor and statin therapy.

Anti-platelets

Unless specifically contraindicated aspirin 75 mg is recommended for all patients after an MI. Newer anti-platelet agents such as clopidogrel have also been shown to be of benefit in secondary prevention. The NSF for CHD (DoH 2000) recommends that 90% of patients should be discharged from hospital taking an anti-platelet therapy.

β Blockers

A number of studies (Yusuf et al. 1985, Packer et al. 1996) have shown that β blockers reduce mortality, sudden death and re-infarction rates after an acute MI. These studies have shown a 20% reduction in risk of death, a 25% reduction in re-infarction and a 30% reduction in risk of sudden death. In the past there has been some contraindication to the use of β blockers in patients with heart failure, although some studies (Packer et al. 1996) have shown that certain β blockers are no longer contraindicated in post-MI patients with stable heart failure. However, these drugs should be used with caution and titrated gradually under supervision.

β Blockers are also useful in the prevention and relief of anginal pain. The NSF for CHD (DoH 2000) indicates that unless otherwise contraindicated 80% of patients with CHD should be discharged from hospital taking a β blocker.

ACE inhibitors

There have been a number of landmark studies (SAVE – Pfeiffer et al. 1992, Acute Infarction Ramipril Efficacy or AIRE 1993, TRACE – Kober et al. 1995) that have shown a significant reduction in the risk of cardiovascular morbidity and mortality. As mentioned above the NSF for CHD (DoH 2000) recommends that, unless otherwise contraindicated 80% of patients should be discharged from hospital taking ACE inhibitors.

Statins

As previously discussed there is overwhelming evidence that lipid-lowering therapy significantly reduces mortality and morbidity in patients with CHD. The NSF for CHD (DoH 2000) recommends that 80% of patients be discharged from hospital taking a statin unless otherwise contraindicated.

Psychological impact of MI and the provision of psychological support

This section considers some aspects of the patient's psychological journey after a cardiac event, to enable the reader to gain insight into how those difficulties may impact on nursing care and the patient's perception of health care provided, e.g. patients stressed during phase I of cardiac rehabilitation often have difficulty comprehending or recalling the information provided to them in hospital. Therefore, nursing care needs to be managed in such a way that the patient feels supported while accessing the same information in different ways, e.g. verbal, written, in group discussions, in consultation with specialist nurse, etc.

Psychological difficulties are common after an acute cardiac event (Jones and West 1995, Thompson et al. 1995, Bergman and Bertero 2001). Increased use of implantable cardioverter defibrillators (ICDs) in patients with ventricular arrhythmias has had a particular impact because these patients experience poor psychosocial adjustment after implantation of the device (Burke et al. 2003). This may be related to the patient's inability to predict when the device would discharge (Samuel et al. 2001). Exploration of the patient's journey during a period of ill-health is an integral part of process mapping in order to improve the quality of care provided within the NHS. Implicit in this process is the knowledge that the patient's experience of the NHS may be very different from the perceptions of the nurses and other health-care professionals caring for that patient.

Stress

For most people having an acute cardiac event is a frightening and unwelcome intrusion which disrupts any sense of control that a person may have of the world. Most patients recall a sense of numbness when recounting their experiences associated with their hospital admission, reminiscent of that experienced by people who undergo post-traumatic stress (Owens et al. 2001). Johnson and Morse (1990) found that patients employed various strategies to regain control and reduce stress, which included seeking reassurance and information from health-care professionals. Stress is a common theme in the patient education material given after an MI, and stress management occurs in 90% of cardiac rehabilitation programmes in the UK (Clark 2003).

Loss and adjustment

Tschudin (1997) described loss as 'an unavoidable and inextricable part of being human'. As a result nurses routinely meet patients experiencing different types of loss, and are aware of the various feelings invoked, e.g. yearning and searching (Bowlby 1981). Loss may also be perceived as a threat, giving rise to feelings of anger or hostility. For many patients having a cardiac event is part of a multiple loss experience (Robinson and McKenna 1998) which includes bereavement, marital breakdown and mental ill-health. For some younger cardiac patients, there was a strong feeling of hostility and anger associated with the anticipated loss of future well-being (Moser and Dracup 1995), and jealousy of older people who have not led a healthy lifestyle, yet have not experienced an acute cardiac event. Patients who had adopted a healthy lifestyle before their acute cardiac event often express anger with their own bodies for failing them. Sometimes the anger and jealousy are projected elsewhere, occasionally on to nurses and other health-care professionals.

The fact that cardiac damage is sustained inside the body means that it is not visible to anyone looking at the patient. Therefore patients are not able to draw attention to the injury in the same way as if they had a broken arm. As a result the significance of the internal damage is often more difficult for the patient and health-care professionals to understand. Adaptation to the changes imposed by this disease process has been thwarted by uncertainty because patients often have to wait for further investigations of the cardiac event before any medical decisions are taken about any future treatment, adding to the sense of disorganization, because patients may feel unable to make any plans for the future. For some patients, trying to live a relatively normal life was difficult when they felt obliged to attend various outpatient appointments, for blood tests, physiological testing, consultations with medical consultants, specialist nurses, etc. This situation was especially problematic when patients with previous chronic ill-health were confronted by a barrage of hospital appointments. Use of process-driven, patient-centred management approaches to scheduling multiple outpatient appointments together enables patients, particularly those with multiple health problems, to gain some sense of normality in their lives. Often patients during one, or all, of the phases of cardiac rehabilitation are on sick leave, unemployed or feel that they are unemployable as a result of their illness. For many people employment holds a central role in life before an MI, bringing with it status and a sense of self-esteem (Jones and West 1995). However, after a heart attack the resultant changes may be associated with a lower standard of living which is perceived by many patients and their families as a loss of status. Many patients experience a sense of loss related to feeling increasingly more dependent on their relatives. This includes those with a previous chronic illness such as diabetes or a respiratory disorder. Such losses require patients to make major psychological adjustments in order to cope, although many patients may experience transient episodes of anxiety or a depressed mood (Goble and Winchester 1999) while making such adjustments to enable them to cope (Moser and Dracup 1995). At least 20% have more persistent symptoms of clinical anxiety or depression that last for a year or more (Jones and West 1995, Moser and Dracup 1995, Thomas 1995, Crowe et al. 1996). Reduction in the incidence of depression in patients after an MI is of particular significance because patients who experience it after an MI have an increased risk of mortality (Frasure-Smith et al. 1995, Crowe et al. 1996).

Anxiety and depression

An anxious patient may complain of physical symptoms such as palpitations, breathlessness or chest pain, which may give rise to panic attacks that are both frightening and debilitating to the patient's psychosocial recovery. Assisting the patient to overcome these symptoms involves helping the patient to understand the experience, and to provide relaxation, or cognitive–behavioural approaches, to cope with the feelings of anxiety in real-life situations (Palmer and Dryden 1995). During cardiac rehabilitation patients need to have the appropriate information available to enable them to participe in the mutual planning of their future treatment. Bergman and Bertero (2001) highlight the use patient education, counselling and behavioural interventions, and Goble and Winchester (1999) advocate the use of these interventions in small groups. However, Wade et al. (2002) found that use of a group cognitive–behavioural intervention for men experiencing psychological difficulties after an MI was problematic because only 30% were interested in attending and, of those, two were not able to complete all the sessions when heart bypass operations became available to them. Although different models of psychological interventions have been used to help such patients, the main focus is on assisting the patient to adapt to change, become self-empowered and regain control (Thomas et al. 2001).

Interpersonal relationships

Many clients describe feelings of isolation during phase II of cardiac rehabilitation. This is the period between discharge from hospital and starting a phase III cardiac rehabilitation programme. This can be particularly marked in patients who were already experiencing difficulties in their interpersonal relationships before the MI, and were distrustful of forming new attachments that risk rejection at a time of vulnerability. This may be related to the level of control that patients feel they have over their life and relationships (Moser and Dracup 1995). Even clients with robust relationships can become frustrated and resentful towards those with whom they have attachments. The unexpected disruption experienced within a family, after a cardiac event, often caused relationships to become strained (Jones and West 1995). The difficulty in providing psychosocial support to cardiac patients is compounded by limited evidence of how the needs of their carers are identified and addressed. The Carers and Disabled Children's Act 2000 requires that the needs of carers be identified when a patient is discharged. One way of improving the emotional support provided to these clients and their families is to develop the role of the clinical psychologist, cardiac liaison nurse or counsellor within the community. Another method may be to provide a psychological support associated with a cardiac support group.

Nurse interventions

A study by Scherck (1992) described how post-MI patients used support seeking, optimism, confrontation, self-reliance, ventilation of feelings and 'thinking things through' as ways of coping with a diagnosis. A nurse needs to listen actively to the cardiac patient in order to understand how he or she is seeking to cope with the new situation. Active listening requires the nurse to pay real attention and not just to the words that a patient may use; the nurse must also attend to her or his tone of voice, facial expression and other non-verbal messages, in order to convey to patients that their feelings are understood. Although active listening skills are essential in establishing a supportive empathic relationship, the nurse may be exposed to the patient's feelings of sadness, anger and hatred which can cause feelings of anxiety within the nurse. Thomas et al. (2001) suggested that acute care nursing staff should maintain a degree of emotional detachment because of the complex range of clinical responsibilities that they hold, and to protect themselves from becoming overwhelmed by anxiety. Therefore time constraints may prevent the nurse from spending sufficient time counselling the patient through any issues. If the nurse has only 10–15 min, it is better to tell the patient how much time is available.

Psychosocial testing

During cardiac rehabilitation, monitoring of the psychological status of patients is part of the role of the multidisciplinary team, although McGee et al. (1999) considered that there is little overall consensus in the literature about a reliable and validated evaluation instrument. The British Heart Foundation provides a range of psychosocial testing tools, which includes the Hospital Anxiety and Depression (HAD) Scale (Zigmond and Snaith 1983). This scale had been used to study the level of anxiety and depression with patients who have had CABG surgery (O'Rourke et al. 1991).

Referral of the patient for counselling

Nursing staff should be able to provide the patient with details of counselling support available. Counselling may be delivered by a range of health-care professionals, such as specialist nurses, occupational therapists, practice nurses and clinical psychologists. Some patients prefer to talk to another expert patient, whom they feel is more able to empathize with their feelings because of shared experiences. Providing the patient with a range of options empowers patients by giving them choice. This facilitates the counselling process, which is concerned with helping a patient to adapt to change and regain a sense of control; this could promote self-empowerment and in some cases leads to a sense of fulfilment within the patient to make the best of the future, which is perceived as precious even when the outcome feels uncertain (Holloway et al. 2000). At times the patient may be concerned with issues that appear to have little to do with the current complaint (Thomas et al. 2001), because patients' current psychological distress may have its origins in previous experiences, which they may not have disclosed even to their most intimate relations. Those experiences may include: childhood experiences of health care, child abuse, death of a parent/sibling/spouse/colleague, separation from a parent and relationship difficulties. Often these earlier events emerge once the counsellor–patient relationship has developed, so that the patient feels sufficiently supported to explore the emotions raised, and the connection between previous experience and the current psychological issues is revealed.

Conclusion

The evidence suggests that a comprehensive cardiac rehabilitation programme can reduce morbidity and mortality in patients with established CHD and that other groups of patients will benefit from taking part in this process. The role of the cardiac rehabilitation specialist is varied and involves close collaboration with other disciplines. There should be clear and concise guidelines to ensure that the patient's journey through the various phases is smooth and that complications are detected and acted on. Cardiac rehabilitation can be delivered in many ways and the key to ensuring that this delivery is comprehensive is good communication.

References

American Association of Cardiovascular and Pulmonary Rehabilitation (AACVPR) (1995) Guidelines for Cardiac Rehabilitation Programs. Champaign, IL: Human Kinetics.

Acute Infarction Ramipril Efficacy (AIRE) investigators (1993) Effects of ramipril on mortality and morbidity of survivors of acute myocardial infarction with clinical evidence of heart failure. Lancet 342: 821.

Association of Charted Physiotherapists Interested in Cardiac Rehabilitation (2002) Standards for the Exercise Component of the Stage III Cardiac Rehabilitation Programme. London: ACPICR.

ASPIRE Steering Group (1996) A British Cardiac Society Survey of the potential for the secondary prevention of coronary heart disease (Action on Secondary Prevention through Intervention to Reduce Events). Heart 75: 334.

Bergman E, Bertero C (2001) You can do it if you set your mind to it: a qualitative study of patients with coronary artery disease. J Adv Nursing 36: 733–41.

Bowlby J (1981) Attachment and Loss: Loss, sadness and depression, Vol. 3. New York: Basic Books.

British Cardiac Society (2001) Guideline for the management of patients with acute coronary syndromes without persistent ECG ST segment elevation. Heart 85:133–142.

British Cardiac Society (2004) Working Group on the definition of myocardial infarction. Heart 90: 603–9.

British Cardiac Society, British Hyperlipidaemia Association, British Hypertension Society Endorsed by the British Diabetic Association (1998) Joint British Recommendations on Prevention of Coronary Heart Disease in Clinical Practice. Heart 80(suppl 2).

Burke JL, Halias CN, Clark-Carter D, White D, Connelly D (2003) The psychosocial impact of the implantable cardioverter defibrillator: An analytic review. Br J Health Psychol 8: 165–70.

Burr ML, Fehily AM, Gilbert F et al. (1989) Effects of changes in fat, fish and fibre intakes on death and myocardial infarction: Diet and Re-infarction Trial (DART). Lancet ii:757.

Cahalin L, Pappoigianopaulos P, Prevost S et al. (1995) The relationship of the six minutes walk test to maximal oxygen consumption in transplant candidates with end stage lung disease. Chest 108: 452–9.

Clark AM (2003) It's like an explosion in your life . . .: lay perspectives on stress and myocardial infarction. J Clin Nursing 12: 544–53.

Coats A, McGee H, Stokes H et al. (1995) British Association for Cardiac Rehabilitation Guidelines. Oxford: Blackwell Science Ltd.

Coats JS, Admaopoulos S, Radaelli A et al. (1992) Controlled trial of physical training in chronic heart failure: exercise performance, haemodynamics, ventilation and autonomic function. Circulation 85: 2119–31.

Collins R et al. (1990) Blood pressure, stroke and coronary heart disease: part 2, short-term reductions in blood pressure: overview of randomised drug trials in their epidemiological context. Lancet 335: 827.

Crowe JM, Runios J, Ebbesen LS, Oldridge, NB, Streiner DL (1996) Anxiety and depression after acute myocardial infarction. Heart Lung 25: 98–107.

Daly LE (1983) Long-term effect on mortality of stopping smoking after unstable angina and myocardial infarction. BMJ 287: 324.

Davidson C, Revel K, Chamberlain D et al. (1995) Report of a working group of the British Cardiac Society: cardiac rehabilitation services in the United Kingdom. Br Heart J 73: 201–2.

De Lorgeril L (1994) Mediterranean alpha-linolenic acid-rich diet in the secondary prevention of coronary hear disease. Lancet 343: 1454.

Department of Health (2000) National Standard Framework for Coronary Heart Disease. London: HMSO.

Department of Health (2000) National Standard Framework for Coronary Heart Disease. London: HMSO.

European Society of Cardiology (2002) Management of acute coronary syndromes in patients presenting without persistent ST-segment elevation. The Task Force on the Management of acute coronary syndromes of the European Society of Cardiology. Eur Heart J 23: 1809–40.

European Society of Cardiology (2003) Management of acute myocardial infarction in patients with ST-segment elevation. The Task Force on the Management of acute myocardial infarction of the European Society of Cardiology. Eur Heart J 24: 28–66.

Fox SM, Naughten JP, Gorman PA (1972) Physical activity and cardiovascular health. The exercise prescription: Frequency and type of activity. Mod Concepts Cardiovasc Dis 41: 25.

Frasure-Smith N, Lesperance F, Talajic M (1995) Depression and 18 month prognosis after myocardial infarction. Circulation 91: 999–1005.

Froelicher V (1988) Cardiac Rehabilitation. Cardiology. Philadelphia: JB Lippincott Co.

Giannuzzi P, Tavazzi L Temporelli PL et al. (1993) Long-term physical training and left ventricular remodelling after anterior myocardial infarction: results of the Exercise in Anterior Myocardial Infarction (EAMI) study group. J Am Cardiol 22: 1821–9.

Goble AJ, Winchester MUC (1999) Best Practice Guidelines for Cardiac Rehabilitation and Secondary Prevention. Melbourne: Department of Human Services.

Holloway I, Sofaer B, Walker J (2000) The transition from well person to 'pain afflicted' patient: the career of people with chronic back pain. Illness, Crisis and Loss 8(4): 373–85.

Horgan J, Bethell H, Carson P et al. (1992) British Cardiac Society Working Party Report on Cardiac Rehabilitation. Br Heart J 67: 412–18.

Johnson JL, Morse JM (1990) Regaining control: the process of adjustment after myocardial infarction. Heart Lung 19: 126–35.

Jones D, West R (1995) Cardiac Rehabilitation. London: BMJ Publishing Group.

Jugdutt BI, Michorowski BL, Kappogoda CT (1988) Exercise training after anterior Q wave myocardial infarction: importance of regional left ventricular function and topography. J Am Cardiol 12: 362–72.

Keteyian SJ, Levine A, Brauner C et al. (1996) Exercise training in patients with heart failure: a randomised controlled trial. Ann Intern Med 124: 1051–7.

Kober L, Tarp-Pederon C, Carlsen J et al. (1995) A clinical trial of angiotensin-converting enzyme inhibitor trandolapril in patients with left ventricular dysfunction after MI. N Engl J Med 333: 1670.

Lanenfold H, Schrieider B, Grimm W et al. (1990) The six minute walk test. An adequate exercise test for pacemaker patients? Pacing Clinical Electrophysiol 12: 30–5.

Lawrence M et al. (1996) Prevention of Cardiovascular Disease. An evidence-based approach. Oxford General Practice Series 33. Oxford: Oxford University Press, pp. 58–63.

Levine S (1944) Some harmful effects of recurrence in the treatment of heart disease. JAMA 126: 80.

Long Term Intervention with Pravastatin in Ischaemic Disease (LIPID) Study group (1998) Prevention of cardiovascular events and death with pravastatin in patients with coronary heart disease and a broad range of cholesterol levels. N Engl J Med 339: 1349.

McGee HM, Hevey D, Horgan JH (1999) Psychological outcome assessments for use in cardiac rehabilitation service evaluation: a 10 year systematic review. Soc Sci Med 48: 1373.

Malmberg K, for the DIGAMI Study Group (1997) Prospective randomised study of intensive insulin treatment on long-term survival after acute myocardial infarction in patients with diabetes mellitus. BMJ 314: 1512.

Moser DK, Dracup K (1995) Psychosocial recovery from a cardiac event: The influence of perceived control. Heart Lung 24: 273–80.

Myers J et al. (2000) Exercise training and myocardial remodelling in patients with reduced ventricular function: one year follow-up with magnetic resonance imaging. Am Heart J 139: 252–261.

Norris RM, on behalf of the UK Heart Attack Study Collaborative Group (1998) Fatality outside hospital from acute coronary events in three British health districts. BMJ 316: 1065.

O'Connor GT, Buriing JE, Fischer ME et al. (1989) An overview of randomised trials of rehabilitation with exercise after myocardial infarction. Circulation 80: 234.

Oldridge NB et al. (1988) Cardiac rehabilitation after myocardial infarction: combined experience of randomised clinical trials. JAMA 260: 945.

Oliver MF (1996) Which changes in diet prevent coronary heart disease? Acta Cardiolog 51: 467.

O'Rourke A, Lewin B, Whitcross, S, Pacey W (1991) The effects of physical exercise training and cardiac education on levels of anxiety and depression in the rehabilitation of coronary bypass graft patients. Int Disability Studies 12: 104–6.

Owens RL, Koutsakis S, Bennet PD (2001) Post-traumatic stress disorder as a sequel of acute myocardial infarction: an overlooked cause of psychosocial disability. Coronary Health Care 5: 9–15.

Packer M, Gheorghiade M, Young J et al., for the US Carvedilol Heart Failure Group (1996) The effect of carvedilol on mortality and morbidity in patients with chronic heart failure. N Engl J Med 334: 1349.

Palmer S, Dryden W (1995) Counselling for Stress Problems. London: Sage Publications.

Pekkanen MD, Linn S, Heiss G et al. (1990) Ten year mortality from cardiovascular disease in relation to cholesterol level among men without pre-existing cardiovascular disease. N Engl J Med 323: 1700.

Pfeiffer MA, Braunwald E, Moye L et al. (1992) Effect of capital on mortality and morbidity in patients with left ventricular dysfunction after myocardial infarction (SAVE). N Engl J Med 327: 669.

Raul G, Germain P, Bareiss P (1998) Does the six minute walk test predict the progress in patient with NYHA class II or III chronic heart failure? Am Heart J 136: 449–57.

Rejski WJ, Foley KO, Woodward CM et al. (2000) Evaluating and understanding performance testing in COPD patients. J Cardiopulm Rehab 20: 79–88.

Robinson DS, McKenna H (1998) Loss: an analysis of a concept of a particular interest to nursing. J Adv Nursing 27: 779–84.

Rossouw JE, Lewis B, Rifkind BM et al. (1990) The value of lowering cholesterol after myocardial infarction. N Engl J Med 323: 1112.

Sack FM et al. (1996) The effect of pravastatin on coronary events after myocardial infarction in patients with average cholesterol levels. N Engl J Med 355: 10001.

Samuel F, Sears JR, Burns JL, Handberg E, Sotile WM, Conti JB (2001) Young at heart: Understanding the unique psychosocial adjustment of young implantable cardioverter defibrillator recipients. J Pacing Clin Electrophysiol 24: 1113–17.

Scandinavian Simvastatin Survival Study Group (1994) Randomised trail of cholesterol lowering in 4444 patients with coronary heart disease: The Scandinavian Simvastatin Survival Study (4S). Lancet 344: 1383.

Scherck KA (1992) Coping with acute myocardial infarction. Heart Lung 21: 327–34.

Scottish Intercollegiate Guidelines Network (2002) Cardiac Rehabilitation: A national clinical guideline. Edinburgh: SIGN.

Shaper AG, Pocock SJ, Walker M et al. (1985) Risk factors for ischaemic heart disease: the prospective phase of the British regional heart study. Journal of Epidemiology 39: 197.

Shaper AG, Wannamethee SG, Walker M et al. (1997) Body weight: implications for the prevention of coronary heart disease, stroke and diabetes mellitus in a cohort of middle aged men. BMJ 314: 1311.

Shepherd J, for the West of Scotland Coronary Prevention Study Group (1995) Prevention of coronary heart disease with provastatin in men with hypercholesterolemia. N Engl J Med 333: 1301.

Silagy C, Mant D, Fowler G et al. and the Working Group for the Study of Transdermal Nicotine in Patients with Coronary Artery Disease (1994) Meta-analysis on efficacy of nicotine replacement therapies in smoking cessation. Lancet 343: 139.

Singh RM, Raslogis S, Verma R et al. (1992) Randomised controlled trial of cardio protective diet in patients with recent acute myocardial infarction results of one year follow-up. BMJ 304: 1015.

Sivers F (1999) Evidence-based Strategies for Secondary Prevention of Coronary Heart Disease. Guildford: A&M Publishing.

Smith D, Song SD, Sheldon TA (1993) Cholesterol lowering and mortality: the importance of considering initial level of risk. BMJ 306: 1367.

Sprafka JM, Burke GL, Folsom AR et al. (1991) Trends in prevalence of diabetes mellitus in patients with myocardial infarction and effect of diabetes on survival: The Minnesota Heart Survey. Diabetes Care 14: 537.

Tang JL et al. (1998) Systematic review of dietary intervention trials to lower blood total cholesterol in free-living Subjects. BMJ 316: 1213.

Taylor H, Henschel A, Brozek J (1949) Effects of bed rest on cardiovascular function and work performance. J Appl Physiol 2: 223.

Thomas JJ (1995) Reducing anxiety during phase 1 cardiac rehabilitation. J Psychosom Res 39: 295–304.

Thomas P, Davidson S, Rance C (2001) Clinical Counselling in Medical Settings. London: Brunner-Routledge.

Thompson DR, Ersser SJ, Webster RA (1995) The experiences of patients and their partners 1 month after a heart attack. J Adv Nursing 22: 707–14.

Tschudin V (1997) Counselling for Loss and Bereavement. London: Baillière Tindall.

Wade T, Birchmore L, Hobby C (2002) Feasibility of a cognitive-behavioural group intervention for men experiencing psychological difficulties after myocardial infarction. Eur J Cardiovasc Nursing 1: 98–114.

Wannamethee SG, Shaper AG, Walker M et al. (1998) Changes in physical activity, mortality and incidence of coronary heart disease in older men. Lancet 351: 1603.

Webster MWI (1997) What cardiologists need to know about diabetes. Lancet 350(suppl 1): 23.

Wilhelmssion C, Vedin JA, Elmfeldt D et al. (1975) Smoking and myocardial infarction. Lancet i: 415.

Wood D, De Backer G, Faergeman O et al. (1998) Prevention of coronary heart disease in clinical practice: Recommendations of the Second Joint Task Force of the European and Other Societies on Coronary Prevention. Eur Heart J.

Wong ND, Cupples LA, Ostfeld AM (1989) Risk factors for long-term coronary prognosis after initial myocardial infarction: The Framingham Study. Am J Epidemiol 130: 469.

World Health Organization (1993) Needs and Actions: Priorities in cardiac rehabilitation and secondary prevention in patients with coronary heart disease. WHO Technical Report Service 831. Geneva: WHO.

Yusuf S et al. (1985) Beta blockade during and after myocardial infarction: an overview of the randomised trials. Prognos Cardiovasc Dis 27: 335.

Zigmond AS, Snaith RP (1983) The Hospital Anxiety and Depression Scale. Acta Psychiatr Scand 67: 361–70.

Zugck C, Kruger S, Berber S et al. (2000) Is the six minute walk test a reliable substitute for peak oxygen uptake in patients with dilated cardiomyopathy? Eur Heart J 21: 540–9.

CHAPTER THIRTEEN

Management of the patient with chronic heart failure

ANNE DORMER

Managing chronic heart failure (CHF) is a formidable challenge for health-care providers in the UK. Current guidelines for the management of heart failure have delivered the framework for evidence-based practice. It is now the remit of local health-care providers to develop integrated care pathways to meet the needs of heart failure patients, from initial diagnosis through to meeting palliative care needs.

Epidemiology of heart failure

Heart failure is a growing problem. It is estimated that the incidence of heart failure in the UK will increase in the future. This projection is made on the basis that the UK has an ageing population and that more people experience myocardial infarction (MI) and hypertension. British Heart Foundation (2003) statistics demonstrate that, for adults under 75, death rates from cardiovascular disease have fallen by 32% in the last 10 years. In addition more patients are being screened for heart failure as a result of European and national guidelines which give guidance about the diagnosis of heart failure and recommend evidence-based treatments and management plans (e.g. Scottish Intercollegiate Guidelines Network or SIGN 1999, Department of Health or DoH 2000, National Institute for Clinical Excellence or NICE 2003).

If not properly managed heart failure places very heavy pressures on hospital beds through emergency admissions and readmissions; in 1999–2000 it accounted for 1.2–2.2% of NHS expenditure, with 70% of costs being related to hospitalization alone (Stewart et al. 2002). In elderly patients with heart failure readmission rates range from 29% to 47% within 3–6 months of the initial hospital discharge (Davies et al. 2000b). It is proposed that half of hospital readmissions caused by heart failure may be preventable (DoH 2000).

The incidence of CHF in the UK is 0.3% per annum (McDonagh and Dargie 1998) (incidence is the number of new cases per year). It is estimated that 760 000 people are presently living with heart failure in the UK, with 63 000 new cases appearing each year (British Heart Foundation 2001). Projected figures estimate that both the incidence and prevalence of heart failure are set to increase over the next 20 years (prevalence is the total number of patients living with heart failure). The prevalence of heart failure increases rapidly with age, with the mean age of the heart failure population being 74 years. Current UK statistics suggest that 1–2% of the population collectively, and 10–20% of the elderly population (> 70 years), have heart failure (SIGN 1999).

Mortality from heart failure

It is difficult to establish the actual number of deaths in the UK from heart failure because guidance on death certificates stipulates that heart failure is not a cause but a mode of death. The aetiology or cause of heart failure is therefore usually listed on the death certificate, e.g. coronary heart disease (CHD) or dilated cardiomyopathy. It is known from epidemiological data that once heart failure is diagnosed the mortality rate is high. Figure 13.1 illustrates the 1-year survival rates for heart failure compared with the major cancers. Heart failure demonstrates mortality rates that compare with many of the common cancers including colon and ovarian cancer.

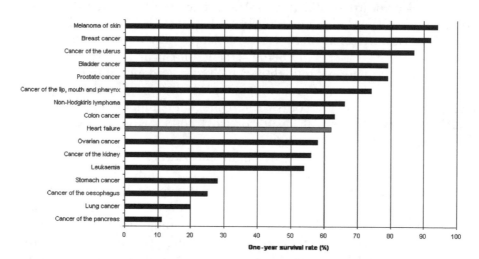

Figure 13.1 One-year survival rates, heart failure and major cancers compared, mid-1990s, England and Wales. Note that patients are diagnosed with heart failure in the Hillingdon Heart Failure Study, 1995–96. (Sources: Cowie et al. 2000.) Reproduced with kind permission of the British Heart Foundation.

Table 13.1 illustrates the findings of the Hillingdon Heart Failure Study (BHF 2003 – see BHF Coronary Heart Disease statistics at www.heart-stats.org). At 18 months after diagnosis of heart failure, 43% of the patients had died.

Table 13.1 Survival after initial diagnosis of heart failure, 1995–98, Hillingdon

	Number	Percentage
All with initial diagnosis of heart failure	220	100
Survive for longer than 1 month	178	81
Survive for longer than 3 months	165	75
Survive for longer than 6 months	154	70
Survive until end of first year	136	62
Survive for longer than 18 months	125	57

From Cowie et al. (2000).

It is widely accepted that the palliative care needs of heart failure patients are largely unmet. Patients with heart failure have a less predictable death trajectory in comparison to dying of cancer, where the physical decline towards death is often seen as a gradual process. In heart failure death can occur suddenly and unpredictably, and frequently without adequate patient and family preparation or palliative care support.

Definitions of heart failure

Heart failure is a complex syndrome that can result from any structural or functional cardiac disorder that impairs the ability of the heart to function as a pump to support a physiological circulation.

NICE (2003, p. 2)

Heart failure has been defined as 'a clinical syndrome caused by an abnormality of the heart and recognised by a characteristic pattern of haemodynamic, renal, neural and hormonal responses' (P Poole-Wilson 1985, cited in Gibbs et al. 2000).

Systolic and diastolic heart failure

There are two distinct subtypes of CHF: systolic and diastolic dysfunction.

The most common cause of heart failure in the UK is ischaemic heart disease, which may lead to impairment of left ventricular (LV) systolic function. Systolic heart failure leads to a progressive deterioration in LV contractibility and accounts for about 70% of all heart failure cases (Gould 2002).

The presence of normal LV function/ejection fraction in a patient with a diagnosis of CHF establishes the diagnosis of diastolic heart failure (in the absence of valvular heart disease) (Vasan and Levy 2003). Diastolic heart failure is defined as overt heart failure caused by the inability of the ventricle to fill adequately at normal filling pressures (Zile and Brutsaert 2002). Diastolic heart failure exists when impaired myocardial relaxation with increased stiffness of the ventricular wall leads to impairment of ventricular filling (Lip et al. 2000).

It is estimated that up to a third of CHF patients have diastolic failure and, although pure forms exist in many patients, both systolic and diastolic failure may be present. Hypertension, CHD and hypertrophic cardiomyopathy are common causes of diastolic failure. Current management strategies include symptom control, e.g. diuretic therapy and treatment of underlying risk factors.

Currently, evidence-based guidelines for heart failure management are directed towards the management of systolic failure. Ongoing randomized controlled trials may help inform guidelines for the diagnosis and management of diastolic heart failure in the future. This chapter is directed at the management of CHF patients with systolic dysfunction.

Aetiology of heart failure

Causes of heart failure include coronary artery disease, hypertension, cardiomyopathy, valve disease, arrhythmias, anaemia and thyrotoxicosis.

The causes of heart failure and the presence of other diseases that may worsen heart failure symptoms should be identified to ensure correct patient management. The most common cause of heart failure in Europe in patients aged under 75 is CHD, usually as a result of MI (European Society of Cardiology 2001). About one person in every three who has MI will show some evidence of heart failure, and approximately one in five will develop heart failure over a 5- to 10-year period. The use of evidence-based medicines will prevent or delay the onset of heart failure; however, in patients with extensive myocardial damage severe heart failure may be difficult to control (Cleland 1999).

Improvements in hypertension management have resulted in a reduction in the incidence of heart failure secondary to hypertension. However, hypertension remains a significant cause of heart failure, particularly in women and black individuals (Lip et al. 2000). Hypertension leads to heart failure by contributing to LV hypertrophy associated with both systolic and diastolic dysfunction. In addition LV hypertrophy increases the risk of cardiac arrhythmias (Lip et al. 2000). Hypertension is an independent risk factor for the development of CHD. Dilated cardiomyopathy exists when the heart enlarges and contracts poorly with no evidence of CHD on cardiac catheterization. Dilated cardiomyopathy may be idiopathic (no known cause), result from alcohol, toxins, drugs, pregnancy or viruses, or be inherited. It can affect any age group and family studies have reported that up to a quarter of cases have a familial basis (Lip et al. 2000). Valve disease, particularly mitral and aortic valve disease, may lead to systolic heart disease if left untreated. Heart failure can also result from systemic diseases that place increased metabolic demands on the heart, e.g. thyrotoxicosis, anaemia and septicaemia (Gould 2002).

Compensatory mechanisms

Compensatory mechanisms are activated in response to a reduced cardiac output. These compensatory mechanisms aim to maintain cardiac output, blood pressure and peripheral perfusion. However, sustained activation of these compensatory mechanisms leads to progression of LV systolic dysfunction and worsening heart failure (Exner and Schron 2001).

The renin–angiotensin–aldosterone system is activated by a fall in cardiac output. Angiotensin I is produced by the effect of renin (produced in the kidneys) on circulating angiotensinogen. Angiotensin I is converted under the influence of angiotensin-converting enzyme (ACE), predominantly in the lungs, to produce angiotensin II, which is itself a powerful vasoconstrictor of the renal and systemic circulation (Jackson et al. 2000); it will help in maintaining systemic blood pressure. Angiotensin II, if left unchallenged, leads to hypertrophy (enlargement) of the left ventricle and further progression of heart failure. It also acts to increase the production of aldosterone from the adrenal cortex, which increases intravascular volume by retaining Na^+ and water. In addition, aldosterone causes K^+ and Mg^{2+} loss through its action on the renal tubules. In CHF a patient's plasma levels of aldosterone may reach 20 times the normal level (Miller and Srivastava 2001).

The sympathetic nervous system is another compensatory mechanism activated to improve and maintain cardiac function. However, sustained activation results in chronic elevation of noradrenaline (norepinephrine) levels that are potentially cardiotoxic (Jackson et al. 2000). A high plasma noradrenaline level in patients with CHF is associated with a poor prognosis (Merck Manual 2004). ACE inhibitors and cardioselective β blockers act to inhibit these compensatory mechanisms and prevent further progression of CHF.

Signs and symptoms

Breathlessness and cough are frequent symptoms of CHF. Breathlessness may occur on exertion and result in a reduced exercise tolerance. Breathlessness may occur as the patient reclines (orthopnoea) or the patient is woken from sleep (paroxysmal nocturnal dyspnoea). Breathlessness may occur as a result of pulmonary oedema; a small increase in pressure in the pulmonary venous system of above 15–20 mmHg may result in fluid congestion in the lungs. Breathlessness in the absence of pulmonary oedema occurs as a result of reduced cardiac output to the respiratory muscles, causing respiratory muscle fatigue (Gould 2002).

Excessive tiredness and fatigue occur as a result of poor circulation to the brain and skeletal muscles. Reduced cerebral blood flow may cause forgetfulness, memory loss and confusion. Fatigue is not helped by poor sleeping patterns which are commonly reported in CHF. Oedema swelling in the feet and legs, can account for weight gain. Oedema may be pitting and patients may complain of tightness/pain in the oedematous limbs.

The New York Heart Association (NYHA, cited in Hatchett and Thompson 2002, p. 196) classification of heart failure is widely used to quantify a patient's functional capacity and is determined by an assessment of symptoms reported by the patient. However, practitioners are reminded that outcomes in heart failure are determined not only by functional class but by also by findings on echocardiography. The following are the four NYHA classes:

- NYHA I: impaired left ventricle but no symptoms
- NYHA II: breathlessness on moderate exertion, e.g. walking up two flights of stairs, walking briskly, walking uphill
- NYHA III: breathless during everyday activities, e.g. walking around the house
- NYHA IV: symptoms at rest, e.g. breathlessness.

Signs

There are limitations in the value of physical examination in relation to the heart failure patient. Some physical signs are difficult to interpret and, if present, may be related to other causes (Watson et al. 2000). Clinical signs of heart failure include: tachycardia, raised jugular venous pressure, pulmonary crepitations, third heart sounds and peripheral oedema (Gould 2002). The Royal College of Physicians (2001) state that a third heart sound is probably the most sensitive and specific physical sign for LV dysfunction.

Diagnosing heart failure: the relevant tests and investigations

Accurate identification of people at high risk of developing heart failure and the assessment and identification of people with suspected heart failure require a systematic approach. The Department of Health (2003) identifies the following groups as being at risk:

- Patients with breathlessness, particularly breathlessness at night, or tiredness
- Patients known to have ischaemic heart disease, or who have had an MI
- Patients who have had a coronary artery bypass graft (CABG) or percutaneous clinical intervention (PCI)
- Hypertensive patients
- Patients with peripheral oedema

If heart failure is suspected a 12-lead ECG and/or brain or B-type natriuretic protein (BNP) or N-terminal pro-BNT (NT-proBNP) test (where available) should be performed. If a patient has a normal 12-lead ECG and BNP or NT-proBNP test then heart failure is an unlikely diagnosis (NICE 2003).

Twelve-lead electrocardiogram

A 12-lead ECG is abnormal in most patients with heart failure, although it can be normal in 10% of cases (Davies et al. 2000a).

Common abnormalities include left bundle-branch block, atrial fibrillation, LV hypertrophy, T-wave inversion and pathological Q waves.

B-type natriuretic protein

The potential value of measuring natriuretic peptides such as BNP and NT-pro BNP is as an exclusion test for heart failure.

Blood measurements of BNP and NT-proBNP have been shown to identify patients with LV dysfunction (Vanderheyden et al. 2004). Cardiac myocytes produce proBNP as a result of cardiac wall stress, and proBNP is split into BNP and NT-proBNP under the influence of the proteolytic enzyme furin (Hall 2004).

Many randomized clinical trials have demonstrated that BNP and NT-proBNP are proven diagnostic markers for heart failure caused by LV systolic dysfunction. An abnormal NT-proBNP concentration is an accurate diagnostic test both for the exclusion of heart failure in the population and in ruling out LV dysfunction in breathless individuals (McDonagh et al. 2004).

Other recommended tests

A chest radiograph may reveal useful information in relation to:

- the size and shape of the heart and whether there is any enlargement (cardiomegaly)
- evidence of lung disease that may cause breathlessness
- evidence of pulmonary oedema.

Although an abnormal chest radiograph may suggest heart failure, a normal one does not exclude heart failure. Cardiomegaly can be absent even in severe LV dysfunction and pulmonary congestion is not always caused by heart disease (National Prescribing Centre 2001).

Routine blood tests and urinalysis are recommended to check for abnormalities. Urea, creatinine and electrolytes check baseline renal function. A full blood count is important to exclude anaemia as a cause of breathlessness, and liver function tests may be abnormal in advanced heart failure secondary to hepatic congestion (Davies et al. 2000a). A thyroid function test is recommended because an overactive gland can cause atrial fibrillation (Cleland 1999). Fasting glucose and lipid profile assesses the patient for hyperglycaemia, and elevated total cholesterol, low-density lipoproteins and triglycerides may contribute to the development of CHD.

Assessment of respiratory function is helpful to exclude lung disease as a cause of breathlessness.

Echocardiography is the present gold standard test for the investigation of heart failure. Transthoracic Doppler two-dimensional echocardiography enables the visualization of the cardiac walls, chambers and valves (McMurray and Dargie 1998). It allows the assessment of systolic and diastolic function (European Society of Cardiology 2001). Enlargement of the left ventricle and impairment of contraction may be seen in systolic dysfunction. In ischaemic heart disease regional wall abnormality may be seen and in dilated cardiomyopathy global impairment of systolic contraction may be observed (Davies et al. 2000a).

Echocardiography also provides assessment of valvular function, identifying aortic, mitral and tricuspid valves and the presence of stenosis or regurgitation. An experienced echocardiographer is skilled to perform 'eyeball' grading of LV systolic dysfunction. The operator estimates LV ejection fraction, correlating to locally agreed categories of mild, moderate or severe impairment of function. If no abnormality is observed then heart failure is unlikely (NICE 2003).

Patients reporting anginal symptoms require assessment to determine whether coronary artery disease is present. An exercise tolerance test may help stratify risk; however, in some patients exercise tolerance is reduced. If the patient is unable to exercise or performs a suboptimal test coronary angiography should be considered. Indeed, coronary angiography should be considered for all patients reporting cardiac pain and for patients with evidence of hibernating myocardium. Stress echocardiography is the means by which myocardial reversibility is assessed.

Pharmacological therapy

In CHF compensatory mechanisms are activated to preserve BP and vital organ perfusion. This neurohormonal activation, if left unchecked, will progress heart failure. Three pharmacological therapies have been found in randomized controlled trials to improve survival by acting to regulate the sympathetic nervous system and the renin–angiotensin–aldosterone system. These therapies include ACE inhibitors, certain β blockers and an aldosterone antagonist.

ACE inhibitors

Angiotensin-converting enzyme inhibitors should be considered for all patients with symptomatic LV systolic dysfunction and are the cornerstone of management of CHF (NICE 2003).

Beneficial effects have been observed in all grades of systolic heart failure from mild to moderate (V-HeFT II) (Cohn et al. 1991) to severe CHF (CONSENSUS 1987). There is good evidence that ACE inhibitors reduce mortality rates and prevent hospital admissions and readmissions (Cleland and MacFadyen 2002). In addition they delay the appearance of symptoms in asymptomatic heart failure (Studies of Left Ventricular Dysfunction or *SOLVD* – *SOLVD* Investigators 1991, 1992) and improve symptoms and exercise tolerance in symptomatic heart failure.

Cough is a common symptom in CHF; it is also a symptom of pulmonary oedema, which should be excluded when a new or worsening cough develops. ACE inhibitor therapy may cause cough as a result of the inhibition of bradykinin within the lung lining (Gould 2002). ACE inhibitor-induced cough should rarely cause the discontinuation of ACE inhibitor therapy (NICE 2003); however, in those patients whose cough cannot be tolerated ACE inhibitor therapy may need to be stopped and an angiotensin II antagonist prescribed in its place. Angiotensin II antagonists do not affect bradykinin metabolism and therefore do not produce cough.

Regular monitoring of renal function is mandatory for patients taking ACE inhibitors. Some rise in urea, creatinine and K^+ may be expected after starting ACE inhibitor therapy. If creatinine increases over 50% above baseline or K^+ to 5.9 mmol/l, adjustment of other therapies impacting on renal

function, e.g. K^+-sparing diuretic therapies or other concomitant therapies, should be considered (NICE 2003). If biochemistry remains unaltered
despite these changes, the dosage of ACE inhibitor therapy should be halved.
If K^+ rises above 6 mmol/l or creatinine increases to 100% above baseline or
to > 350 μmol/l, the ACE inhibitor should be stopped (NICE 2003).

Hypotension may occur as a result of the vasodilatory effect of ACE inhibition. If the patient experiences dizziness or postural hypotension, loop
diuretic therapy and other concomitant medication need review. In addition
the patient's fluid intake is checked to ensure adequate daily intake. Advice
may be given for the ACE inhibitor to be taken in the evening (if a once-daily
dose); in some cases a reduction in ACE inhibitor dose may be required.

A number of patients taking ACE inhibitors may complain of loss of
taste or taste disturbance; if this is intolerable one ACE inhibitor may be
changed for another and the symptom observed for improvement.

Diuretic therapy

Diuretic therapy is essential for the symptomatic relief of CHF when a
patient presents with fluid overload: acute pulmonary oedema or peripheral oedema. Loop diuretics have a powerful action by inhibiting the
reabsorption of Na^+ and Cl^- from the ascending loop of Henle in the renal
tubule. Urine output is increased for 4–6 h after administration of
furosemide (frusemide) or bumetanide therapy as a result of increased salt
and water loss. Blood chemistry should be checked after dose increases
because loop diuretics cause K^+ loss. Loop diuretics also promote hyperuricaemia (high uric acid in the blood) (Gould 2002) and gout may therefore
develop as a result of therapy. The use of diuretic therapy results in a rapid
improvement in breathlessness and exercise tolerance (European Society of
Heart Failure 2001). The lowest dose possible to relieve symptoms should be
used to avoid side effects, e.g. hypotension, and because of the fact that loop
diuretics also increase activation of the sympathetic nervous system and the
renin–angiotensin–aldosterone system, which progresses heart failure.

Thiazide diuretics, e.g. bendrofluazide, are mild in action and act on
the distal convoluted tubule, reducing Na^+ reabsorption. Thiazide therapy may be less effective in elderly people as a result of the age-related and
heart failure-mediated reduction in the glomerular filtration rate (Davies
et al. 2000b). Side effects of thiazide therapy include hyponatraemia and
hypokalaemia.

Metolazone is a powerful thiazide-like diuretic that may be used in combination with loop diuretic therapy. This double nephron blockade leads to
a greater diuretic effect, but requires close supervision and monitoring of
biochemistry. Davies et al. (2000) advise that combination therapy should,
initially, be considered on a twice-weekly basis.

There is no randomized controlled trial evidence that loop or thiazide diuretics improve the prognosis of patients with CHF and so diuretics should be prescribed in combination with ACE inhibitors if possible.

β Blockers

β Blockers licensed for use in heart failure should be initiated in patients with heart failure caused by LV systolic dysfunction after diuretic and ACE inhibitor therapy (NICE 2003). Over the past decade clinical trials have shown that β blockers have beneficial effects on death rates and quality of life. Previously the use of β blockers in heart failure was contraindicated because of the widely held view that they contributed to worsening of heart failure symptoms by reducing myocardial contractility. However, the use of β blockers evaluated in almost 10 000 patients with CHF in over 20 randomized controlled trials has shown that they reduce mortality rates and hospital admissions and improve patients' clinical status (Lonn and McKelvie 2000). β Blockers in CHF reduce the toxic effects of the sympathetic nervous system, improving time for filling of the ventricles during diastole, and thereby increasing the stroke volume.

Currently, in the UK carvedilol and bisoprolol are the only two β blockers licensed for use in heart failure. There is evidence to support the use of metoprolol but it is currently not licensed for use.

The Metoprolol in Dilated Cardiomyopathy Trial (Waagstein et al. 1993) demonstrated improvements in LV ejection fraction (LVEF) and exercise tolerance in patients taking metoprolol, resulting in a reduction in death rates and need for cardiac transplantation in patients with idiopathic dilated cardiomyopathy.

The first Cardiac Insufficiency Bisoprolol Study (CIBIS I – Lechat et al. 1994) recruited 641 patients, demonstrating a 34% reduction in hospital admissions for people with heart failure and major improvements in functional status.

The larger CIBIS II study (1999) enrolled 2647 stable heart failure patients, who were NYHA III–IV with LVEF < 35%. Ischaemic heart disease was the prominent shared characteristic, although 12% of the patients enrolled had dilated cardiomyopathy with normal coronary arteries demonstrated on angiography. The trial was stopped prematurely because there was a highly significant difference in mortality in favour of bisoprolol. The trial demonstrated a 32% reduction in all-cause mortality rate and a 32% reduction in heart failure hospitalizations.

The largest randomized trial to demonstrate a mortality benefit was published in 2001. MERIT-HF (MEtoprolol CR/XL Randomised Intervention Trial of congestive Heart Failure) Study Group (1999) enrolled 3991 patients of NYHA functional class II–IV with an ejection fraction of < 40% to metoprolol with controlled/extended release or place-bo. All-cause mortality rate was reduced 34% with metoprolol over 1 year.

The benefits of carvedilol were demonstrated by the US Carvedilol Heart Failure Program (Packer et al. 1996a), which demonstrated survival benefit in four different studies with similar inclusion criteria and design. Patients with an ejection fraction (EF) of < 35% were randomized to carvedilol or placebo. The trials were terminated early because of significant survival benefit.

The COPERNICUS (Carvedilol Prosective Randomised Cumulative Survival) trial enrolled 2289 patients with advanced heart failure, LVEF < 25%, patients reporting symptoms at rest or on minimal exertion. Patients were randomized to carvedilol or placebo, the carvedilol arm demonstrating a reduced mortality rate of 35% in comparison to placebo (Packer et al. 2001).

The results of these trials demonstrated that certain β blockers could substantially reduce death rates in patients with symptomatic heart failure in addition to ACE inhibitors.

Aldosterone antagonists

Spironolactone is a K^+-sparing diuretic and aldosterone antagonist. Patients with heart failure caused by LV systolic dysfunction who remain moderately to severely symptomatic despite optimal therapy should be prescribed spironolactone at a dose of 12.–50 mg/day (NICE 2003).

The RALES study compared spironolactone (mean dose 25 mg daily) with placebo in 1663 patients with severe heart failure (NYHA III–IV, LVEF < 35%) who had symptoms despite taking loop diuretics, ACE inhibitors and/or digoxin. Results demonstrated a 35% reduction in mortality rate compared with placebo; in addition, the frequency of hospitalizations was reduced by 35% and symptoms improved (Pitt et al. 1999).

Hyperkalaemia and renal failure should be excluded before starting spironolactone and at regular intervals thereafter. Blood chemistry checks are recommended at 1, 4, 8 and 12 weeks, 6, 9 and 12 months, and 6-monthly thereafter (NICE 2003).

Gynaecomastia is a common side effect of spironolactone therapy; if it becomes intolerable to the patient spironolactone may be discontinued.

Digoxin

Digoxin is used to control ventricular rate in atrial fibrillation and to allow more effective filling of the ventricle. Digoxin is also used in symptomatic CHF caused by LV systolic dysfunction, in sinus rhythm, where it acts as an inotrope (Gibbs et al. 2000).

The Digitalis Intervention Group (1997) studied the effect of digoxin on mortality and morbidity in patients with heart failure (LVEF < 45%). This double-masked, placebo-controlled trial randomized 6800 patients to digoxin 125–500 μg once daily or placebo in addition to other standard therapies, mainly ACE inhibitors and diuretics.

The study found that digoxin has no overall effect on survival but reduced hospital admissions. NICE (2003) guidelines therefore recommend that digoxin should be considered for patients with severe or worsening heart failure in addition to ACE inhibitor, diuretic and β-blocker therapy.

Angiotensin II receptor antagonists

All angiotensin receptor antagonists are an option for patients who do not tolerate ACE inhibitor as a result of the side effect of persistent dry cough. Unlike ACE inhibitors, angiotensin receptor antagonists do not increase bradykinin, which causes cough.

The Evaluation of Losartan in the Elderly or ELITE II trial (Pitt et al. 1997) was designed to assess whether losartan was superior to captopril in improving survival: 3152 patients (NYHA II–IV, LVEF < 40%) were randomized to losartan 50 mg once daily or captopril 50 mg three times a day. No difference in all-cause mortality was demonstrated; the results did not clarify whether angiotensin receptor antagonists were as effective as ACE inhibitors in reducing mortality rates.

The Candesartan in Heart failure Assessment in Reduction of Mortality and morbidity programme (CHARM 2003) investigated the role of Candesartan in patients with CHF. CHARM Alternative investigated the use of Candesartan in patients with LVEF<40% and ACE intolerant. Results demonstrated that despite prior intolerance to another inhibitor of the renin angiotensin aldosterone system, candesartan was well tolerated. CV death or CHF hospitalisation was reduced by 23% and treatment effects began early after 3-6 months. In patients with symptomatic chronic heart failure and ACE inhibitor intolerance, candesartan reduces cardiovascular mortality and morbidity. Candesartan is currently the only angiotensin II receptor antagonist to be licensed in the UK for the treatment of chronic heart failure.

Isosorbide/Hydralazine combination

There is no evidence from randomized controlled trials to suggest that nitrates improve symptoms or prognosis in heart failure. The combination of isosorbide dinitrate and hydralazine were tested in the first and second Veterans' Administration Heart Failure Trials, compared with enalapril (Cohn et al. 1991). The isosorbide/hydralazine combination was not shown to improve mortality; however, there was some evidence that the combination improved symptoms and moderately improved exercise capacity (Cohn et al. 1991).

An isosorbide/hydralazine combination may be considered in patients with heart failure who are intolerant of ACE inhibitors or angiotensin II antagonists (NICE 2003).

Calcium channel blockers

Short-acting or dihydropyridine Ca^{2+} antagonists should be avoided in heart failure, because they are associated with worsening of heart failure symptoms.

Amlodipine is the only Ca^{2+} channel blocker considered safe for the medical management of chest pain and hypertension in heart failure as demonstrated in the Prospective Randomised Amlodipine Survival Evaluation (PRAISE) study (Packer et al. 1996b). NICE guidelines (2003) recommend that amlodipine should be considered for the treatment of co-morbid hypertension and/or angina in patients with heart failure.

Anticoagulants

Oral anticoagulants reduce the risk of stroke in heart failure patients with atrial fibrillation. In patients with heart failure in sinus rhythm, anticoagulation should be considered for patients with a history of thromboembolism, LV aneurysm or intracardiac thrombus (NICE 2003).

Amiodarone

Amiodarone is the only anti-arrhythmic drug with no clinically relevant negative inotropic effects. Amiodarone is effective against most supraventricular and ventricular arrhythmias. It may restore and maintain sinus rhythm in patients with heart failure and atrial fibrillation even in the presence of enlarged left atria (European Society of Cardiology 2001).

Aspirin

Aspirin 75–150 mg should be prescribed for patients with heart failure and atherosclerotic arterial disease, including CHD (NICE 2003).

Oxygen

O_2 therapy is prescribed to treat acute heart failure but at present has no evidence base to support its use in CHF. O_2 therapy may lead to haemodynamic deterioration in severe heart failure (European Society of Cardiology 2001).

Invasive procedures and the role of surgery in CHF

Some patients with CHF may benefit from invasive procedures and/or surgical interventions. Valve disease causes heart failure as a result of pressure and volume overload. Valve repair or replacements to treat cardiac valve stenosis or insufficiency had some of the earliest cardiac surgery successes.

Coronary heart disease is the most common cause of heart failure. For patients reporting angina, cardiac cathetcrization will determine the extent of atherosclerosis. In addition cardiac catheterization may be used for patients with suspected dilated cardiomyopathy as a means of excluding coronary artery disease and confirming the diagnosis of dilated cardiomyopathy, although it is known that coronary artery disease will be found on angiography in about 50% of patients thought to have dilated cardiomyopathy (Cleland and MacFayden 2002).

Revascularization

NICE (2003) guidelines state that only patients who have refractory angina should be routinely considered for revascularization. Coronary artery bypass surgery or occasionally PCI should be considered for patients with anginal symptoms. In 1985, Raihimtoola reviewed the results of coronary artery bypass trials and identified patients with LV dysfunction and coronary artery disease which improved on revascularization. CABG surgery offers symptomatic improvement but is associated with higher mortality rates in the operative and postoperative period. Young (2003) discusses how one of the problems in offering CABGs to patients with angina and heart failure is determining postoperative benefits. Controlled case studies have demonstrated that the identification of viable myocardium that can be reperfused is essential for a good outcome. Perfusion studies identify heart muscle that has become dormant (hibernating) as a result of chronic reductions in coronary blood flow. The gold standard technique for identifying hibernating myocardium is positron emission tomography (PET) (see Chapter 9). Study outcomes of CABG surgery in patients with angina and CHF reported that revascularization improved symptoms, exercise tolerance and psychological well-being.

Implantable cardioverter defibrillators and cardiac resynchronization therapy

Implantable cardioverter defibrillators (ICDs) are used to treat ventricular tachycardia (VT) and ventricular fibrillation (VF) (see Chapter 10). An ICD system is made up of a pulse generator and an electric lead. Modern ICDs are small and light (weighing about 75 g). The ICD continually monitors heart rhythm. If the ICD detects an arrhythmia, it will deliver therapy to the heart. The type of therapy received by patients is determined by program settings that may be set to meet individual demands.

Anti-tachycardia pacing (ATP)

If the ICD detects a fast regular heart rate, delivery of a series of rapid pacing pulses may interrupt the tachycardia to restore normal heart rhythm.

Cardioversion

When necessary the ICD will provide an electrical shock to reinstate normal heart rhythm. Impaired LV systolic function is a strong risk factor for sudden cardiac death. In the 1990s randomized controlled trials demonstrated the mortality benefit of implantable defibrillators over anti-arrhythmic drug therapy. The AVID Trial (Antiarrhythmics versus Implantable Defibrillaiton Investigations 1997) was the first large randomized study, which compared ICD therapy with class III anti-arrhythmic drug therapy for sudden death survivors and other patients with life-threatening tachyarrhythmias. The all-cause mortality rate was reduced in the ICD group by 39% at 1 year, 27% at 2 years and 31% at 3 years. Two other studies – the Canadian Implantable Defibrillator study (CIDS – Connelly et al. 2000) and the Cardiac Arrest Study Hamburg (CASH – Kuck et al. 2000) – also demonstrated mortality rate benefits of 37 and 20%, respectively. The MADIT (Multicenter Automatic Defibrillator Trial – Moss et al. 1996) trial found that, in patients with prior MI who are at high risk for ventricular tachyarrhythmia, prophylactic therapy with an implanted defibrillator improved survival compared with conventional medical therapy. The MADIT II (Moss et al. 2002) trial randomized 1232 patients with previous MI and LV systolic dysfunction. Results concluded that in patients with previous MI and advanced LV systolic dysfunction implantation of a defibrillator improved survival.

Current NICE guidance on the insertion of ICDs states that ICD therapy should be considered for secondary prevention in patients with the following:

- Cardiac arrest caused by either VT or VF
- Spontaneously sustained VT causing syncope or significant haemodynamic compromise
- Sustained VT without syncope/cardiac arrest, and an associated reduction in EF (< 35%) but no worse than NYHA III.

It can also be used as primary prevention in patients with a history of previous MI and all of the following:

- Non-sustained VT on Holter 24-h ECG monitoring
- Inducible VT on electrophysiological testing
- LV systolic dysfunction with an EF <.35% and no worse than NYHA III.

Cardiac resynchronization therapy (CRT) is used to restore proper timing (synchrony) of ventricular contraction and therefore improve pump efficiency. CRT is delivered by means of biventricular pacing to the heart, which is similar to a standard pacemaker implantation. CRT involves a small device being implanted below the skin of the upper chest and three leads (two into the right ventricle and one into the coronary sinus which enables pacing of left ventricle) inserted to the heart via the *venous system*. CRT has been demonstrated to increase the net cardiac output of the heart without increasing O_2 consumption. The patients best suited to receive CRT will have:

- symptomatic heart failure with NYHA III–IV despite optimal drug therapy
- LV systolic dysfunction
- wide QRS on ECG reflecting LV dysynchrony.

Studies to date with cardiac resynchronization therapy have shown improved LV systolic function, improved symptoms, improved quality of life, improved exercise tolerance and reverse re-modelling. In addition CRT has been shown to reduce hospitalizations by 80% (European Society of Cardiology 2001). The MIRACLE study (www.medtronic.com.newsroom) evaluated 453 patients NYHA III–IV with a QRS wider than 130 ms and an EF ≤ 35%. Results demonstrated an increase in exercise capacity, NYHA functional class and quality-of-life scores. In addition improvements were found on echocardiography, with a reduction in systolic and diastolic volumes and increase in LVEF. Patients suitable for CRT therapy and at high risk of sudden death may be offered a CRT device with defibrillator back-up. The COMPANION investigators (Bristow et al. 2004) tested the hypothesis that prophylactic cardiac resynchronization therapy with or without a defibrillator would reduce the risk of death and hospitalization among patients with advanced CHF and intraventricular conduction delays. The study enrolled 1520 patients who had advanced heart failure (NYHA III–IV) caused by ischaemic or non-ischaemic cardiomyopathies and widened QRS. Patients were randomized to receive optimal pharmacological therapy alone or in combination with cardiac resynchronization therapy, with either a pacemaker or a pacemaker defibrillator. CRT was found to reduce the all-cause mortality rate and when combined with a defibrillator significantly reduced the mortality rate. The COMPANION study was the first to demonstrate mortality benefit in dilated cardiomyopathy patients treated with an ICD.

Partial left ventriculotomy and cardiomyoplasty

Partial left ventriculotomy (Bastista operation) involves reducing the size of the left ventricle by removal of a wedge of myocardium. Current guidelines do not at present recommend this operation because in recent studies a number of patients undergoing it subsequently required LV assist device or transplantation when surgery failed (European Society of Cardiology 2001).

Cardiomyoplasty involves wrapping of the latissimus dorsi muscle around the failing left ventricle which is then electrically stimulated to aid LV contraction. It is also not currently recommended in guidelines because the procedure has been applied only to a small number of patients (European Society of Cardiology 2001). Both of these procedures are now largely abandoned; emerging approaches currently being evaluated include ACORN cardiac restraining/support device and a MyoSplint LV re-modelling device. The ACORN cardiac support device is a mesh of surgically compatible elastic material that wraps around the left and right ventricles (Young 2003). The MyoSplint aims to reduce LV dilatation and re-modelling. It consists of three splints that are placed across the LV chamber which can be adjusted to decrease the LV radius. Both new procedures are to be evaluated in larger-scale, randomized clinical trials (Young 2003).

LV assist devices

The short-term use of LV assist devices has been studied in a small number of patients. Results have demonstrated sustainable improvements in heart function in some of those patients. It is not possible to know before implantation whether myocardial recovery will be sufficient to allow explantation of the device. Further research is required.

Increasing numbers of LV assist devices are being implanted as a bridge to transplantation; however, the use of long-term implants is currently being tested in clinical trials. The REMATCH (Rose et al. 1999) study revealed that patients not suitable for transplantation because of age or other illnesses (co-morbidities) have a survival benefit and improved quality of life from implantation of a mechanical circulatory support device. The trial involved patients with end-stage heart failure (mean LVEF of 17%) and the results found that the 1-year survival rate in the LV device insertion group was almost doubled.

Cardiac transplantation

Recent results in heart transplant recipients on triple immunosuppressive therapy have shown a survival rate of about 70–80% at 5 years (European Society of Cardiology 2001). The identification of heart transplant recipients is based on the expected gain in survival and quality of life over other medical and surgical options (Deng 2002). Cardiac transplantation is the treatment of choice for patients with severe heart failure who remain symptomatic despite optimal medical treatment, and whose 1-year estimated life expectancy is less than 50% (Gould 2002). The main problems associated with cardiac transplantation include a shortage of donor organs and rejection of the donor organ after surgery. Patients have to take long-term immunosuppressive drugs to prevent rejection, but long term these drugs are associated with hypertension, renal failure and increased cancer rates.

Cell transplantation

The concept of regenerating the failing heart is in experimental stages. Cells from a variety of sources have been considered, e.g. embryonic cardiomyocytes, neonatal cardiac myocytes, skeletal myoblasts and smooth muscle cells.

Xenotransplantation theoretically provides an unlimited supply of cells, tissues and organs from another animal, e.g. the pig. Deng (2002) suggests that cell transplantation and xenotransplantation must be tested using appropriately designed studies.

Non-pharmacological and lifestyle measures

Over recent years the concept of self-management strategies for patients within chronic disease management programmes have been advocated and indeed form a key part of The NHS Plan (DoH 2001). Empowerment of patients to self-manage aspects of their care and then access health services requires effective communication strategies between health professional and patient. Effective communication with the patient, family and/or carer is essential in order to educate, counsel, empower and reassure. A full explanation of heart failure and how to manage symptoms may alleviate patient anxiety and improve quality of life. If patients are taught how to recognize signs of worsening failure, they can act immediately to access heart failure services. Information should be given in a patient-centred way, ensuring that information is given at the patient's request or need. Information should be given in such a way that the individual understands it, taking into account cognitive abilities and language barriers. Information giving empowers the patient to make decisions with regard to compliance with medicines, accessing health-care services and making healthy lifestyle changes. Ethnic minorities may experience communication difficulties. Ensuring effective verbal and written communication for ethnic minority patients requires consideration and planning by heart failure service providers. In CHF lifestyle changes can alleviate symptoms, slow disease progression and improve quality of life.

Smoking

Stopping smoking can be a difficult lifestyle change; smokers who stop smoking are more likely to see their heart failure symptoms improve. Smoking has adverse haemodynamic effects in patients with congestive heart failure (Gibbs et al. 2000). Lifetime smokers often need help to stop smoking and smoking cessation services should be offered.

Diet and nutrition

Being overweight puts extra strain on the heart. Overweight patients are more likely to be breathless on exertion. Reduction in saturated fat and cholesterol intake in the diet is recommended as a step towards weight reduction to within 10% of optimal body weight. Advanced heart failure and/or poor nutrition can lead to cardiac cachexia which is observed by weight loss and muscle wasting. A nutritional assessment by the dietitian is indicated in this group of patients to maintain nutritional requirements and improve quality of life.

Reduction in salt intake

A high-salt diet can lead to fluid retention (oedema). Patients are advised about tips to limit their salt intake such as:

- Never add salt at the table, try adding herbs, spices, pepper or mustard instead
- Try cooking with less or no salt.

Low-salt substitutes are not recommended because they still contain salt and are higher in K^+. Patients are advised to avoid high-salt foods and choose low-Na^+ alternatives; convenience foods are often higher in salt and should be limited. The following foods are examples of some of the foods usually high in Na^+:

- Canned soups and dry soup mixes
- Ham, bacon and sausage
- Salted nuts and peanut butter
- Processed meats, e.g. salami, hot dogs
- Snack foods, e.g. crisps
- Fast food
- Pre-packed frozen dinners.

Fluid intake

Fluid restriction may be recommended for patients with severe symptoms. A high fluid intake may reduce the effectiveness of diuretic therapy and contribute to congestion. Severely symptomatic patients may be advised to limit their fluid intake to 1.5–2.0 l daily.

Reduction in alcohol intake

Alcohol is a myocardial depressant (Gibbs et al. 2000). Drinking alcohol may exacerbate symptoms of heart failure. Patients are encouraged to limit their alcohol intake to no more than 2 units/day. Patients diagnosed with alcohol-induced cardiomyopathy are advised not to drink alcohol; the prognosis is poor if consumption continues and subsequent referral to the alcohol team may be necessary.

Exercise

NICE guidelines (2003) recommend that heart failure patients be encouraged to adopt regular exercise, which has been found to benefit them by improving symptoms and increasing energy levels. Regular exercise may also help regulate BP, improve circulation, promote weight loss and lower cholesterol levels. Regular exercise does not improve LV function but helps to prevent loss of muscle mass and physical deconditioning. Stable heart failure patients should be offered supervised exercise programmes that are tailored to meet individual capabilities. Patients should be encouraged to be active in their daily lives, finding a balance between exercise and rest. Rest and relaxation are important and patients are advised to 'listen to their bodies' and rest when necessary.

Immunization

Heart failure can be worsened by flu or a chest infection which is a frequent cause of admission to hospital. Patients should be offered an annual influenza immunization and a once-only pneumococcal immunization.

Contraceptive advice

Contraceptive advice should be given to women of child-bearing age because the maternal mortality rate is high with pregnancy and childbirth, and particularly in those with symptomatic heart failure.

Sexual activity

Sexual activity is an important part of an individual's overall physical and emotional well-being. Most patients with stable heart failure can continue normal sexual relations; however, in symptomatic patients with poor exercise tolerance, less demanding ways to express love and affection should be explored. Some men will report erectile dysfunction which may occur as a result of either reduced cardiac output or pharmaceutical measures. A range of treatment options is available for erectile dysfunction and CHF patients should be referred as per local guidelines.

Anxiety and depression

Feelings of stress, anxiety and depression are common and may adversely affect libido. Anxiety and depression tend to be more common in patients with heart failure than in the general population. Heart failure patients who score positively for anxiety and/or depression on the Hospital Anxiety and Depression Scale or who are diagnosed as having anxiety and depression by a doctor should be referred to the appropriate services. Patients diagnosed with depression should be managed following the NICE (2004) guidelines.

A variety of booklets is published for the benefit of heart failure patients, e.g. *Living with Heart Failure* (British Heart Foundation at www.bhf.org.uk) and *Management of Heart Failure, Understanding NICE guidance – information for people with heart failure, their carers, and the public* (www.nice.org.uk).

The role of the heart failure specialist nurse

The role of the heart failure specialist nurse has emerged as an invaluable factor in the planning of services for heart failure patients. The National Service Framework (NSF) for CHD (DoH 2000, Chapter 6) sets out how the NHS and others can help:

- people with heart failure live longer and achieve a better quality of life
- people with unresponsive heart failure and other malignant presentations of CHD receive appropriate palliative care support.

The publication of this Framework and the work of local CHD implementation groups have led to an increased number of heart failure specialist nurses working across primary and secondary care. The evidence base for their effectiveness has been researched by a number of studies undertaken in the UK, the USA, Australia and Sweden, and have concluded that heart failure specialist nurse interventions improve quality of life, reduce hospital admissions, reduce costs and possibly improve mortality rates.

Blue et al. (2001) performed a randomized controlled trial to investigate whether specialist nurse interventions improve outcomes in patients with CHF: 165 patients admitted to hospital as a result of LV systolic dysfunction received heart failure nurse intervention before discharge and after, with regular home visits for up to 1 year thereafter. The results demonstrated that heart failure nurse interventions can substantially reduce the risk of readmission to hospital for heart failure. Blue concluded that regular contact for review of treatment and patient education is likely to contribute to this effect.

Appleton et al. (2002) performed a randomized controlled trial to investigate the benefit of specialist nurse-led interventions in an outpatient population with stable congestive heart failure: 55 patients were randomized. Patients in the intervention group received comprehensive CHF education, individual dietary advice and regular review of medications. Regular follow-up in the clinic, provision of a daytime telephone helpline and home visits (if necessary) were provided. The results demonstrated that, in a population of outpatients with stable CHF, a specialist nurse-led management programme reduces total and CHF-related hospital admissions and is cost-effective. Stewart et al. (2002) examined the economic consequences of applying a specialist nurse-mediated, post-discharge management service for heart failure within a whole population. They concluded that such a service would reduce readmissions to hospital, reduce costs, and improve patients' quality of life and also the efficiency of the health-care system.

Grady et al. (2000) produced a statement to health-care professionals from the cardiovascular nursing council of the American Heart Association. This statement listed components of successful management programmes for heart failure patients (see box).

Components of successful management programmes for CHF patients

- Follow-up post discharge:
  Home visit
  Telephone follow-up
  Nurse-managed clinic visit
- Increased accessibility of a health-care provider
- Patient education
- Physical examination by a heart failure nurse
- Medication adjustment by a heart failure nurse:
  Independent
  Under direct supervision of the physician
- Clinic visit to a cardiologist
- Coordination of care
- Exercise programme

Many heart failure specialist nurses work as advanced practitioners coordinating the care of heart failure patients, and working across primary and secondary care settings. Assessment of the patient's physical, psychological and social needs is central to the role, followed by planning and implementing interventions that are based on best practice guidelines. Communication with heart failure patients aims to provide the information that patients need to self-manage their heart failure symptoms, taking control of their disease management (as cognitive abilities allow), e.g. competency in self-adjustment of diuretic therapies. Other core components of the role may incorporate teaching and training of other health professionals, research and audit, and contributions towards clinical governance.

The heart failure specialist nurse assesses the patient's physical and psychological status as well as social support mechanisms. Cardiovascular assessment of the patient's clinical status determines whether heart failure symptoms are stable with no evidence of decompensation (worsening of heart failure). Many secondary care heart failure clinics have been organized so that the advanced nurse practitioner has access to a cardiologist with expertise in managing heart failure. The heart failure specialist nurse plays a pivotal role, acting as a coordinator of care in the referral of patients within the multidisciplinary team. The multidisciplinary approach has been found to improve quality-of-life outcomes for heart failure patients (Moser and Riegel 2001).

Clinical assessment of the patient in the heart failure clinic

Clinical assessment of the heart failure patient includes eliciting patient history to determine recent symptomatic status, a cardiovascular examination and an assessment of patient compliance with lifestyle and pharmacological regimens.

The cardiovascular examination includes a general inspection of the patient, observing for breathlessness at rest and/or cyanosis. Heart rate and rhythm are assessed through examination of the radial pulse, at the wrist, or through auscultation of the heart at the apex. If an abnormality of heart rate or rhythm is noted, an ECG may be necessary to document heart rhythm and determine whether medical intervention is necessary. Sitting and standing BP measurements are recorded. Standing BP is measured to exclude postural hypotension, which may result from drug therapies.

Signs of cardiac failure may be found in other systems, and so the legs and abdomen are examined for signs of oedema. Some nurses with advanced practice competencies auscultate the heart and lungs to check for abnormality of breath and heart sounds. Rhonchi are wheezes often heard as a consequence of asthma (medium-to-high pitch on expiration) or bronchitis (medium-to-low pitch on inspiration and expiration).

Crepitations are crackling sounds heard as a result of secretions (which may clear if the patient is asked to cough), pulmonary oedema, inflammation or fibrosis. Crepitations increase towards the end of inspiration and are not affected by coughing. Severe pulmonary oedema may occur in the absence of crepitations (Ford and Munro 2000). Cardiac auscultation is a difficult skill to acquire and competence is gained from experience and repeated performance. Understanding of the electrical and mechanical events that occur in the heart is essential to the appreciation of heart sounds and murmurs (Gould 2002).

Palliative care

In 1990, the World Heath Organization defined palliative care as:

> . . . the active total care of patients whose disease no longer responds to curative treatment. Control of pain, of other symptoms and of psychological, social and spiritual problems is paramount. The goal of palliative care is achievement of the best quality of life for patients and their families.
>
> WHO (1990, cited in Kinghorn and Gamlin 2001, p. 7)

NICE guidelines (2003) acknowledge that there is substantial unmet palliative care need for heart failure patients and their carers and recommend that:

- the palliative care needs of patients and their carers should be identified, assessed and managed at the earliest opportunity
- patients with heart failure and their carers should have access to professionals with palliative care skills within the heart failure team.

To provide a supportive care environment for heart failure patients, health professionals need to adopt a palliative care approach. There is a need for nurses and doctors working with heart failure patients to access available skills and resources and to develop palliative care skills in conjunction with the support and expertise of specialist palliative care professionals. The basic principles of palliative care include good communication, symptom management, supportive care and optimal terminal care. Heart failure and cancer patients share many similar physical, psychological and social problems. Twycross (1997), investigating symptoms reported by patients in the advanced stages of cancer, found that physical symptoms included pain, fatigue, dry mouth, drowsiness, nausea and anorexia. Psychological symptoms included worry, feelings of sadness or nervousness, irritability and difficulty concentrating. It is widely acknowledged that worsening symptoms of heart failure are often poorly managed, yet palliative care specialists have developed treatment strategies that effectively control many of the distressing symptoms reported (Kendall 2003). Team working or a partnership approach between cardiology health professionals and specialist palliative care requires innovation. The unpredictable death trajectory in CHF must not detract from strategies to develop supportive services for heart failure patients at all stages along this chronic disease pathway.

Patients with heart failure often receive inadequate communication and have unmet psychosocial need, as uncovered in studies performed by McCarthy et al. (1997) and Rogers et al. (2000). The information needs of heart failure patients are broad and include a need for information and advice about their condition, information about medicines or invasive interventions and preparation for end of life. Communication that allows patients to express their feelings, fears and hopes in order to support the patient living with uncertainty is a skill that expert palliative care specialists need to share with cardiology health professionals, who often feel uncomfortable and unsure in this role. Feelings of hopelessness have an adverse effect on an individual's ability to cope; palliative care encompasses consideration of the human spirit and an individual's need for hope.

Chaplin and McIntyre (2001, p. 143) state that 'In essence, hope is about the inner human potential to cope with adversity and to grow as a person'. They identify that the challenge for nurses is to integrate their approaches to fostering hope with their other activities in providing palliative care.

Conclusion

Chronic heart failure is associated with high mortality and morbidity rates. The incidence of chronic heart failure in the UK is set to rise as the elderly population increases and many more patients survive myocardial infarction and hypertension. Accurate identification of people at high risk of developing heart failure and the assessment and identification of people with suspected heart failure require a systematic approach. Once diagnosed, the ability to deliver evidence-based care through the provision of coordinated management strategies is the challenge facing health-care providers. Empowering patients to self-manage aspects of their care is a key component of chronic disease management advocated in *The NHS Plan* (DoH 2001). Finally the palliative care needs of patients and their carers should be identified, assessed and managed at the earliest opportunity.

References

Antiarrhythmics versus Implantable Defibrillators (AVID) Investigators (1997) A comparison of antiarrhythmic drug therapy with implantable defibrillators in patients resuscitated from near fatal ventricular arrhythmias. N Engl J Med 337: 1576–83.

Appleton B, Palmer ND, Rodrigues EA (2002) Study to evaluate specialist nurse-led intervention in an outpatient population with stable congestive heart failure (The SENIF trial). Aintree Cardiac Centre, University Hospital Aintree Liverpool.

Blue L, Lang E, McMurray JJV et al. (2001) Randomised control trial of specialist nurse intervention in heart failure. BMJ 323: 715–18.

Bristow MR, Saxon LA, Boehmer J et al. (2004) Cardiac-resynchronisation therapy with or without an implantable defibrillator in advanced chronic heart failure (COMPANION Investigators). N Engl J Med 350: 2140–50.

British Heart Foundation (2001) Coronary Heart Disease Statistics: Morbidity supplement. London: British Heart Foundation: www.heartstats.org.

British Heart Foundation (2003) Survival after initial diagnosis of heart failure, 1995–98, Hillingdon. One year survival rates, heart failure and the major cancers compared, mid 1990s, England and Wales: www.heartstats.org.

Chaplin J, McIntyre R (2001) Hope: the heart of palliative care. In: Kinghorn S, Gamlin R (eds), Palliative Nursing Bringing Comfort and Hope. London: Baillière Tindall.

CHARM (2003) The CHARM programme. Lancet 362: 759–66, 767–71, 772–6, 777–81.

CIBIS Investigators and Committees (1999) The cardiac insufficiency bisoprolol study II (CIBIS-II): a randomised trial. Lancet 353: 9–13.

Cleland JGF (1999) Understanding Heart Failure. Poole: Family Doctor Publications.

Cleland GF, MacFadyen RJ (2002) An Illustrated Guide to Heart Failure. London: Current Medical Literature Ltd.

Cohn JN, Johnson G, Ziesches S et al. (1991) A comparison of enalapril with hydralazine-isosorbide dinitrate in the treatment of chronic congestive heart failure (V-HeFT II). N Engl J Med 325: 303–10.

Connelly SJ, Gent M, Roberts RS et al. (2000) Canadian Implantable Defibrillator Study (CIDS): a randomised trial of the implantable cardioverter defibrillator against amiodarone. Circulation 101: 1297–302.

CONSENSUS Trial Study Group (1987) Effects of enalapril on mortality in severe congestive cardiac failure: results of the Cooperative North Scandinavian Enalapril Survival Study (CONSENSUS). N Engl J Med 316: 1429–35.

Cowie MR, Wood DA, Coats AJS et al. (2000) Survival of patients with a new diagnosis of heart failure: a population based study. Heart 83: 505–10.

Davies RC, Hobbs FDR, Lip GYH (2000a) History and epidemiology. In: Gibbs CR, Davies MK, Lip GYH (eds), ABC of Heart Failure. London: BMJ Books, p. 1.

Davies RC, Gibbs CR, Lip GYH (2000b) Investigation. In: Gibbs CR, Davies MK, Lip GYH (eds), ABC of Heart Failure. London: BMJ Books, p. 17.

Deng MC (2002) Cardiac transplantation. Heart 87: 177–84.

Department of Health (2000) National Service Framework for Coronary Heart Disease. London: HMSO.

Department of Health (2001) The NHS Plan: An action guide for nurses, midwives and health visitors. London: HMSO.

Department of Health (2003) Developing Services for Heart Failure. London: DoH.

Digitalis Intervention Group (DIG) (1997). The effect of digoxin on mortality and morbidity in patients with heart failure. N Engl J Med 336: 525–33.

European Society of Cardiology (2001) Task Force Report Guidelines for the diagnosis and treatment of chronic heart failure. Eur Heart J 22: 1527–60.

Exner DV, Schron EB (2001) Impact of pharmacologic therapy on health related quality of life in heart failure: findings from clinical trials. In: Moser D, Riegel B (eds), Improving Outcomes in Heart Failure: An interdisciplinary approach. Gaithersburg, MA: Aspen Publication.

Ford MJ, Munro JF (2000) Introduction to Clinical Examination, 7th edn. Edinburgh: Churchill Livingstone.

Gibbs CR, Davies MK, Lip GYH (eds) (2000) ABC of Heart Failure. London: BMJ Books.

Gould M (2002) Chronic heart failure. In: Hatchett R, Thompson D (eds), Cardiac Nursing: A comprehensive guide. London: Churchill-Livingstone.

Grady KL, Dracup K, Kennedy G et al. (2000) Team management of patients with heart failure. A statement of health care professionals from the cardiovascular nursing council of the American Heart Association. Circulation 102: 2443–256.

Hall C (2004) Essential biochemistry and physiology of (NT-pro)BNP. Eur J Heart Fail 6: 257–20.

Hatchett R, Thompson D (2002) Cardiac Nursing – A comprehensive guide. Edinburgh: Churchil-Livingstone.

Jackson G, Gibbs CR, Davies MK, Lip GYH (2000) Pathophysiology In: Gibbs CR, Davies MK, Lip GYH (eds), ABC of Heart Failure. London: BMJ Books, p. 9.

Kendall M (2003) Palliative care – an elitist concept? Nurse2Nurse Magazine 3(7): 22–3.

Kinghorn S, Gamlin R (2001) Palliative Nursing: Bringing comfort and hope. London: Baillière Tindall.

Kuck KH, Cappato R, Siebels J et al. (2000) Randomised comparison of antiarrhythmic drug therapy with implantable defibrillators in patients resuscitated from cardiac arrest: the Cardiac Arrest Study Hamburg (CASH). Circulation 102: 748–54.

Lechat P, the CIBIS Investigators (1994) A randomised trial of beta-blockade in heart failure: the Cardiac Insufficiency Bisoprolol Study. Circulation 90: 1765–73.

Lip GYH, Gibbs CR, Beevers DG (2000) Aetiology. In: Gibbs CR, Davies MK, Lip GYH (eds), ABC of Heart Failure. London: BMJ Books, p. 5.

Lonn E, McKelvie R (2000) Clinical review: Drug treatment in heart failure. BMJ 320: 1188–92.

McCarthy M, Addington-Hall JH, Ley M (1997) Communication and choice in dying from heart disease. J R Soc Med 90: 128–31.

McDonagh TA, Dargie HJ (1998) Epidemiology and pathophysiology of heart failure. Medicine 26: 111–15.

McDonagh TA, Holmer S, Raymond I, Luchner A, Hildebrant P, Dargie HJ (2004) NT-proBNP and the diagnosis of heart failure: a pooled analysis of three European epidemiological studies. Eur J Heart Fail 6: 269–73.

McMurray J, Dargie H (1998) Chronic Heart Failure, 2nd edn. London: Martin Dunitz.

Merck Manual (2004) Heart Failure. Section 16 Chapter 203 (www.merck.com)

MERIT-HF Study Group (1999) Metoprolol CR/XL Randomised Intervention Trial (MERIT-HF). Lancet 353: 2001–7.

Miller AB, Srivastava P (2001) Angiotensin receptor blockers and aldosterone antagonists in chronic heart failure. Cardiol Clin 19: 195–202.

Moser DK, Riegel B (2001) Improving Outcomes in Heart Failure: An interdisciplinary approach. Gaithersburg, MA: Aspen.

Moss AJ, Jackson Hall W, Cannom DS et al. (1996) Improved survival with an implantable defibrillator in patients with coronary disease at high risk for ventricular arrhythmia (MADIT). N Engl J Med 335: 1933–40.

Moss AJ, Zareba W, Jackson Hall W et al. (MADIT II Investigators) (2002) Prophylactic Implantation of a defibrillator in patients with myocardial infarction and reduced ejection fraction. N Engl J Med 346: 877–83.

National Institute for Clinical Excellence (2003) Management of Chronic Heart Failure in Primary and Secondary Care. London: NICE (www.nice.org.uk).

National Institute for Clinical Excellence (2004) Depression: The management of depression in primary and secondary care. London: NICE.

National Prescribing Centre (2001) MeReK BRIEFING Issue No 15: www.npc.ppa.nhs.uk.

Packer M, Fowler MB, Roecker EB, for the US Carvedilol Study Group (1996a) The effects of carvedilol on morbidity and mortality in patients with chronic heart failure. N Engl J Med 334: 1349–55.

Packer M, O'Connor M, Ghali JK et al. (1996b) Effect of amlodipine on morbidity and mortality in severe chronic heart failure. N Engl J Med 335: 1107–14.

Packer M, Coats AJS, Fowler MB et al. (2001) Effect of carvedilol on survival in severe chronic heart failure. N Engl J Med 344: 1651–8.

Pitt B, Segal R, Martinez FA et al. (1997) Randomised trial of losartan versus captopril in patients over 65 with heart failure (Evaluation of Losartan In the Elderly Study, ELITE). Lancet 349: 747–52.

Pitt B, Zannad F, Remme WJ et al. (1999) The effect of spironolactone on morbidity and mortality in patients with severe heart failure. Randomised Aldactone Evaluation Study Investigators. N Engl J Med 341: 709–77.

Quinn M, Babb P, Brock A, Kirby L, Jones J for Office for National Statistics (2001) Cancer trends in England and Wales 1950 1999. London: The Stationery Office.

Raihimtoola SH (1985) A perspective on the three large multicentre randomised trials of coronary artery bypass surgery for chronic stable angina. Circulation 72(suppl V): 123–35.

Rogers A, Addington-Hall JM, Abery A (2000) Knowledge and communication difficulties for patients with chronic heart failure: qualitative study. BMJ 321: 605–7.

Rose EA, Moskowitz AJ, Packer M (1999) The REMATCH trial: rationale, design and endpoints. Randomised evolution of mechanical assistance for treatment of congestive heart failure. Ann Thorac Surg 67: 723–30.

Royal College of Physicians (2001) Medical Masterclass: Cardiology and respiratory medicine. London: Blackwell Science.

Scottish Intercollegiate Guidelines Network or SIGN (1999) Diagnosis and treatment of heart failure due to left ventricular systolic dysfunction. A national clinical guideline. Edinburgh: SIGN.

SOLVD Investigators (1991) The effect of enalapril on survival in patients with reduced left ventricular ejection fractions and congestive heart failure. N Engl J Med 352: 293–302.

SOLVD Investigators (1992) Effect of enalapril on mortality and the development of heart failure in asymptomatic patients with reduced left ventricular ejection fraction. N Engl J Med 327: 685–91.

Stewart S, Blue L, Walker A, Morrison C, McMurray JJ (2002) An economic analysis of specialist heart failure nurse management in the UK. Eur Heart J 23: 1369–78.

Twycross R (1997) Symptom Management in Advanced Cancer, 2nd edn. Oxford: Radcliffe Medical Press.

Vanderheyden M, Bartunek J, Goethals M (2004) Brain and other natriuretic peptides: molecular aspects. Eur J Heart Fail 6: 261–8.

Vasan RS, Levy D (2003) Heart failure due to diastolic dysfunction: Definition, diagnosis and treatment. In: McMurray JJV, Pfeffer MA (eds), Heart Failure Updates. London: Martin Dunitz, pp. 1–13.

Waagstein F, Bristow MR, Swedberg K et al. (1993) Metoprolol in Dilated Cardiomyopathy (MDC) Trial Study Group. Beneficial effects of metoprolol in idiopathic dilated cardiomyopathy. Lancet 342: 1441–50.

Watson RDS, Gibbs CR, Lip GYH (2000) Clinical features and complications. In: Gibbs C, Davies MK Lip GYH (eds), ABC of Heart Failure. London: BMJ Books.

World Health Organization (1990) Cancer Pain Relief and Palliative Care. Technical Report Series 804. Geneva: WHO.

Young JB (2003) Innovative surgery for heart failure: A new era? In: McMurray JJV, Pfeffer MA (eds), Heart Failure Updates. London: Martin Dunitz, pp. 241–60.

Zile MR, Brutsaert DL (2002) New concepts in diastolic dysfunction and diastolic heart failure. Part 1 diagnosis, prognosis and measurements of diastolic function. Circulation 105: 1387–93.

Index